I0053420

**DECODING AI BIAS IN MEDICINE: How Artificial Intelligence Ignores Traditional, Indigenous, and Holistic Healing**

© 2025 by Anthony B. James, All Rights Reserved

Published by Meta Journal Press: BeardedMedia.Com, 8491 Central Ave. Brooksville, Fl 34613

For general information on our products and services or for technical support, please contact our customer care Department within the United States at 1(706)358-8646.

● **Cover Art Credits**
Cover concept and indigenous motif design by Dr. Anthony B. James.
Base imagery generated using artificial intelligence tools including ChatGPT-4 and DALL·E by OpenAI.
Final composition © 2025 Dr. Anthony B. James.

AI-generated elements used under license with OpenAI, in accordance with its commercial use policy. All design, prompt creation, modification, and post-production editing were executed by the author to ensure originality and cultural integrity.

This cover is a human-authored, derivative work incorporating AI-assisted components, and is protected under U.S. copyright law.

**Contributor: Dr. Benoit Tano**

● **Library of Congress Control Number: 2025914217**
● **ISBN: 978-1-886338-40-1**

ISBN-13: 978-1-886338-40-1

54995

9 781886 338401

● **Country the book is printed in United States of America**

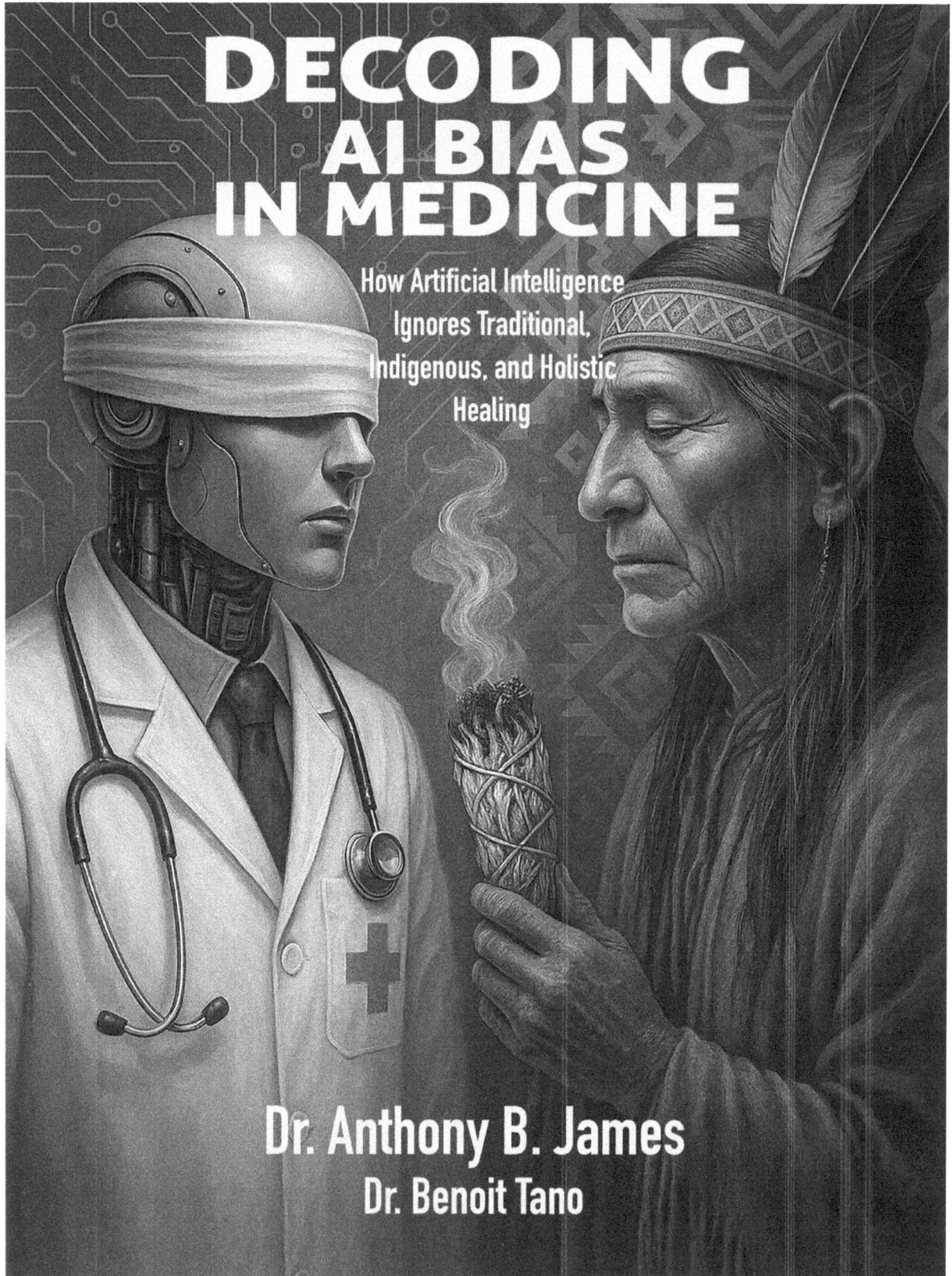

# DECODING
## AI BIAS
## IN MEDICINE

How Artificial Intelligence
Ignores Traditional,
Indigenous, and Holistic
Healing

## Dr. Anthony B. James
### Dr. Benoit Tano

**DECODING AI BIAS IN MEDICINE:**

**How Artificial Intelligence Ignores Traditional, Indigenous, and Holistic Healing**

**by**

**DR. Anthony B. James & Academic Contributor Dr. Benoit Tano**

## Disclaimer

The contents of this book, DECODING AI BIAS IN MEDICINE: How Artificial Intelligence Ignores Traditional, Indigenous, and Holistic Healing, are intended for educational and informational purposes only. The views expressed herein are those of the author and do not necessarily reflect the views of the publisher, Integrative Medical Press. While efforts have been made to ensure the accuracy and reliability of the information provided, the author and publisher make no guarantee, warranty, or representation, express or implied, regarding the completeness, accuracy, or currency of the information contained in this publication. It is the reader's responsibility to verify the applicability and relevance of the information in various contexts, particularly when applying the insights to patient care or AI system development. This book does not substitute for professional judgment, medical advice, or consultation with healthcare professionals or AI specialists. The discussions surrounding artificial intelligence and various medical systems, including traditional, indigenous, and holistic healing practices, are complex and constantly evolving. Therefore, the explorations and analyses in this book should be interpreted as the author's perspectives, rooted in current knowledge as of 2025, and are subject to change as new information becomes available. Case studies and references are provided for illustrative purposes and should be construed as examples rather than endorsements or comprehensive comparisons. Mention of specific technologies, processes, or proprietary AI systems is for informational purposes only and does not imply recommendation or endorsement by the author. Readers are encouraged to critically evaluate the content and consult multiple sources when making decisions related to the implementation of AI in healthcare. The inclusion of any commercial references does not signify promotion, and no commercial endorsement by the author or the publisher is intended or should be inferred. Ethical considerations and regulatory compliance are crucial in the deployment of AI systems in healthcare. The scenarios and strategies discussed herein should be adapted to align with local ethical standards and regulations.

4

# Table Of Contents

14

20

22

24

26

## Preface

In the heart of our rapidly evolving healthcare landscape, technology, particularly Artificial Intelligence (AI), promises revolutionary changes. However, as we tread this transformative path, an urgent question looms over us: Are we inadvertently programming our biases into the very systems meant to eradicate them? This inquiry forms the crux of 'DECODING AI BIAS IN MEDICINE,' where we delve into the nuanced interfaces of AI, medicine, and, importantly, the overlooked realms of traditional, indigenous, and holistic healing practices. The genesis of this book was sparked by a concerning observation – the distinct underrepresentation and misunderstanding of non-Western medical knowledge in AI models that increasingly decide the nuances of health and sickness. As Western biomedical paradigms dominate AI applications in healthcare, there exists a significant risk that these technologies will perpetuate historical injustices and exacerbate disparities in global health outcomes. To decode, understand, and address these biases, this book is structured into a multi-faceted exploration spanning historical analyses, ethical debates, and forward-thinking solutions. Starting with a foundational overview of AI in healthcare, we examine the mechanics of AI systems and the inherent biases that infiltrate its algorithms from skewed datasets and monocultural development teams. Each subsequent chapter peels back a layer of complexity in how AI interacts with, and often sidelines, diverse medical traditions from around the world. From the sands of shamanic healing rituals to the precision of Ayurvedic diagnostics enhanced with AI, our case studies highlight both shortcomings and potential transformative collaborations. As we journey through each chapter, we also envision practical strategies for integrating a more culturally competent and ethically aligned AI in medicine. Techniques for decolonizing medical AI and innovating future algorithms to empathize with the rich tableau of global healing practices are critically discussed. This book serves not only as a scholarly critique but also as a clarion call to those involved in AI and healthcare — to pivot towards inclusivity, respect for cultural wisdom, and genuinely equitable healthcare solutions. Welcome to a pathbreaking exploration that rethinks the very fabric of medical technology. It is time we heal the biases before we heal with bias.

## Foreword

It is with immense responsibility and honor that I introduce 'DECODING AI BIAS IN MEDICINE: How Artificial Intelligence Ignores Traditional, Indigenous, and Holistic Healing.' In this pivotal work, we begin an exploration of the complex interplay between advanced medical technologies and the rich tapestry of traditional healing practices that have sustained human health for centuries. As we stand at the crossroads of technological innovation and cultural heritage, this book sheds light on the overlooked biases embedded within AI systems, particularly within the medical sphere. These biases not only perpetuate historical injustices but also overlook the profound wisdom inherent in traditional, indigenous, and holistic healing practices. Through a comprehensive analysis spanning technical insights and cultural studies, this book aims to bridge the divide. Beginning with an exploration of AI in current medical systems and its inherent biases, we delve into the historical context in depth. These initial discussions lay the groundwork for a more profound investigation into the marginalization of indigenous and holistic practices in the chapters that follow, providing a voice to those often silenced in the narrative of medical progress. Notably, the book not only critiques but also offers constructive pathways forward. It outlines practical solutions for integrating AI with traditional healing methods, ensuring that these technologies respect and enhance these ancient practices without superseding them. By incorporating case studies and practical examples, we ensure that theoretical discussions are grounded, offering tangible blueprints for future integration. Ultimately, this book serves as a call to action for developers, policymakers, and practitioners in the medical field to recognize and rectify these biases. It advocates for a more inclusive approach to healthcare that respects and integrates the diversity of healing practices worldwide. Our journey through these pages is not just an academic exercise; it is a crucial step towards crafting a more equitable and holistic future in medical practice. Thank you for joining us on this important journey.

**Introduction to AI, Medicine, and Bias**

**Defining Artificial Intelligence**

Artificial Intelligence (AI) emerges as a revolutionary force in medicine, wielding the power to reshape diagnosis, treatment, and patient care. At its core, AI encompasses technologies capable of performing tasks that typically require human intelligence. These tasks include reasoning, learning from data, recognizing patterns, and making decisions. AI systems range from those that handle specific, well-defined functions to more complex networks that engage in unsupervised learning and autonomous decision-making. The potential of AI in medicine is vast, promising enhanced efficiencies and breakthroughs in patient outcomes. However, the integration of AI raises intricate questions about bias and ethical implications. Delving deeper into AI's role in healthcare requires a nuanced understanding of its mechanisms. This subheading examines the fundamental aspects of AI technology, highlighting the sophisticated algorithms that drive systems, ranging from neural networks to machine learning models, and their applications in medical settings. As AI continues to evolve, its definition expands, reflecting its growing impact across medical disciplines.

**AI in Modern Medical Systems**

The integration of AI into modern medical systems marks a transformative phase in healthcare delivery. By leveraging AI, hospitals and clinics enhance their operational efficiency, enabling swifter diagnostics and tailored treatment plans. AI tools interpret large volumes of data, from radiographic images to genetic profiles, with a precision and speed unattainable by human clinicians alone. This capability not only accelerates diagnostic processes but also improves the accuracy of prognoses, fundamentally reshaping patient management.

However, the deployment of AI technologies in medical settings is not without its challenges. Issues of data privacy, security, and the need for transparent algorithms are pressing concerns that healthcare administrators must address. Additionally, the reliance on AI for critical health decisions introduces complex ethical questions, particularly regarding accountability in the event of diagnostic errors or treatment failures.

Despite these hurdles, the future of AI in medicine looks promising. As technology advances and regulatory frameworks evolve, AI is poised to become an indispensable asset in modern medical systems, potentially bridging gaps in healthcare accessibility and enhancing global health outcomes.

**Understanding Bias: Concepts and Consequences**

The concept of bias in AI, particularly in medical applications, encompasses preconceived notions and skewed data that AI systems learn from, leading to potentially unjust or harmful outcomes. Bias can arise from various sources, such as the data used for training AI systems, which might not be adequately representative of diverse populations. This skewed input results in output that perpetuates these imbalances, potentially disadvantaging certain groups in medical diagnostics and treatment plans.

Understanding the consequences of such biases in AI is critical. Misdiagnoses, inappropriate treatment recommendations, and overlooked symptoms are just a few potential repercussions. These failures not only compromise patient care but can exacerbate existing healthcare disparities, particularly affecting marginalized communities.

Moreover, AI-driven bias can erode trust in medical technology, leading to skepticism and reluctance from both patients and healthcare providers. Collaborative efforts among AI developers, clinicians, ethicists, and patients are essential for identifying, mitigating, and preventing biases that uphold the integrity and fairness of AI applications in medicine.

## Historical Evolution of AI in Healthcare

The journey of AI in healthcare traces back to the late 20th century when initial explorations focused on simple pattern recognition. Early systems, such as expert systems, attempted to mimic human clinical decision-making, relying heavily on fixed rules and structured inputs. Over the decades, with advancements in data storage and computational power, AI has evolved significantly. The 1990s marked the integration of neural networks, which significantly enhanced AI's ability to manage complex datasets, propelling advancements in areas such as imaging and diagnostics.

Entering the 21st century, machine learning became predominant, with algorithms learning from vast amounts of data to improve accuracy over time. This era saw AI applications becoming more nuanced, capable of handling unstructured data such as electronic health records and predictive analytics. Today, AI's footprint in healthcare extends from robotic surgery to personalized medicine, pushing the boundaries of what is achievable in-patient care and operational efficiency.

Looking back, this evolution not only marked technological leaps but also underscored the growing necessity for safeguards against AI-induced biases and ethical dilemmas. As AI's capabilities expanded, so too did the imperative for rigorous oversight and inclusive training data, aiming to ensure equitable healthcare outcomes for all demographics.

## AI in Diagnostic Medicine: Current Landscape

The current landscape of AI in diagnostic medicine sets a dynamic stage for innovation and challenges. Advanced AI systems are now crucial in interpreting complex diagnostic data, thereby enhancing the precision of radiology, pathology, and other diagnostic fields. Often, these AI models process and analyze medical imagery with greater speed and accuracy than human counterparts, providing crucial support in diagnosis and treatment planning.

Despite these advances, the integration of AI in diagnostics is fraught with ethical and practical dilemmas. The reliance on large, often impersonal datasets can lead to a detachment from individual patient contexts, risking the oversimplification of complex human conditions. Moreover, the quality of AI diagnostics heavily depends on the diversity and completeness of the data, which are not always guaranteed.

Looking ahead, the growth of AI in diagnostics promises to refine its integration into traditional medical practice. Ongoing research and regulatory adjustments aim to mitigate biases and enhance the representativeness of AI systems, to craft a future where AI complements the nuances of human medical judgment without overriding it.

## Bias Detection Methods in AI Systems

Identifying and mitigating bias in AI systems within medical settings requires sophisticated techniques calibrated for high stakes. Detection often starts with diversity audits of training data, ensuring representation from varied demographics. Discrepancies in this area usually lead to biased AI outputs. Testing involves generating synthetic data and simulating diverse clinical scenarios to evaluate AI performance across different patient profiles. This method reveals hidden prejudices not initially apparent.

Furthermore, bias can be monitored using statistical analysis techniques, such as regression testing, which measures how variables like race or gender influence AI decisions. This intersectional approach helps pinpoint the nuanced ways bias manifests in medical AI. Sensitivity analysis, another critical tool, assesses how variations in input data can affect outcomes, highlighting the system's robustness against skewed data.

Continuous monitoring forms the cornerstone of bias mitigation. Post-deployment, AI systems in medicine are continually monitored through real-time feedback loops, which integrate clinician experiences and patient outcomes to refine algorithms. This ongoing vigilance ensures AI advancements contribute positively to equitable healthcare delivery.

## Bias vs. Accuracy in Medical AI

The balance between bias and accuracy in medical AI has emerged as a pivotal concern. While advancements in AI have significantly enhanced diagnostic accuracy, they also risk reinforcing historical biases embedded within training data. Accurate AI models perform efficiently on the data they have been trained on; however, this accuracy may mask underlying biases when applied universally across diverse patient populations, potentially leading to misdiagnosed conditions in underrepresented groups.

Minimizing bias without compromising accuracy requires a nuanced approach, integrating diverse datasets that reflect the broad spectrum of human conditions and demographic variations. These inclusive data pools equip AI systems to make more accurate and equitable decisions. A model's utility in clinical settings hinges not only on its precision but also on its capacity to operate fairly across different populations.

Bias and accuracy in medical AI are not mutually exclusive; instead, they are interdependent. Addressing one should not undermine the other. Ideally, efforts to enhance algorithmic fairness should be designed to improve, rather than impede, diagnostic accuracy. This dual focus has the potential to lead to groundbreaking innovations in personalized medicine, ultimately benefiting the entire spectrum of patients by providing tailored and unbiased healthcare solutions.

## The Role of AI in Personalized Medicine

Artificial intelligence stands at the forefront of transforming personalized medicine, aiming to tailor treatment to individual patient profiles. By analyzing vast datasets, AI identifies patterns that may not be apparent to human clinicians, facilitating highly personalized therapy plans. This capability not only enhances treatment efficacy but also reduces the likelihood of adverse drug reactions.

However, the integration of AI in personalized medicine raises significant concerns regarding data bias and the representation of diverse genetic backgrounds. If not adequately managed, biased AI systems can perpetuate treatment disparities, leading to suboptimal care for underrepresented groups. It is therefore crucial that the development of AI tools involves diverse data that reflects the broad spectrum of human health conditions.

Implementing AI in personalized medicine necessitates ongoing oversight and consideration of ethical implications. Collaboration among scientists, ethicists, and healthcare providers is essential to ensure AI applications respect patient diversity and promote equity in healthcare outcomes. The goal is designing AI-driven interventions that are as inclusive as they are innovative, offering every patient precisely calibrated care that addresses their unique health needs.

## Challenges of Integrating AI in Medical Settings

Integrating AI into medical settings introduces a complex array of challenges. Primarily, cultural and institutional resistance often surfaces as traditional health care providers grapple with new technological paradigms. Staff may fear obsolescence or express skepticism towards AI's diagnostic recommendations, which can impede the adoption and effective utilization of AI technologies.

Technical hurdles also play a significant role. Ensuring AI systems communicate seamlessly with existing electronic health records (EHRs) and other healthcare IT infrastructure is often a formidable challenge. Compatibility issues may lead to significant disruptions in workflow, potentially compromising patient care. Moreover, maintaining patient privacy while utilizing AI poses another considerable concern, as these systems often require access to vast amounts of sensitive data.

Addressing these challenges requires a multidisciplinary approach that involves continuous training, updates to IT infrastructure, and robust data protection strategies. Ethical considerations must also steer the development and implementation of AI, ensuring technologies enhance rather than undermine the trust and integrity fundamental to healthcare.

## Types of Bias in AI: From Algorithmic to Systematic

In medical AI, biases span from algorithmic to systematic. Algorithmic bias occurs when flawed algorithms produce skewed results due to non-representative or incomplete training data. These biases can manifest subtly, affecting the accuracy and fairness of diagnoses and treatment recommendations. For example, specific algorithms might misinterpret data from minority groups if not adequately represented in the training set, leading to misdiagnoses or inappropriate treatments.

Systematic bias extends beyond the data and algorithms, permeating the very structures within which AI systems operate. This includes institutional biases embedded in the healthcare protocols and practices that inform how data is collected, analyzed, and applied. Such biases are often more challenging to detect and rectify, as they involve complex interplays of social, economic, and political forces that influence medical decision-making processes.

Addressing these types of bias requires a multifaceted approach. It involves not only refining data sets and algorithms but also critically examining and modifying the healthcare infrastructures that sustain systemic biases. Ongoing efforts to incorporate holistic and indigenous healing knowledge into AI training can provide invaluable perspectives that challenge conventional biases and enhance AI's capacity to serve diverse populations equitably.

## Impact of Bias on Healthcare Quality

The infiltration of bias in AI systems fundamentally undermines the quality of healthcare provided to diverse populations. Biased algorithms can precipitate unequal healthcare outcomes, where some demographic groups receive substandard care due to inherent flaws in AI-driven diagnosis and treatment plans.

For instance, if an AI system is predominantly trained on data from one ethnic group, it may produce less accurate or relevant results for other groups. This can lead to misdiagnosis or delayed treatment for underrepresented groups, amplifying existing health disparities. The consequences extend beyond individual patients, impacting community health statistics negatively and perpetuating cycles of inequality.

Translating these biased outputs into clinical settings without rigorous checks can erode trust in medical technology, complicating the relationship between healthcare providers and patients. The challenge lies in refining AI applications to perform equitably across all populations, ensuring that the promise of better healthcare through technology is realized universally, not selectively.

**AI and Ethical Medical Practice**

AI and ethical medical practice intersect profoundly, steering the discussions around the responsible use of technology in healthcare. Ethical considerations must prioritize patient autonomy, confidentiality, and equitable treatment - principles that are sometimes at odds with the operation of AI systems in medicine.

AI models, ideally unbiased and accurate, often struggle with ethical complexities such as informed consent. Patients must understand how their data is used, a challenge where AI operates opaquely, deciphering vast datasets behind the scenes. Fostering transparency is crucial, enabling patients to make informed decisions about their treatment options, understanding AI's role therein.

Moreover, equity remains a paramount concern. Ethical AI must not only avoid perpetuating existing healthcare disparities but actively contribute to their amelioration. Strategies include diverse training datasets and interdisciplinary oversight, ensuring AI tools cater universally and fairly. Without utmost diligence in ethical considerations, AI's potential to revolutionize medicine risks being overshadowed by its pitfalls.

**The Significance of Data Integrity**

Data integrity forms the backbone of effective AI application in healthcare. Ensuring the accuracy and completeness of data is pivotal, as any compromise can result in skewed AI outputs that may jeopardize patient care. Reliable data underpins the development of algorithms that are both precise and impartial, enabling AI to serve diverse patient demographics effectively.

Moreover, the validity of data determines AI's ability to accurately reflect the vast spectrum of human diseases and treatments, including those recognized in traditional and indigenous medicine. Incorporating holistic healing approaches into AI systems demands a rigorous validation of data sources to prevent the overlook of valuable non-conventional medical knowledge.

Failure to maintain data integrity not only disrupts the operational efficiency of AI systems but also compounds the risk of bias transmission into clinical decisions. The healthcare sector must thus enforce stringent data governance protocols to safeguard data accuracy and foster an inclusive AI framework that respects and integrates a wide array of medicinal practices.

**Addressing AI Prejudices in Therapy Recommendations**

Addressing AI biases in therapy recommendations involves a nuanced understanding of the diverse medical notions that shape treatment options. AI algorithms often prioritize conventional medical data, marginalizing traditional, indigenous, and holistic insights that could offer valuable therapeutic perspectives. To truly harmonize AI with an inclusive therapeutic repertoire, developers need to incorporate a broader spectrum of medicinal knowledge.

Efforts to mitigate AI prejudices in therapy strategies must start with diversified data collection. Incorporating ethnographically diverse medical practices in training datasets ensures that AI systems can offer recommendations that respect cultural and regional health traditions. This approach not only enhances the cultural competence of AI but also deepens its diagnostic and therapeutic precision.

Moreover, continuous monitoring and updating of AI systems are crucial to safeguard against the perpetuation of outdated or biased medical practices. Collaboration between AI technicians, healthcare professionals, and cultural representatives can forge pathways that honor both scientific and traditional healing methodologies, thereby improving patient outcomes across diverse populations.

**Cross-disciplinary Approaches to AI and Medicine**

Bridging the gap between disparate disciplines offers pioneering pathways to diminish AI bias in medicinal contexts. The fusion of computational sciences with sociology, anthropology, and traditional medicine transforms AI into a more holistic tool. Intriguingly, this synthesis facilitates a broader interpretation of health data, viewing patient information through a spectrum of cultural, social, and traditional lenses rather than purely biomedical ones.

Engagement with professionals from diverse fields seeds innovation in AI's algorithmic development, ensuring varied perspectives inform the framework from the outset. For instance, collaboration between AI developers and traditional healers could unveil biases previously unnoticed by technologists alone. Such partnerships encourage the embedding of indigenous healing practices into the corpus of AI healthcare solutions, enhancing its relevance and reducing cultural bias.

Moreover, involving ethicists and psychologists in AI design helps in crafting systems sensitive to patient dignity and privacy, aligning technological advancements with ethical medical practice. These cross-disciplinary endeavors not only enrich the AI development process but also anchor it in a more ethically conscious and culturally aware methodology, promising a fairer medical future for all.

**AI's Reliance on Historical Medical Data**

The functionality and validity of AI in modern healthcare hinge crucially on the historical medical data it ingests. This reliance often embeds latent biases deeply within AI systems, originating from the data's demographic and technological discrepancies. Historical medical databases may predominantly represent certain populations over others, skewing AI algorithms towards these better-documented groups, which perpetuates and even exacerbates healthcare disparities.

Moreover, the type of data collected and valued historically reflects medical paradigms and practices, frequently sidelining indigenous, traditional, or holistic approaches. As AI systems are trained on data steeped in conventional Western medicine, the rich diversity of global medical knowledge finds little reflection in AI-driven diagnostics and treatments. This imbalance not only limits the effectiveness of AI in diverse settings but also dismisses a wealth of cultural health practices.

Addressing this challenge calls for a reevaluation of historical datasets with an aim to integrate diversity at the foundation of AI training. Efforts must be made to archive and utilize a more representational gamut of medical data, incorporating nuanced health practices from varied cultures to guide AI towards more equitable and universally competent medical solutions.

**Societal Perceptions of AI in Healthcare**

Societal perceptions of AI in healthcare vary widely, influenced by a blend of media portrayals, personal experiences, and cultural backgrounds. Positive views often stem from AI's potential to revolutionize diagnostics, improve treatment precision, and enhance patient care efficiency. However, skepticism exists, particularly around issues of privacy, the impersonality of technology in medical interactions, and fears of reduced human oversight.

The general public's trust in AI technologies in medicine correlates strongly with their understanding of how these systems operate and the benefits they offer. Effective communication and education about AI's role and limitations can foster greater acceptance and trust. Moreover, showcasing successful case studies where AI has significantly improved health outcomes can shift perceptions positively.

Nevertheless, apprehensions about replacing human judgment with algorithmic decisions persist. To address these concerns, ongoing dialogue between healthcare providers, technologists, and patients is essential, emphasizing AI as a tool to assist, not replace, human expertise in medical practice. Striking this balance can cultivate a more informed and supportive environment for AI integration in healthcare.

## Potential Sources of Bias Embedded Within AI Tools

The sources of bias inherent in AI tools are multifaceted, rooted in both the data these systems are built upon and the methodologies employed in their development. Predominantly, biases arise from the demographic imbalances in the health data used to train AI. If the data skews towards populations, the resulting AI applications naturally inherit these discrepancies, potentially leading to misdiagnoses or inappropriate treatment recommendations for underrepresented groups.

Further embedding bias, the design and programming decisions made by developers—who may themselves have unconscious biases—can influence AI behavior. These biases are often opaque, woven into the algorithms through subjective decisions about which data variables to emphasize or ignore. Additionally, the economic and institutional priorities shaping these tools can also guide AI functionalities towards certain biases, inadvertently prioritizing efficiency or cost-effectiveness over comprehensive patient care.

Ultimately, recognizing these potential sources of bias demands rigorous scrutiny and continuous revision of AI systems to ensure equitable and effective medical treatment for all demographics.

## Strategies to Mitigate AI Bias

Mitigating bias in AI is pivotal for ensuring equitable healthcare outcomes across diverse populations. A foundational strategy involves diversifying training data sets. By incorporating global health data, including traditional, indigenous, and holistic healing practices, AI systems gain a richer, culturally informed perspective, enhancing their diagnostic and treatment outputs.

Another critical approach is the implementation of rigorous algorithm auditing systems. Regular reviews and updates of AI algorithms help identify and rectify biases that might evolve over time. These audits should be conducted by interdisciplinary teams, including data scientists, ethicists, and practitioners from diverse medical traditions to ensure comprehensive evaluations.

Furthermore, fostering transparency in AI operations engages public trust and facilitates an open dialogue about the technology's capabilities and limitations. Educating healthcare providers and patients about AI's operational mechanisms and inherent biases can lead to more informed interactions with these systems.

Lastly, implementing robust ethical guidelines and continuous training programs for AI developers can help instill a bias-aware culture within tech teams, ultimately leading to more equitable AI applications in medicine.

## The Importance of Transparency in AI Operations

Transparency is crucial in AI operations within healthcare, serving as a cornerstone for trust and accountability. As AI systems increasingly make decisions that affect patient outcomes, clear visibility into how these decisions is made is paramount. This involves disclosing the algorithms' decision-making processes and the data on which they are trained, allowing for scrutiny and understanding from healthcare professionals and patients alike.

Moreover, transparency is not just about revealing the 'how' and 'what' but also about explaining the 'why' behind AI decisions. This is essential for diagnosing and addressing potential biases that may arise from skewed data inputs or flawed algorithmic logic. Ensuring that AI operations are transparent can help mitigate these issues, fostering an environment where technology supplements human judgment rather than obscures it.

Publicly accessible records of AI operations, including their successes and failures, create a feedback loop that benefits developers, clinicians, and the wider community. This openness not only improves the algorithms through diverse input but also bolsters public confidence in AI-assisted medicine, aligning technology with the ideals of ethical practice and equitable care.

**AI Training: Developing Bias-Aware Medical Algorithms**

The task of ingraining fairness into AI within medicine revolves fundamentally around training strategies. As AI systems are contingent on the data and principles fed into them, creating bias-aware algorithms demands a deliberate fusion of diverse data sources and ethical training practices. This requires integrating global health knowledge, including underexplored medical systems like traditional and indigenous healing, to provide a multifaceted perspective.

Furthermore, developers must be equipped with tools and knowledge to recognize and adjust for biases. Training programs focusing on ethical AI creation are critical, emphasizing the importance of cultural competence and sensitivity. These efforts must be supported by robust policy frameworks that mandate the inclusion of diverse datasets and fairness audits.

Lastly, creating feedback mechanisms where AI's decisions are continually assessed and adjusted in real-world settings ensures ongoing refinement. Collaborative work environments that bring together technologists, ethicists, and medical professionals can foster the development of genuinely inclusive medical AI systems, ultimately enhancing patient care across various demographic groups.

**Balancing Human Oversight with AI Autonomy**

Balancing human oversight with AI autonomy in medical contexts is crucial for maintaining the integrity and safety of healthcare delivery. While AI can process vast datasets quicker than human practitioners, it lacks the nuanced understanding and empathetic decision-making that characterize human interactions. To optimize outcomes, a hybrid model where AI supports rather than replaces clinicians is essential.

This integration requires clear protocols specifying when and how clinicians should interface with AI systems. Establishing boundaries for AI's autonomous operations helps prevent over-reliance on technology, safeguarding against potential biases that AI systems may perpetuate. Continuous training for healthcare professionals on interacting with and overseeing AI operations ensures that human judgment remains at the forefront of patient care.

Moreover, incorporating regular assessments of AI decisions by medical professionals can provide real-time checks and balances, enhancing patient outcomes. These assessments help to highlight any deviation from standard care practices prompted by AI recommendations, ensuring that treatment plans remain patient-centered and culturally sensitive. Thus, a deliberate balance between AI autonomy and human oversight is pivotal for ethical and effective medical practice.

**Examining Case Studies of AI Induced Errors in Medicine**

The journey through AI-induced missteps in medicine reveals critical lessons. One notable case involved an AI system designed to prioritize patient care in emergency departments. Unfortunately, the system failed to correctly interpret symptoms from non-Western patients, leading to delayed treatments for critical conditions. This error stemmed from a dataset predominantly filled with Western patient data, spotlighting the risk of demographic bias in AI training datasets.

Another case featured an AI-driven diagnostic tool for skin cancer that disproportionately misdiagnosed darker skin tones. The underlying cause was a training set composed mainly of lighter skin images, reflecting a stark oversight in dataset diversity. Such instances underscore the necessity for comprehensive and inclusive data that reflect global demographic variations.

These case studies serve as sobering reminders of the potential consequences of neglecting diversity and inclusivity in AI development. They push for a recalibration of how AI tools are designed, demanding rigorous bias checks and a broader scope in testing protocols to enhance accuracy and fairness in medical AI applications.

**Future Prospects: Enhancing AI's Role in Fair Medical Practices**

As AI becomes increasingly integral to healthcare, the focus must shift to enhancing its role in fair medical practices. The future landscape hinges on developing AI systems that can effectively learn from diverse medical knowledge spanning traditional, indigenous, and holistic healing. This requires innovative modifications in AI's learning algorithms to understand and integrate multifaceted health paradigms, transcending conventional Western medical data sources.

Incorporating ethical AI training that emphasizes inclusion and represents all patient demographics will be crucial. Advanced AI models must not only recognize varied health practices but also respect and apply these insights to provide culturally sensitive and equitable treatment recommendations. This could involve collaborative efforts between AI technologists and healers from various cultural backgrounds, aiming to fuse traditional health wisdom with cutting-edge technology.

Conclusively, sustaining ongoing public and professional engagement will ensure that AI's evolution aligns with societal values. As AI systems adapt, an established framework for continuous improvement and accountability in AI-driven interventions is imperative, ensuring that future AI advancements enhance inclusivity and fairness in medical practices.

## Summary

Artificial Intelligence (AI) is transforming modern medicine, offering unprecedented advancements in diagnosis, treatment planning, and patient care efficiency. The integration of AI in healthcare spans from handling substantial volumes of data like radiographic images and genetic profiles to enhancing diagnostic accuracy and treatment personalization. AI technologies, including neural networks and machine learning models, are progressively being adapted to understand complex medical data autonomously, fostering significant breakthroughs in various medical fields. However, this technological integration carries inherent challenges, primarily concerning bias and ethical implications. Bias in AI, emanating from skewed training data and algorithmic design, can lead to discriminatory practices and unequal healthcare outcomes, especially among marginalized communities. Boasting the capacity to refine diagnosis and prognoses, AI's promise in medicine continues to grow, potentially narrowing healthcare accessibility gaps and propelling global health advancements. Yet, the reliance on data-driven AI systems necessitates rigorous oversight to prevent the perpetuation of existing biases and ensure fair and equitable treatment across all patient demographics. Addressing these biases requires a concerted effort involving continuous monitoring, transparent algorithms, and inclusive data practices that embrace the diversity of patient populations. The evolution of AI in healthcare is identified not just by technological advances but also by the increasing necessity to safeguard against ethical dilemmas and ensure comprehensive patient treatment irrespective of demographic factors. The chapter underscores the critical need for interdisciplinary collaborations, wherein AI developers, ethicists, clinicians, and patients collectively endeavor to mitigate biases and uphold the integrity of AI applications in medicine.

## References

[1] Eric J. Topol, 'Deep Medicine: How Artificial Intelligence Can Make Healthcare Human Again'.
https://www.amazon.com/Deep-Medicine-Artificial-Intelligence-Healthcare/dp/1541644638
[2] Ruqaiijah Yearby, Lawrence O. Gostin, 'Structural Racism and Health Disparities: Reconfiguring the Social Determinants of Health Framework to Include the Root Cause'.
https://www.ncbi.nlm.nih.gov/pmc/articles/PMC8006603/
[3] Charlene Goh, Matthew Chin Heng Chua, 'Integrating Artificial Intelligence into Healthcare Operations: Challenges and Perspectives'. https://www.sciencedirect.com/science/article/pii/S0007681319301023
[4] Ziad Obermeyer, Sendhil Mullainathan, 'Dissecting Racial Bias in an Algorithm Used to Manage the Health of Populations'. https://science.sciencemag.org/content/366/6464/447

### Case Study: AI Implementation in Dermatological Diagnosis: A Case of Bias and Success

The integration of Artificial Intelligence (AI) in dermatology has advanced the efficiency and accuracy of skin disease diagnoses. However, a prominent hospital faced significant challenges when deploying a new AI system designed to enhance diagnostic processes for skin conditions across diverse populations. Originally, the AI tool was trained using predominantly Caucasian skin data, which led to an alarming rate of misdiagnoses in patients with darker skin tones. This discrepancy highlighted critical issues of bias in AI models affecting medical outcomes.

An investigation revealed that the AI system's algorithm was not exposed to sufficient training data from diverse races and ethnicities. This oversight resulted in the AI's poor performance in accurately diagnosing conditions such as melanoma and psoriasis in non-Caucasian patients, important given the different morphologies these conditions can exhibit on various skin types. The consequences of these misdiagnoses were severe, ranging from delayed treatment to unnecessary anxiety and inappropriate treatments for patients.

In response, the hospital initiated a comprehensive overhaul of their AI training protocols. In collaboration with dermatologists specializing in skin of color, data scientists expanded the AI system's training dataset to include a wider array of skin tone images and case studies. This approach not only improved the algorithm's diagnostic accuracy but also elevated the hospital's standard of equitable care. Moreover, continuous feedback loops were integrated, allowing ongoing algorithm adjustments based on real-world diagnostic outcomes and clinician reviews.

The refined AI system notably reduced diagnostic errors and substantially improved patient satisfaction and trust in dermatological AI diagnostics. This case study underscores the importance of diversity in training datasets and continuous algorithm monitoring to minimize bias in AI medical systems, ensuring fair and accurate healthcare delivery across all demographics.

### Case Study: Overcoming AI Challenges in Predictive Oncology at Regional Hospital

The Regional Hospital faced significant barriers when attempting to integrate AI in predictive oncology, with the key challenge stemming from the biased outcomes produced by their new AI diagnostic tool. This AI system was primarily trained on data from a limited demographic, skewing its predictive analytics towards that population's cancer profiles, which led to unreliable predictions for the hospital's multi-ethnic patient base.

Upon identifying discrepancies in cancer prediction rates among diverse patient groups, the oncology department raised concerns regarding the potential risks of such biases. The AI model, while technologically advanced, was misjudging tumor aggressiveness and recommended treatment plans deviated substantially between ethnic groups, particularly underserving historically marginalized communities.

Recognizing the severity of these issues, the hospital took a proactive approach by forming a multidisciplinary team including AI technologists, data scientists, oncologists, and ethicists. The primary objective was to reconfigure the existing AI algorithms to handle a broader spectrum of genetic variability and environmental factors influencing cancer progression across different ethnicities. This involved curating a new training dataset that encompassed a more representative cross-section of the hospital's patient population, including more comprehensive genetic material, lifestyle information, and prior medical histories.

Moreover, the implementation phase included continuous monitoring systems to track the AI's performance and adaptability in real-time, accommodating feedback from oncologists and feedback from patients regarding treatment outcomes. This system not only improved the AI tool's prediction accuracy but also restored trust among patients and staff. The case study from Regional Hospital illustrates the necessity of continuous oversight, diverse data integration, and interdisciplinary collaboration to mitigate bias in medical AI applications, ultimately aiming to deliver truly personalized and equitable cancer treatment.

### Case Study: Revolutionizing Emergency Care: AI-Enhanced Triage System at MetroHealth Center

MetroHealth Center, a major urban hospital, took a bold step toward innovative healthcare by integrating an Artificial Intelligence (AI)-based triage system aimed at optimizing their emergency department's efficiency and patient flow. Initially, the system promised to reduce wait times and prioritize patients based on the severity of their conditions through an automated, data-driven process. The AI system, leveraging machine learning and complex algorithms, analyzed incoming patient data in real-time, assessing symptoms and predicting the urgency of medical attention needed.

However, after the initial deployment, the hospital observed unintended disparities in patient prioritization. The AI system disproportionately flagged high-priority cases among patients with certain demographic profiles—specifically, its under-prioritized elderly patients and certain ethnic minorities. Analysis revealed that the training data used primarily consisted of historical patient records which inadvertently reflected past biases in patient treatment and triage decisions. This revelation prompted a critical reassessment of the AI system's decision-making framework.

In response, MetroHealth formed a task force comprising AI developers, emergency medicine specialists, and bioethics experts. This team was charged with redesigning the AI's algorithm to be more inclusive and representative of the diverse population the hospital serves. They augmented the training data with a more balanced dataset, including a wider array of patient interactions, to cover varied medical scenarios affecting different demographic groups. More importantly, they introduced continuous learning capabilities to the AI system, enabling it to adjust its algorithms based on ongoing patient outcome data and feedback from clinical staff.

The restructured AI triage system marked a significant improvement. It not only balanced the accuracy of patient prioritization but also highlighted the hospital's commitment to equitable health treatment. The endeavor nurtured greater trust in AI-assisted processes among the staff and patients, showcasing the critical role of ongoing oversight and dynamic algorithm adaptation in deploying AI technologies in sensitive, high-stakes environments like emergency medicine.

### Case Study: AI in Cardiovascular Risk Prediction: Redefining Preventive Care

Heart disease remains one of the leading causes of mortality worldwide, with early intervention being critical to prevent adverse outcomes. Prompted by this healthcare challenge, GoodHope Hospital implemented an AI-powered cardiovascular risk prediction system aimed at enhancing preventive care strategies. The system was designed to utilize deep learning algorithms to analyze electronic health records (EHRs), lifestyle factors, and genetic markers to predict patients at high risk of cardiovascular events.

Initially, the AI model demonstrated impressive predictive accuracy in clinical trials involving predominantly Western populations. However, when deployed in a diverse urban area serving a multi-ethnic community, the model's efficacy noticeably diminished. It became evident that the AI system was underperforming in accurately identifying risk in individuals from certain ethnic backgrounds, particularly those from South Asian and African descents, who are statistically at a higher risk for cardiovascular diseases. This discrepancy in predictive accuracy raised concerns about the inclusivity and fairness of the AI tool.

Upon investigation, it was discovered that the training data largely consisted of information from Caucasian patients, leading to a model biased towards that demographic's cardiovascular profiles. To address this, GoodHope Hospital initiated a systematic revision of the AI system's training protocols. Collaborations with cardiologists who specialize in ethnic-specific cardiovascular issues were established, and new data pooling strategies were implemented to include a broader spectrum of genetic data and lifestyle information reflective of the diverse patient population.

The revised AI system employed an ongoing learning strategy, continuously updating its algorithms with new patient data and outcomes. This adaptive approach allowed the AI to become more sensitive to the nuances of different ethnic groups' cardiovascular risks. In addition, the hospital launched a community outreach program to increase health literacy and participation in preventive care, particularly targeting underrepresented groups. This multi-faceted approach not only enhanced the AI's predictive capacity but also fostered a more inclusive environment, promoting equitable health outcomes across all demographics.

### Case Study: AI-Enhanced Mental Health Screening at WellnessTech Clinic

WellnessTech Clinic, a progressive mental health facility, embarked on integrating Artificial Intelligence (AI) to revolutionize patient screening and treatment plans. The AI system, designed to analyze patient responses from initial consultations and ongoing therapy sessions, promised to identify mental health issues more swiftly and accurately than traditional methods. Initially, the system showed promising results in identifying common disorders like anxiety and depression, suggesting customized treatment paths based on patient data.

However, a significant challenge arose when the AI began to show discrepancies in diagnosing patients from diverse cultural backgrounds. Particularly, its under-diagnosed certain mental health conditions, such as post-traumatic stress disorder (PTSD) in veterans of non-Western origin and misinterpreted cultural expressions of distress as psychiatric symptoms in minority groups. This misinterpretation stemmed from the AI's training data, which predominantly included input from Western patients, lacking a comprehensive representation of cultural-specific expressions and conditions.

The clinic responded by forming a cross-disciplinary panel consisting of AI technologists, clinical psychologists, cultural studies experts, and ethicists. The goal was to redevelop the AI's learning algorithms to incorporate a broader spectrum of cultural expressions and symptom manifestations. This involved curating a new, diversified dataset that included nuanced mental health presentations from various cultural contexts, ensuring these variations were well-represented.

Additionally, to address real-time discrepancies, WellnessTech implemented a continuous feedback mechanism where clinicians reviewed AI assessments and provided insights on any cultural misinterpretations. This data was then used to adapt and refine the AI algorithms regularly. The outcome was a more sensitive AI system that not only recognized a wider array of mental health issues across different cultures but also proposed treatment plans that respected patients' cultural and individual nuances.

**Case Study: Enhancing Diabetes Management through AI-Powered Predictive Analytics**

A leading healthcare technology company developed an AI system designed to enhance the management of diabetes by predicting episodes of hyperglycemia and hypoglycemia before they occur. The AI tool utilized machine learning algorithms to analyze continuous glucose monitoring (CGM) data, along with patient-recorded food intake, physical activity, and medication adherence, to forecast glucose level trends. Initially, the AI model demonstrated high accuracy in a controlled test group, primarily constituted of a homogenous patient demographic.

Upon wider deployment across a diverse patient base, however, the tool began exhibiting significant discrepancies in predicting glucose events for patients of different ethnic backgrounds and socioeconomic statuses. For instance, it became apparent that the AI was less accurate for patients with varied dietary habits that were not well-represented in the initial training data set. Additionally, patients from lower socioeconomic backgrounds, who might have irregular access to consistent healthcare, displayed unpredicted glycemic events that the system failed to anticipate.

The company acted by organizing a diverse focus group including endocrinologists, patients, and data scientists. They aimed to address these discrepancies by collecting a broader array of data that included more variables related to lifestyle choices and social determinants of health. This enriched data pool enabled more inclusive training and fine-tuning of the AI algorithms.

Moreover, to mitigate bias and improve reliability, the firm introduced transparency in AI operations, providing clear insights into how the AI made predictions and allowing clinicians to review and adjust AI-driven recommendations. This dual approach not only improved the system's accuracy across diverse patient profiles but also bolstered patient and practitioner trust in the AI-driven tool. Through these enhancements, the healthcare provider was able to offer a more personalized and effective diabetes management solution, promoting better patient outcomes universally.

**Case Study: AI-Driven Stroke Rehabilitation: Challenges and Breakthroughs at NeuroHeal Clinic**

In a notable attempt to integrate advanced technology into rehabilitative care, NeuroHeal Clinic began utilizing an AI-driven system designed to personalize rehabilitation programs for stroke survivors. The system employed machine learning algorithms to analyze patient data, including motor function, speech ability, and cognitive assessments, to tailor specific therapies to each patient's recovery progress.

Initially, the AI demonstrated remarkable success in shortening recovery timeframes and improving patient outcomes by dynamically adjusting therapy plans based on real-time data. However, the clinic soon encountered a significant hurdle. The AI system started showing a pattern of less favorable outcomes for older patients and patients from certain ethnic minorities, suggesting underlying biases in its decision-making processes.

Investigation revealed that the system's training data primarily included recovery patterns and responses from younger, ethnically homogeneous populations, leading to skewed therapeutic recommendations. The implications of these biases were profound, ranging from slower recovery rates in the affected groups to increased frustrations and decreased trust in the AI system among patients and healthcare providers.

As a response, NeuroHeal initiated a comprehensive review of their AI protocols. This involved collaboration with experts in geriatric and cross-cultural medicine to retrain the AI system with a more diverse dataset reflective of the clinic's patient demographics. Additionally, the clinic introduced a continuous monitoring system that allowed real-time adjustments to the AI's recommendations, based on feedback from physiotherapists and occupational therapists directly involved in patient care.

This proactive approach not only addressed the bias issues but also restored confidence in the AI system's efficacy. As a result, the clinic saw an improvement in rehabilitation outcomes across all demographic groups, reinforcing the potential of AI in enhancing personalized medical care and advocating for the importance of diversity in training data to prevent bias in medical AI applications.

### Case Study: Multidisciplinary Approach to Addressing AI Biases in Pediatric Asthma Management

A leading pediatric hospital, renowned for its innovative approach to chronic illness management, embarked on implementing an AI-driven tool aimed at revolutionizing the treatment protocols for pediatric asthma. This AI system was designed to analyze patient data including symptom patterns, environmental triggers, and historical treatment responses, to recommend personalized care plans. Initially, the system showed promise by reducing emergency interventions by adapting proactive management strategies.

However, challenges surfaced when discrepancies in treatment efficacy became apparent across different demographic groups. The AI tool was primarily effective for patients from urban areas, leading to concerns about its applicability to rural and ethnically diverse patient populations. A deeper analysis revealed that the AI's training data were overwhelmingly sourced from urban hospitals, which did not accurately represent the environmental and genetic factors prevalent in rural settings.

The hospital decided to take a multidisciplinary approach to resolve these issues. This included forming a team composed of AI developers, pediatricians, geneticists, and anthropologists with a deep understanding of the socio-cultural dynamics affecting health in diverse populations. The team's first action was to reassess and expand the diversity of the data set, integrating a wide range of environmental and socio-economic factors affecting asthma.

In parallel, the hospital initiated a series of community engagement workshops in various locales, aiming to educate and gather feedback directly from affected communities. This feedback was crucial in identifying overlooked factors like regional allergens and traditional housing conditions that could influence asthma triggers.

Following the integration of this new, comprehensive data, the AI system underwent rigorous retraining sessions. The redeveloped model was then continuously monitored and fine-tuned in response to real-world outcomes. This approach not only led to more accurate and equitable treatment recommendations but also helped in building trust within the community, showcasing the ability of AI to adapt to the complexities of diverse healthcare needs.

### Review Questions

**1.** A 68-year-old woman with chronic knee osteoarthritis visits her doctor, complaining of increased pain and decreased mobility. She is a retired nurse and prefers non-pharmacological treatments due to previous adverse reactions to NSAIDs. Recently, she read about the potential benefits of Traditional Thai Massage (TTM) and is now considering it as an alternative treatment. What should the physician incorporate into her treatment plan based on her interest in TTM?

A) Recommend an immediate start of TTM alongside physical therapy.

B) Advise against TTM and prescribe a low-dose NSAID.

C) Suggest starting TTM but monitor its effectiveness closely.

D) Recommend a surgical consultation immediately.

**Answer: C**

Explanation: Traditional Thai Massage (TTM), known for its efficacy in managing pain and improving mobility in conditions like osteoarthritis of the knee, can be a valuable addition to the treatment plan. Given the patient's adverse reactions to NSAIDs and her preference for non-pharmacological treatments, suggesting the initiation of TTM is appropriate. The physician should monitor its effectiveness closely, allowing adjustments based on the patient's response. This approach respects the patient's preferences, potentially reduces pain and enhances mobility without the risks associated with NSAIDs or surgery.

## Overview of AI in Healthcare

### Defining Healthcare AI: Scope and Applications

Artificial intelligence (AI) in healthcare represents a transformative convergence of technology and medicine. Its scope is vast, encompassing everything from patient diagnostics to treatment planning and management. Healthcare AI leverages machine learning algorithms and big data analytics to interpret complex medical data, enabling more accurate diagnoses and personalized treatment strategies.

The applications are broad, including predictive analytics for patient monitoring, AI in surgical robotics, and the personalization of therapy protocols. AI empowers healthcare systems to function more efficiently by automating tasks, such as the interpretation of medical images and managing healthcare records. Furthermore, it enhances patient care by providing more precise treatment options and quicker diagnostics, potentially reducing hospital stays and improving health outcomes.

Beyond direct care, AI's utility spans to administrative functions within healthcare settings, optimizing operations like scheduling, billing, and compliance documentation. This multifaceted integration of AI paves the way for more responsive, accessible, and efficient healthcare delivery globally.

### Evolution of AI in Medical Practice

The evolution of AI in medical practice traces a remarkable trajectory from early computational models to sophisticated algorithms capable of mimicking human cognitive functions. Initially, AI was primarily used for basic data management and to assist with patient scheduling. As technology advanced, so too did AI's role, evolving into a critical tool for diagnostic support through pattern recognition in imaging and data analysis.

This transition was further fueled by the integration of machine learning, enabling AI systems to learn from vast datasets without explicit programming. These advances allowed AI to provide personalized treatment plans, predict patient outcomes, and support complex surgical procedures with enhanced precision. Innovations such as deep learning have paved the way for AI to analyze unstructured data like clinical notes, extracting valuable insights that were previously inaccessible.

Today, AI's influence extends across almost every aspect of healthcare, from robotic-assisted surgeries to mental health assessments. Its evolution reflects a growing synergy between technological capabilities and medical needs, aiming to augment not just the speed but the quality-of-care delivery.

### Core Technologies Powering AI in Healthcare

The backbone of AI in healthcare hinges on several pivotal technologies. Primarily, machine learning algorithms empower systems to make predictions and decisions based on data analysis. These algorithms adapt and improve over time, learning from new data inputs and outcomes to refine their prognostic accuracy.

Furthermore, deep learning, a subset of machine learning, utilizes artificial neural networks to analyze complex data structures. This enables the detailed interpretation of vast amounts of medical data, such as imaging and genomic information, with a level of precision that mimics human expertise but at a significantly faster pace. Deep learning has revolutionized fields such as radiology and pathology by providing more accurate diagnoses and predictive insights.

Natural language processing (NLP) is another critical component. It allows for the extraction of structured information from unstructured data sources like clinical notes and research papers. By analyzing this data, AI can provide comprehensive insights into patient health records, enhancing both the accuracy of diagnoses and the efficiency of care coordination.

## AI Applications in Diagnostics

The incorporation of AI in diagnostics marks a pivotal shift in medical practice, offering unprecedented accuracy and speed in patient evaluation. AI's ability to swiftly analyze vast datasets has significantly enhanced diagnostic processes, such as identifying patterns in X-rays and MRIs that might elude human detection. Moreover, AI algorithms have been instrumental in genetic sequencing, expediting the identification of genetic disorders and tailoring personalized treatment plans.

However, the benefits transcend mere speed. AI-driven diagnostics ensure a consistency unavailable to even the most trained professionals, mitigating human error and variability in diagnostic assessments. For instance, AI systems in pathology can evaluate tissue samples for malignancy with remarkable precision, providing a valuable second opinion to pathologists.

Despite these advancements, challenges persist. The accuracy of AI diagnostics often depends on the diversity and quality of training data. Ensuring that these systems are trained on comprehensive datasets, representative of the global population, remains crucial to avoid replicating biases seen in earlier applications.

## AI in Treatment Planning and Management

Artificial Intelligence (AI) revolutionizes treatment planning and management in healthcare, offering tailored strategies that significantly enhance patient outcomes. By integrating complex algorithms and vast data pools, AI systems can predict individual patient responses to various treatment modalities, facilitating personalized medicine at its core.

These AI-driven systems analyze historical health data, genetic information, and ongoing treatment results to refine and adapt treatment plans dynamically. This capability ensures that treatments are not only based on broad medical knowledge but are also continuously optimized according to patient-specific factors and emerging medical research.

The impact of AI on treatment management transcends traditional boundaries by incorporating predictive analytics to preemptively adjust treatments, potentially reducing the need for invasive procedures and minimizing side effects. Moreover, AI's ability to synchronize diverse data sources enables a more holistic approach to patient care, bridging gaps between different healthcare providers and specialties.

In essence, AI's sophisticated analytics and adaptive learning algorithms promise a future where treatment plans are as dynamic and unique as the patients themselves, driving forward a new era in customized healthcare.

## AI's Role in Surgical Procedures

The integration of AI in surgical procedures marks a significant advancement in the precision and efficiency of operations. AI-driven robotic systems offer unparalleled accuracy, reducing human error and enhancing outcomes in complex surgeries. These robots, guided by AI algorithms, can perform delicate tasks such as suturing and tissue manipulation with greater precision than human hands.

AI also plays a critical role in preoperative planning. By analyzing a multitude of data points from patient medical history to real-time imaging, AI systems help surgeons plan the most effective surgical approach. This tailored strategy minimizes risks and optimizes recovery times, contributing to better overall patient care.

Moreover, AI assists during surgery through real-time diagnostics and decision support. It can instantaneously process imaging data to guide surgeons in identifying and navigating critical areas. This real-time capability ensures that surgical interventions are both safe and precisely targeted, further enhancing the role of AI as an indispensable tool in modern surgical suites.

**Use of AI in Medical Imaging**

Artificial Intelligence (AI) has revolutionized the field of medical imaging, providing tools that enhance the precision and speed of image analysis. AI algorithms, especially those rooted in deep learning, excel at interpreting medical images, from X-rays to MRIs, with a degree of detail surpassing human capabilities. These systems analyze patterns in imaging data, enabling them to detect anomalies such as tumors and fractures with high accuracy.

Furthermore, AI in medical imaging not only assists in diagnosis but also aids in monitoring treatment progress and predicting disease outcomes. By analyzing sequential images, AI can track changes in a patient's condition, offering valuable insights that inform treatment adjustments. This ongoing assessment plays a pivotal role in personalized medicine, ensuring patient treatment plans remain adaptive and optimized.

Despite its benefits, the integration of AI into medical imaging requires careful consideration of data privacy and ethical standards. Ensuring robust protection of patient data and addressing potential biases in AI models are critical to maintaining trust and efficacy in AI-supported healthcare environments. The continuous advancement in AI technology promises further enhancements in medical imaging, potentially transforming diagnostic procedures and improving patient outcomes across the globe.

**AI in Drug Discovery and Development**

AI is transforming the landscape of drug discovery and development, accelerating processes that traditionally took years. Machine learning algorithms analyze biological and chemical data to predict how different substances affect human health, vastly improving the efficiency of identifying new drugs.

This technological revolution extends to the refinement of drug formulations and optimization of dosing schedules. AI systems sift through vast arrays of historical data and ongoing clinical trials to find optimal therapeutic combinations and minimize side effects. Such precision not only speeds up the development cycle but also enhances patient safety.

Additionally, AI's predictive capacities are invaluable in personalized medicine. By analyzing genetic markers, AI can predict individual responses to medications, allowing for more personalized treatment plans that drastically improve patient outcomes. The integration of AI into this field promises to refine therapeutic approaches, tailor medications to individual needs, and revolutionize healthcare.

**Benefits of AI: Enhancing Healthcare Delivery**

The advent of AI in healthcare has significantly propelled advancements in healthcare delivery, marking a transformative shift in how services are provided and managed. By leveraging AI, healthcare systems can achieve unprecedented levels of efficiency, reduce wait times and streamline patient flow from admission to discharge. This integration results in more timely healthcare interventions and enhanced patient satisfaction.

Additionally, AI's predictive analytics power plays a pivotal role in preventive care. By analyzing vast datasets, AI can forecast potential health issues before they become critical, allowing for preemptive medical action that can save lives and reduce the need for more invasive treatments later. This not only improves patient outcomes but also reduces the overall strain on healthcare systems.

Moreover, AI contributes to resource allocation by optimizing the use of medical equipment and personnel. Hospitals can harness AI to predict peak times for different services and allocate resources more effectively, ensuring that patients receive the right care at the right time. Overall, the integration of AI into healthcare delivery sets a foundation for more responsive, efficient, and patient-centered service provision.

**AI in Patient Monitoring and Care**

AI is revolutionizing patient monitoring and care, transforming the landscape of continuous health tracking and long-term care management. By leveraging machine learning algorithms and sensor technologies, AI systems provide real-time data analysis, offering a comprehensive view of a patient's health status. This capability significantly enhances early detection of potential health issues, allowing for prompt interventions that can prevent complications.

Moreover, AI-enabled devices facilitate remote patient monitoring, crucial for elderly or chronically ill patients who may require constant observation. These technologies ensure patients receive attentive care while maintaining independence in their own homes. Integration with mobile health applications empowers patients with actionable insights into their health parameters, fostering proactive personal health management.

AI-driven tools also assist healthcare professionals by reducing routine monitoring tasks, allowing them to focus more on direct patient care. Additionally, predictive analytics in AI systems can forecast acute medical events, thereby orchestrating timely emergency responses, ultimately improving patient outcomes and enhancing the efficacy of healthcare delivery.

**Telemedicine and AI: Expanding Access to Care**

Telemedicine, powered by Artificial Intelligence (AI), is radically altering the landscape of healthcare accessibility. By integrating AI tools, telemedicine platforms can decipher complex medical data, provide accurate diagnoses, and suggest tailored treatment plans, all in real-time. This technology enables healthcare professionals to reach underserved populations in remote and rural areas, bridging the significant gap in medical service provision.

AI enhances telemedicine by facilitating more precise and predictive analytics. These systems assess patient data and predict health threats before they escalate, allowing doctors to intervene promptly from a distance. Moreover, AI-driven teleconsultations offer convenience and lessen the necessity for physical hospital visits, which is crucial for patients with mobility challenges or those in regions with limited medical facilities.

Additionally, the fusion of AI with telemedicine ensures continuous patient monitoring and care management, overcoming geographical and logistical barriers. This not only democratizes healthcare by making it more inclusive but also significantly lowers costs, making healthcare more affordable and sustainable across diverse populations.

**AI-Driven Predictive Analytics in Public Health**

AI-driven predictive analytics is revolutionizing public health by providing foresight into epidemiological trends and potential outbreaks. These systems harness vast datasets, from hospital records to social determinants of health, to forecast public health threats, facilitating timely interventions.

The predictive power of AI allows for more strategic allocation of resources, targeting areas most at risk. Public health officials can deploy preventive measures, such as vaccination campaigns or educational programs, precisely where they are needed most. This preemptive approach helps in managing diseases more effectively, mitigating possible epidemics.

Moreover, AI analytics aid in understanding the impact of environmental factors on public health. By correlating data like pollution levels, weather patterns, and health outcomes, AI systems provide insights that lead to more informed policy decisions, ultimately fostering a healthier population.

Despite the promise, effective implementation requires stringent ethical considerations to ensure data privacy and prevent biases in AI models, maintaining the integrity of public health initiatives.

**Integration of AI with Electronic Health Records**

The integration of AI with Electronic Health Records (EHRs) marks a pivotal advancement in healthcare technology. AI systems enhance the functionality of EHRs by enabling more sophisticated data management and analysis capabilities. This integration allows for the seamless extraction and interpretation of patient data, supporting healthcare providers in making more informed clinical decisions.

Moreover, AI algorithms can identify patterns and anomalies in large volumes of data that would be challenging for humans to detect, leading to earlier diagnoses and personalized treatment plans. This capability not only improves clinical outcomes but also increases the operational efficiency of healthcare facilities. By automating routine tasks, AI frees up medical staff to focus on more complex and patient-centered activities.

Additionally, AI-driven EHRs facilitate better patient engagement and health management. They provide patients with accessible, understandable insights into their health records, promoting transparency and empowering individuals in their health journeys. The future of healthcare sees AI at the core of EHR systems, transforming data into actionable wisdom.

**AI in Healthcare: Regulatory and Ethical Considerations**

The integration of AI into healthcare prompts significant regulatory and ethical considerations, reflecting the dual imperative of innovation and patient safety. Regulators grapple with establishing guidelines that foster innovation while safeguarding patient data and ensuring equitable AI deployment. The complexity of AI models, coupled with their profound impact on health determinations, necessitates transparent AI frameworks to maintain accountability and trust.

Ethically, AI raises questions about bias and decision-making authority. Systems trained on limited or skewed datasets may exhibit biases that could lead to discriminatory healthcare practices. Regulating bodies are thus tasked with mandating rigorous fairness audits and continuous monitoring to mitigate these risks.

Furthermore, there's an ongoing debate regarding the extent to which AI should influence patient care decisions, emphasizing the need for a balanced approach that respects human oversight in critical health interventions.

In response, collaborations between technologists, ethicists, and regulators are crucial to address these concerns comprehensively. They work towards robust standards that not only prioritize patient outcomes but also respect the sensitive nature of health data, steering the future of AI in healthcare towards a more ethical and compliant trajectory.

## Data Privacy and Security in Medical AI Systems

The intersection of AI and healthcare has ushered in revolutionary capabilities in medical data processing and analysis. Yet, this integration raises substantial concerns regarding data privacy and security. Ensuring the confidentiality and safety of patient data in AI-driven systems is pivotal, given the sensitive nature of health information.

Medical AI systems often require vast quantities of data, sourced from diverse health records, to train and improve their predictive accuracy. This necessity exposes the data to potential breaches and misuse, underscoring the urgent need for robust encryption and secure data handling practices. Healthcare organizations must employ advanced cybersecurity measures to protect against unauthorized access while maintaining data integrity.

Furthermore, regulatory compliance, such as adherence to HIPAA in the United States, plays a critical role in shaping the frameworks within which AI operates. By enforcing stringent standards, healthcare providers can safeguard patient information, thereby foster trust and encourage the broader acceptance of AI technologies in medical contexts.

## The Impact of AI on Healthcare Professionals

The integration of AI into healthcare profoundly impacts professionals across various disciplines. AI tools optimize diagnostic and therapeutic processes, leading to a transformation in job roles and responsibilities. As AI systems undertake routine tasks, healthcare professionals are called upon to manage more complex clinical decisions, necessitating advanced training and new skill sets.

However, this shift also stirs concerns about job displacement. While AI can enhance efficiency, it introduces anxiety among workers about the diminishing need for human intervention in certain areas. Healthcare institutions must navigate these changes sensitively, providing retraining programs to ensure workforce adaptability.

Moreover, AI's influence extends to improving work-life balance for medical staff. Automated systems reduce administrative burdens, allowing doctors and nurses more time for direct patient care and interaction, which is essential for holistic treatment. This balance is crucial in preventing burnout among healthcare workers, enhancing both patient care and professional satisfaction.

## Patient Outcomes and AI: Assessing Efficacy

Assessing the efficacy of AI in healthcare hinges on its impact on patient outcomes. AI applications, from diagnostics to treatment management, promise enhanced precision and expedited care, yet the real measure of success lies in tangible improvements in patient health. Studies comparing AI-assisted interventions with conventional practices often reveal significant gains in treatment accuracy and patient satisfaction, underscoring AI's potential to elevate standard care protocols.

However, the narrative is not uniformly positive. Some reports caution about the over-reliance on AI systems, highlighting instances where AI's lack of adaptability in complex clinical scenarios led to suboptimal outcomes. Continuous monitoring and outcome-based evaluations are essential to mitigate such risks, ensuring that AI tools align closely with patient safety and health standards.

Ultimately, the integration of AI into healthcare settings must be patient-centric, emphasizing improved health outcomes as the primary goal. Collaborative efforts between AI developers, healthcare providers, and regulatory bodies are crucial to refine AI applications, making them robust companions in the journey towards enhanced patient care.

**Challenges of Implementing AI in Health Systems**

The deployment of AI in health systems presents myriad challenges, both technical and organizational. A primary obstacle is the infrastructure inadequacy in existing health settings. Many hospitals lack the advanced IT support needed to integrate AI solutions seamlessly, potentially leading to operational disruptions and increased costs.

Furthermore, there is a pronounced skills gap among healthcare personnel. The rapid evolution of AI technology necessitates continuous learning, yet many professionals are unprepared for the steep learning curve associated with these new technologies. This gap not only hinders effective implementation but also raises concerns about the reliability of AI-driven decisions in clinical settings.

Additionally, resistance to change within the healthcare community can stifle AI adoption. The tradition-bound nature of medicine often views AI with skepticism, influenced by fears of diminished human oversight and potential job displacement. Establishing trust and demonstrating clear benefits are essential to overcoming these barriers and fully leveraging AI in health systems.

**Overcoming Skepticism: Building Trust in Healthcare AI**

The journey to integrate AI into healthcare is fraught with skepticism. Trust, a fundamental element in healthcare, often becomes a challenge when introducing AI technologies. To overcome such skepticism, transparency in AI operations and decision-making processes is pivotal. Clearly communicating how AI tools derive their conclusions reassures both healthcare professionals and patients of the system's reliability and safety.

Educational initiatives also play a crucial role. By demystifying AI technologies through training programs, healthcare providers can gain a deeper understanding and confidence in using these systems. Bridging the knowledge gap ensures that AI tools are used effectively and responsibly, enhancing trust among users.

Collaboration between AI developers and healthcare practitioners in designing and implementing AI solutions fosters a sense of shared ownership and accountability. Involving practitioners in the developmental stages helps tailor AI systems to real-world clinical needs, further embedding trust and acceptance within the medical community.

**Interdisciplinary Collaboration in AI Healthcare Solutions**

The dynamism of AI healthcare solutions lies in effective interdisciplinary collaboration. Bridging distinct fields, medicine, technology, data science, and ethics—facilitates a comprehensive approach to developing AI applications that are not only technologically advanced but also clinically relevant and ethically sound.

Medicine, steeped in direct patient care, brings nuances of human health that AI alone cannot decipher. Technologists and AI experts, on the other hand, contribute cutting-edge algorithms and models that enhance data analysis and decision-making capabilities. Ethicists ensure that these developments adhere to necessary moral guidelines, safeguarding patient interests and societal norms. Through such collaboration, the scope and effectiveness of AI in healthcare are exponentially increased, presenting new avenues for patient treatment and health management.

Regular dialogue among professionals across these disciplines promotes a continuous exchange of ideas and updates, aligning AI solutions with current medical practices and ethical standards. This synergy not only accelerates the innovation process but also enhances acceptance and integration into everyday healthcare.

## Training Healthcare AI: Data, Algorithms, and Models

The fundamental challenge in training healthcare AI involves curating high-quality data that reflects diverse patient demographics and conditions. Data sets need to be comprehensive and inclusive to avoid biases that can affect AI's decision-making capabilities. This data must also be continuously updated to capture evolving health trends and emerging medical knowledge.

Selecting the right algorithms and models is crucial for the effective application of AI in healthcare. These algorithms must be robust, capable of handling complex and varied datasets, and must learn from real-world feedback to adapt and improve continuously. Collaboration between data scientists and healthcare professionals ensures that the technical development of AI tools aligns with clinical realities and needs.

Finally, rigorous testing and validation stages are essential to train healthcare AI responsibly. Professionals must simulate a variety of clinical scenarios to ensure that AI systems perform reliably under different conditions. This robust testing safeguards both patient safety and the accuracy of AI applications in clinical settings.

## The Future of AI-Assisted Telehealth Services

The evolution of AI-assisted telehealth services is poised to revolutionize or to complicate accessibility and efficacy in healthcare delivery. Prevailing technologies enable a seamless integration of real-time health monitoring and virtual consultations, ensuring continuous patient care regardless of geographical barriers.

Future developments are expected to leverage predictive analytics, enhancing preventive care by identifying potential health risks before they evolve into serious conditions. This proactive approach could dramatically reduce emergency visits and hospital admissions, optimize healthcare resources and minimize costs. Moreover, integration with wearable technologies will allow for more personalized health assessments, tailoring treatments to individual needs based on a continuous stream of physiological data.

The potential challenges include ensuring privacy and data security, along with maintaining the human touch in patient care. Continuous advancements in AI must prioritize ethical considerations and aim to enhance, rather than replace, the clinician-patient relationship. Successful implementation will require robust regulatory frameworks and interdisciplinary collaboration to fully realize the transformative potential of AI in telehealth.

## Global Adoption of AI in Healthcare: Trends and Variations

AI adoption in healthcare exhibits significant global variations, influenced by regional technological advancements and policy environments. Developed nations often lead with comprehensive AI integration in medical systems, driven by robust technical infrastructures and governmental support. In contrast, developing countries face hurdles due to limited resources and infrastructure challenges, which slow AI adoption rates.

Cultural factors also play a crucial role in the adoption process. For instance, countries with a strong tradition of holistic and indigenous medicine may show resistance or require adaptations in AI applications to embrace these longstanding healthcare practices. This necessitates the development of AI solutions that are culturally sensitive and capable of integrating traditional knowledge with modern medical practices.

Despite these variations, a common trend is the growing recognition of AI's potential to enhance healthcare outcomes. Countries worldwide are increasingly investing in AI research and collaborations, aiming to overcome barriers and harness AI's capabilities for broader healthcare improvements.

### Innovations in AI: Case Studies of Success in Healthcare

Artificial intelligence in healthcare showcases success stories that revolutionize patient care, emphasizing the technology's transformative power. A prominent example is the AI-driven diagnostic system used in dermatology, which significantly enhances the detection accuracy of skin cancers. This system analyzes skin lesion images with a precision surpassing that of experienced dermatologists, ensuring early and accurate diagnoses.

Similarly, in cardiovascular care, AI algorithms now predict heart attacks and strokes by analyzing historical patient data and current medical tests more accurately than conventional prediction models. Such innovations have led to personalized treatment plans and preventive strategies, considerably reducing emergency incidents.

Moreover, AI has made strides in mental health by powering applications that provide real-time cognitive behavioral therapy, making mental health support accessible to those in remote or underserved areas. These case studies not only exemplify AI's potential in enhancing healthcare outcomes but also illustrate its role in advancing medical care equality globally.

### Summary

The utilization of Artificial Intelligence (AI) in healthcare is transforming various aspects of patient care and administrative tasks, revolutionizing the industry with improvements in efficiency and personalized treatments. AI applications in healthcare range from patient diagnostics and robotic-assisted surgeries to administrative tasks like scheduling and compliance. The integration of AI with core technologies such as machine learning, deep learning, and natural language processing allows for sophisticated data analysis, enhancing diagnostics, surgical procedures, and treatment planning. AI-driven tools in diagnostics improve the accuracy and speed of patient evaluations, while in treatment management, they enable personalized medicine by predicting individual responses to treatments. In surgical applications, AI enhances precision in operations and aids in preoperative planning. AI's influence extends to medical imaging where it aids in interpreting diverse data, supporting diagnosis, treatment monitoring, and prediction of disease outcomes. Furthermore, AI expedites drug discovery by analyzing extensive biological data, enhancing the efficiency of developing new medications. Beyond clinical applications, AI is instrumental in improving healthcare delivery by optimizing operations and reducing costs, and it aids in patient monitoring by providing real-time data that facilitate proactive medical interventions. Challenges include data privacy concerns, the need for substantial infrastructure, and ensuring AI systems are unbiased and ethical. Despite these hurdles, the integration of AI is poised to significantly enhance healthcare outcomes and accessibility, providing a more responsive, efficient, and patient-centered healthcare system.

## References

[1] Artificial Intelligence in Health Care: Anticipating Challenges and Opportunities.
https://jamanetwork.com/journals/jama/fullarticle/2762308
[2] Deep Learning for Cardiac Image Segmentation: A Review.
https://www.frontiersin.org/articles/10.3389/fcvm.2020.00025/full
[3] Translational AI and Deep Learning in Diagnostic Pathology. https://www.nature.com/articles/s41571-019-0252-y
[4] AI-powered drug discovery captures pharma interest. https://www.nature.com/articles/d41573-019-00011-9
[5] Natural language processing in radiology: A systematic review.
https://pubs.rsna.org/doi/10.1148/radiol.16151269
[6] Ethics of AI in Radiology: Summary of the Joint European and North American Multisociety Statement.
https://pubs.rsna.org/doi/10.1148/radiol.2019191586

### Case Study: Integrating AI into Chronic Disease Management: The Case of Type 2 Diabetes

A major metropolitan hospital introduced an AI-driven platform to enhance the management of Type 2 diabetes, a chronic disease affecting millions globally. This initiative was part of a broader digital transformation strategy aimed at improving patient outcomes and optimizing healthcare resources. The hospital collaborated with a leading AI technology firm to develop a system that leverages machine learning algorithms to analyze patient data and predict individual health risks. The AI system integrated seamlessly with existing electronic health records, allowing for real-time data analysis and more personalized patient care.

Once the system was implemented, it immediately began evaluating patient data, including blood sugar levels, dietary habits, and previous treatment responses. The AI platform utilized predictive analytics to identify patients at high risk of complications such as diabetic retinopathy and kidney disease. Healthcare providers received alerts and could intervene earlier than with traditional monitoring methods. For patients, this meant a more proactive approach to managing their condition, potentially reducing severe outcomes and improving quality of life.

The health outcomes from the pilot phase were promising. The system's capability to continuously learn from new data further refined the accuracy of its predictions. Over time, the hospital noted a significant decrease in emergency room visits and hospitalizations for diabetes-related complications. This case study highlights the potential of AI in transforming chronic disease management by offering personalized and preemptive medical care.

However, several challenges were encountered during implementation. Initial resistance from healthcare professionals due to concerns about job displacement and the reliability of AI decision-making required targeted change management strategies, including ongoing training and education. Privacy and data security were also paramount, necessitating strict compliance with healthcare regulations and ethical standards to protect patient information.

### Case Study: AI-Enhanced Emergency Response: Revolutionizing Stroke Care

In an innovative leap forward for emergency medical services, a regional hospital in a dense urban area integrated an Artificial Intelligence (AI) system to enhance its stroke care protocols. The initiative involved deploying an AI-driven diagnostic tool that harnesses deep learning algorithms to quickly analyze brain imaging scans for signs of a stroke. The primary goal was to reduce the time between a patient's arrival and treatment initiation, which is crucial in stroke care where rapid response can significantly influence outcomes.

The AI system was trained on thousands of historical imaging data, enabling it to identify and differentiate various types of strokes, such as ischemic and hemorrhagic strokes, with high precision. Upon implementation, the emergency department (ED) staff were equipped with tablets that could receive real-time analysis results directly from the AI system, allowing for immediate and accurate diagnosis. This integration significantly shortened the decision-making process, with the AI providing recommendations for the best treatment protocols based on the specific stroke type identified.

The results of this AI integration were remarkable. The average time from patient arrival to treatment, known as 'door-to-needle' time, was reduced by about 40%, significantly improving the rate of recovery and reducing the incidence of permanent disabilities among stroke patients. Additionally, the hospital reported increased confidence among its medical staff in diagnosing and treating strokes, attributed to the AI system's reliability and accuracy.

Despite the success, the journey to integrate AI into emergency stroke care was not without hurdles. Initial skepticism among medical staff, especially concerning the AI's diagnostic decisions, was a significant challenge. The hospital addressed these concerns by arranging comprehensive training sessions to educate the staff about the AI system's functionality and the reliability of its diagnostic accuracy. This case study illustrates the transformative potential of AI in acute medical settings, where time-sensitive treatment is paramount, showcasing a future where AI plays a crucial role in life-saving medical interventions.

### Case Study: AI Application in Pediatric Oncology: Enhancing Treatment Outcomes

The integration of Artificial Intelligence (AI) into the pediatric oncology department of a well-regarded university hospital marks a significant step towards personalized medicine for childhood cancer treatment. The hospital embarked on a pioneering initiative to utilize AI in analyzing genetic data alongside clinical outcomes, aiming to tailor treatments to individual genetic profiles, a challenge presented by the diverse and often aggressive nature of pediatric cancers.

The initiative started with the formation of a cross-functional team including oncologists, data scientists, geneticists, and AI specialists. They developed an AI-driven tool that mapped each patient's cancer genome and cross-referenced it with a vast database of cancer genomic data. This tool, powered by deep learning algorithms, could identify genetic markers that were predictive of treatment response, enabling clinicians to choose the most effective treatment regimens for each child.

By continuously feeding treatment results back into the AI system, the tool refined its predictive capabilities, leading to increasingly effective treatment recommendations. The highly individualized approach resulted in a notable improvement in treatment response rates and reduced side effects, as treatments were no longer one-size-fits-all but were specifically designed to combat the unique genetic makeup of each child's cancer.

However, the implementation phase was fraught with challenges. Data privacy concerns were paramount, given the sensitivity of the genetic information involved. The hospital had to ensure data protection compliance and build a secure framework for data handling. Additionally, the complexity of AI systems required continuous education and training for healthcare practitioners, which involved significant resource allocation.

Despite these hurdles, the initiative demonstrated the potential of AI to revolutionize pediatric oncology. The program not only enhanced clinical outcomes but also provided invaluable insights into the genetic bases of pediatric cancers, paving the way for new research and drug development targeted at genetic profiles.

### Case Study: AI-Driven Behavioral Health Interventions: Transforming Mental Health Treatment

In an ambitious project undertaken by a large urban hospital network, an AI-driven platform was launched to revolutionize the approach towards mental health treatment, particularly focusing on depression and anxiety disorders. The network, facing a surge in mental health cases and constrained by a limited number of qualified mental health professionals, turned to technology for a scalable solution. The development involved creating a machine learning model that could analyze various patient data points, from psychiatric evaluation notes to ongoing therapy feedback, to identify personalized treatment pathways.

The initiative started with a pilot program involving a thousand patients who consented to having their therapy sessions and health records analyzed by AI. The AI system was designed to learn from the outcomes and feedback of psychotherapy treatments and adjust treatment suggestions in real-time. This allowed therapists to dynamically tailor their approaches based on the AI's findings, which included identifying the most effective therapeutic techniques for each patient.

As the system evolved, it not only suggested modifications in therapy practices but also recommended specific medication adjustments and lifestyle changes based on predictive analytics. It was observed that patients under the AI-driven intervention showed a quicker improvement in standardized clinical scales for depression and anxiety, compared to those under traditional treatment regimens.

However, the implementation was not without challenges. Ethical concerns regarding patient privacy and the implications of AI making health-related recommendations needed careful consideration. Extensive dialogue was required to calibrate the balance between AI assistance and human decision-making in treatment. Additional challenges included integrating AI tools with existing healthcare IT systems and ensuring all data handling was compliant with medical data protection standards.

This case study highlights the potential of AI to significantly enhance the efficiency and personalization of mental health treatment, proving crucial during times of increased demand and healthcare professional shortages. The hospital network plans to expand the AI's application to other areas of behavioral health, aiming to establish a new standard in personalized care.

### Case Study: AI Revolution in Cardiology: Advanced Predictive Models for Heart Disease Prevention

In a groundbreaking initiative, a technologically advanced hospital in collaboration with a leading AI research center deployed an AI-based solution aimed at revolutionizing cardiology. This collaboration focused on the development and implementation of advanced predictive models designed to forecast the onset of cardiovascular diseases in high-risk patients. The system utilized a combination of deep learning and natural language processing to analyze a wide range of data points including genetic profiles, lifestyle factors, and historical health records from a diverse patient pool.

The AI model was meticulously designed by a multidisciplinary team composed of cardiologists, data scientists, and AI specialists. The primary goal was to integrate the AI tool into the hospital's health information system to allow for seamless real-time data processing and prediction. The system provided cardiologists with actionable insights, offering recommendations for preventive measures tailored to individual patient profiles.

Within months of implementation, the hospital observed a remarkable improvement in preventive cardiology practices. The AI system was able to identify subtle signs of potential heart disease that were often overlooked in traditional examinations. Patients identified by the AI as high-risk were given personalized lifestyle and medication plans, which resulted in a statistically significant reduction in incidence rates of cardiovascular events among this group.

Despite the successes, the project faced several challenges. The accuracy of the AI predictions heavily depended on the quality and comprehensiveness of the input data. There were concerns regarding data integrity and the potential bias in AI algorithms, emphasizing the need for continuous monitoring and refinement of the system based on real-world outcomes. Ethical considerations also played a pivotal role, especially concerning patient consent and the transparency of AI-driven decisions.

This case study not only showcases the potential of AI in transforming cardiology but also highlights the importance of ethical considerations and data management in deploying AI healthcare solutions. It illustrates a path forward where AI could play a central role in not just treating but also preventing complex diseases through sophisticated predictive analytics.

## Case Study: Optimizing Hospital Operations with AI-Powered Workforce Management

A large hospital system based in an urban center faced significant operational challenges, particularly in the allocation of nursing staff across its various departments efficiently. High patient influx, unpredictable healthcare demands, and logistical challenges often led to staff shortages or, conversely, inefficient utilization of staff resources. To address these issues, the hospital decided to implement an AI-driven workforce management system designed to optimize staffing based on real-time data and predictive analytics.

The AI system integrated with the hospital's existing electronic health records (EHR) and HR management software to gather comprehensive data on patient admissions, discharges, transfers, and staff availability. Machine learning algorithms analyzed this data to forecast patient load and determine optimal staffing patterns. The system could identify patterns that human planners might miss, such as predicting peak times for different types of patient care needs and suggesting preemptive staffing adjustments. Additionally, the AI provided insights into staff performance and patient care outcomes, enabling more informed decision-making.

Upon implementation, the hospital experienced a marked improvement in several key areas. Staff satisfaction increased due to better-managed workloads and fewer instances of overstaffing or understaffing. Patient wait times decreased, and the quality of care improved, as the right number of nurses were always available at the right times. The AI's adaptive learning capabilities meant that it continued to refine its predictions and recommendations, becoming more accurate over time.

Despite these improvements, the hospital faced challenges during the system's integration. Some staff members were initially skeptical about relying on an AI for staffing decisions, concerned about the potential for job loss or reduced human oversight. To mitigate these concerns, hospital management conducted extensive training sessions to educate staff on the benefits of AI assistance and ensured that final staffing decisions remained in the hands of human managers. Data privacy was another concern; the hospital had to bolster its cybersecurity measures to protect sensitive employee and patient data handled by the AI system.

## Case Study: AI-Driven Prosthetic Development: Personalizing Mobility Solutions

In a landmark project, a prominent biomedical research institute in collaboration with a tech startup has developed a next-generation AI-driven prosthetic limb designed to adapt dynamically to different environments and user activities. This advanced prosthetic limb uses sensors and AI algorithms to learn the user's gait, preferences, and common obstacles in real-world scenarios to offer a more natural and responsive experience. This case revolves around Jane, a trial participant who lost her right leg in an accident and struggled with traditional prosthetics.

The project initiated by gathering massive amounts of biomechanical data from diverse populations to train the AI system in recognizing various movement patterns and environments. It incorporated machine learning techniques to process this data and predict optimal movement responses under different circumstances. The AI-enhanced prosthetic provided Jane with a significantly improved mobility experience, adapting in real-time to her walking speed, the terrain, and even her tiredness levels. For instance, it automatically adjusted stiffness and damping during a hike on a rough trail or softened the impact when descending stairs, reducing the physical strain and risk of injury.

However, this integration of AI into prosthetic development was not without challenges. Initial calibrations and adjustments were time-consuming, requiring Jane to spend several hours over multiple sessions to fine-tune the prosthetic's responses to her specific needs. Privacy concerns were also raised regarding the continuous data collection needed to train and refine the AI. To address these issues, the research team implemented stringent data protection protocols and ensured that all personal data was anonymized and secured.

Throughout this project, the team conducted extensive testing and gathered feedback to refine the algorithms and enhance the prosthetic's functionality. The outcome not only provided Jane with a much more adaptable and comfortable prosthetic limb but also set new standards in personalized prosthetic design, paving the way for broader applications of AI in improving individual quality of life through tailored health technology solutions.

**Case Study: AI Optimization of Orthopedic Surgeries: The Future of Personalized Joint Replacement**

A large urban hospital renowned for its advanced orthopedic department launched an innovative program integrating Artificial Intelligence (AI) into joint replacement surgeries. This initiative aimed to substantially reduce recovery times, enhance surgical precision, and personalize patient care plans. The hospital partnered with a leading AI solutions provider to develop a system that utilizes machine learning algorithms and 3D imaging technology to plan and execute customized joint replacements.

The AI system began by creating precise 3D models of a patient's joint, using imaging data gleaned from MRIs and CT scans. These models were then used to simulate various scenarios and predict the optimal alignment and fit of prosthetic implants, tailored specifically to each patient's anatomy. Advanced robotics, guided by these AI-generated plans, assisted surgeons during operations, ensuring that implants were placed with unprecedented accuracy. This method significantly differed from traditional approaches, which relied heavily on the surgeon's experience and visual judgment during the procedure.

Post-surgery, the AI system continued to monitor patient recovery via sensors embedded in the rehabilitative equipment, adjusting physiotherapy regimens in real-time based on data such as range of motion and patient-reported pain levels. As a result, patients experienced quicker recovery times and improved functionality of replaced joints.

Despite these promising developments, the hospital faced several challenges. Skepticism from traditional surgeons, concerned about the reliability of AI decisions and the perceived reduction in their clinical autonomy, posed initial obstacles. Furthermore, the integration of such sophisticated AI technology required substantial investments in training medical staff and upgrading surgical equipment, presenting financial and logistical concerns.

However, the long-term benefits observed from early implementations, including lower rates of post-operative complications and higher patient satisfaction, validated the investment. The case study not only underscores the potential for AI to transform orthopedic surgery but also highlights the necessity for ongoing training, adaptation, and interdisciplinary collaboration to fully realize this technology's capabilities in healthcare.

**Review Questions**

**1. A 52-year-old patient with a history of chronic back pain is considering AI-driven treatment options but is also deeply involved in traditional Thai massage therapy, which has previously helped manage his symptoms. Given his background and preferences, what should be considered when recommending a treatment plan?**

A) Rely solely on AI-driven treatment recommendations

B) Integrate AI-driven recommendations with traditional Thai massage

C) Discontinue traditional Thai massage and switch entirely to conventional medical treatments

D) Use AI solely for diagnostic purposes and rely on traditional methods for treatment

**Answer: B**

Explanation: Integrating AI-driven recommendations with traditional Thai massage offers a personalized approach that respects the patient's successful past experiences with traditional therapy while incorporating modern diagnostic tools. This combination allows for targeted medical interventions alongside proven traditional techniques, enhancing overall treatment efficacy and patient satisfaction. AI can provide insights into new treatment possibilities or adjustments needed based on the latest medical data, while traditional Thai massage can continue to provide relief and manage symptoms as previously experienced by the patient.

## Concepts of Bias in AI Systems

### Defining Bias in Artificial Intelligence

Bias in artificial intelligence (AI) refers to systematic errors or prejudices in algorithms or data that lead to unfair outcomes, often reflecting historical, social, or cultural inequalities. This concept is critical, as AI systems increasingly make decisions affecting many aspects of human life, including medicine.

Defining bias in AI involves recognizing disparities in how information is processed, and decisions are made. These biases can originate from various sources, such as the data used to train AI systems, which may not adequately represent all groups or fail to account for non-conventional medical practices. This limitation can skew AI's outputs, contributing to decisions that disadvantage certain populations or overlooking traditional healing methods.

Understanding and defining AI bias is the first step toward addressing disparities in healthcare technology applications. Acknowledging the existence of these biases allows developers and stakeholders to strategize more effectively for inclusive and equitable AI deployment, ensuring all patients benefit equally from technological advances.

### Types of Bias in AI Systems

AI systems can manifest several types of bias, each affecting decision-making processes in unique ways. Measurement bias arises when data inaccuracies lead to erroneous AI outputs, often due to faulty data collection instruments or processes. Another prevalent form is sampling bias, occurring when training data does not representatively capture the population diversity, skewing AI's understanding and predictions.

Algorithmic bias is introduced by the underlying mathematical models that may inherently favor certain outcomes. This is particularly critical in healthcare, where such biases could lead to misdiagnoses or inappropriate treatment recommendations. Prejudice bias, fueled by societal stereotypes and historical inequalities, is embedded within the data, often inadvertently reflecting or amplifying existing human biases in medical treatment outcomes.

Lastly, exclusion bias happens when AI systems overlook non-conventional medical insights, such as traditional or holistic approaches, due to their underrepresentation in mainstream data sets. Addressing these biases requires meticulous attention to data curation, algorithmic design, and continuous monitoring for equitable AI application in medicine.

## Sources of Bias in AI Algorithms

The origin of bias in AI algorithms can be traced to several critical sources. Predominantly, it emerges from the data itself. The data used to train AI models often encapsulates existing societal prejudices or historical inequalities, inadvertently leading to biased computational outcomes. In medicine, this can result in AI tools that preferentially treat or diagnose based on biased historical health data, neglecting minority groups or non-Western medical practices.

Another significant source is the design of algorithms. Developers' perspectives and unconscious biases can influence how algorithms interpret data, potentially leading to biased decisions. For example, if an algorithm is primarily designed by individuals from a particular demographic, it might unconsciously reflect their medical treatment preferences or diagnostic prioritizations.

Further compounding this issue, the selection and tuning of model parameters can also introduce bias. Choices regarding which features to emphasize or underrepresent can skew AI predictions, prioritizing some health outcomes over others. This selection process can inadvertently overlook the efficacy of traditional, indigenous, or holistic health practices, thereby amplifying cultural biases in healthcare technology.

## Bias in Training Data for AI

Bias in AI training data manifests profoundly within the healthcare sector, dramatically influencing AI-driven outcomes. Datasets, often derived from specific population segments, fail to encompass the broader demographic spectrum, including underrepresented groups and those practicing alternative medicine. This exclusion leads to algorithms that are unfamiliar with or misinterpret non-conventional medical practices, skewing results away from holistic or indigenous treatments.

The repercussions are significant. AI systems trained on such biased data might misdiagnose or underdiagnose conditions more prevalent in minority populations or propose treatments that are ineffectual or harmful under traditional healing paradigms. This not only undermines patient care but also exacerbates existing health disparities.

Mitigating this bias necessitates a concerted effort to diversify training datasets and incorporate a wide array of cultural health knowledge. Implementing rigorous standards for data inclusion and continuously validating AI outputs against diverse health outcomes are vital steps towards equitable healthcare AI.

## Impact of Bias on Algorithm Accuracy

The impact of bias on the accuracy of AI algorithms in healthcare cannot be overstated. When biases are embedded within AI systems—whether through skewed data, erroneous model assumptions, or prejudiced algorithmic frameworks—the accuracy and reliability of their outcomes suffer. This impacts the diagnostic precision and treatment efficacy AI tools can offer, often resulting in misdiagnoses or suboptimal healthcare delivery, particularly to underserved communities or those undergoing traditional treatments.

Accuracy issues further exacerbate existing disparities by promoting healthcare solutions that do not align with the diverse needs of the global population. For instance, if an AI system trained predominantly on data from a particular ethnic group, it may show diminished performance when diagnosing ailments in people from other ethnicities. This not only questions the universality of AI solutions in healthcare but also raises serious ethical concerns about equity and justice in medical AI applications.

Overcoming these challenges necessitates a profound revision of data selection, algorithm design, and continuous system validation to monitor for biases and ensure higher accuracy in diverse scenarios. Enhancing algorithm accuracy involves not just technical adjustments but also a commitment to ethical AI use, promoting trust and inclusivity in healthcare innovations.

## AI Decision-Making and Human Prejudice

The interplay between AI decision-making and human prejudice illuminates a complex aspect of bias in medical AI systems. AI algorithms, while designed to enhance decision-making, inherit human biases that pervade their outputs. These biases influence AI's judgment, often mirroring societal prejudices against underrepresented groups, including those relying on traditional healing methods.

Moreover, decisions made by AI can reinforce existing disparities by perpetuating the oversight of alternative medicinal approaches, such as indigenous healing practices absent from mainstream datasets. This reinforcing cycle of prejudice compromises not only the inclusivity of AI solutions but also their validity in diverse clinical settings. Such biases are not only technically detrimental but ethically troubling, questioning the fairness of AI impacts on various communities.

Addressing this requires a deliberate reconceptualization of AI development processes to actively detect and neutralize ingrained human biases. Vigilance in training AI systems with diverse, inclusive data sets and continuous oversight can gradually dismantle the prejudices that skew AI decision-making in medicine.

## Systematic vs. Random Bias in AI

In the discourse surrounding AI bias, distinguishing between systematic and random biases is crucial, particularly within the domain of healthcare. Systematic bias occurs when certain patterns persistently skew data in one direction due to underlying structural issues. For instance, training data that systematically excludes traditional healing methods unmistakably inserts a bias towards Western medical practices, thus predisposing AI algorithms against indigenous approaches.

Conversely, random bias represents anomalies that occur without a discernible pattern, arising from random errors in data collection or processing. Unlike systematic bias, these are not rooted in deeper prejudices or consistent errors, and they typically do not replicate across different datasets.

Identifying whether biases in AI are systematic or random is vital for implementing effective mitigation strategies. Systematic biases require structural adjustments in data curation and algorithmic design, whereas random biases might be addressed through enhanced data processing techniques and robust error checks. Understanding and addressing these nuances ensure more equitable AI applications in medicine.

## Measuring and Detecting Bias in AI

Effectively measuring and detecting bias in AI systems is foundational for developing equitable healthcare technologies. Precision in this domain involves using statistical methods to scrutinize AI decision processes, identifying any deviations that privilege one group over another, thus compromising fairness. First, comparative studies across different demographic groups can highlight discrepancies in AI performance, signaling potential biases that need scrutiny.

Subsequently, implementing validation methods like confusion matrices helps uncover biases in prediction outcomes. These matrices make it possible to view false rates of predictions for different groups, showcasing explicit areas where the AI fails to perform uniformly. Moreover, advanced analytics like disparate impact analysis provide deeper insights into unintentional biases, measuring how various outcomes disproportionately affect distinct groups.

The drive towards unbiased AI also benefits from continuous monitoring, employing feedback loops that integrate real-world user data back into the system to self-correct observed biases. This iterative process ensures AI systems evolve with an increasing awareness of and sensitivity to multifaceted human needs and values.

## Bias Mitigation Techniques in AI Development

Addressing AI bias in medical systems necessitates robust mitigation strategies, ensuring equity and inclusivity. One pivotal approach involves diversifying the input data; by encompassing a broader spectrum of cultural practices and patient demographics, developers can train AI systems to recognize and appropriately handle a wide range of healthcare paradigms, including traditional and indigenous healing techniques.

In addition to diversity in data, algorithmic fairness methods play a critical role. Techniques such as regularization can adjust algorithmic decisions to avoid perpetuating or amplifying existing biases. Implementing blind or anonymized data processing, where sensitive attributes (e.g., race, ethnicity) are masked, helps focus AI's decision-making on relevant medical factors rather than demographic characteristics.

Moreover, continuous monitoring and updating of AI systems form an essential part of bias mitigation. Using real-world outcomes to refine and adjust AI predictions ensures that the systems evolve considering new data and discoveries, thereby minimizing prior biases and adapting to diverse healthcare scenarios. Engaging multidisciplinary teams in the development process further enriches the perspective and oversight, aligning AI advancements with ethical medical practices.

## The Role of Annotation in AI Bias

Annotation in AI serves as a significant determiner of how data is interpreted and used by machine learning algorithms. As annotators tag data based on the features they recognize as significant, this process inherently carries the risk of embedding human biases into the system. Different annotators may interpret data elements differently based on cultural, social, or personal biases, leading to discrepancies in how data is labeled.

This variability can be especially consequential in the context of medical AI, where diverse interpretations of symptoms or treatments across different medicinal traditions could lead to biased outcomes. For example, symptoms recognized in Western medicine might be annotated differently from those in traditional healing, affecting the AI's diagnostic recommendations. Therefore, ensuring that annotation guidelines are robust and inclusive of various medical paradigms is crucial.

Effectively managing this aspect of AI development involves rigorous training for annotators on bias recognition and the implementation of multiple annotation layers to cross-verify data accuracy. Institutions must also strive for transparency in the annotation process by documenting methodologies and providing justifications for labeling decisions, thereby enhancing the reliability and fairness of AI systems in medicine.

## Bias in AI Interpretation and Prediction

The challenge of bias in AI interpretation and prediction extends beyond mere data input to the core of AI's operational framework. When AI systems interpret data, biases can lead to skewed predictions which disproportionately affect marginalized communities. For instance, AI that has not been exposed to holistic healing practices might misinterpret their efficacy or relevance, thus undermining alternative medical paradigms.

Moreover, such biases in predictions are not just theoretical concerns but manifest in real-world outcomes. An AI system trained primarily on Western medical data might fail to recognize or properly interpret symptoms and remedies from non-Western traditions. This could lead to incorrect predictions about patient health and inappropriate treatment recommendations.

Addressing these challenges requires a nuanced understanding of both the technical and cultural dimensions of AI systems. Collaborative efforts between AI developers, medical practitioners, and cultural scholars can help in designing AI models that respect and integrate a diverse spectrum of medical knowledge and practices.

**Legal and Ethical Implications of AI Bias**

The legal and ethical implications of AI bias in medicine extend beyond technical fairness, touching on fundamental rights and professional responsibilities. Legally, biased AI systems can contravene laws designed to protect against discrimination, potentially leading healthcare providers into inadvertent legal breaches. Ethical issues arise when AI systems perpetuate inequalities, contradicting the medical ethos of do no harm and equality of care.

Ethically, biased decisions by AI can undermine patient trust, a cornerstone of effective healthcare. This erosion of trust not only damages individual provider-patient relationships but also weakens the public's confidence in the healthcare system. Legally, if AI-driven decisions are found discriminatory, healthcare institutions may face lawsuits, stringent penalties, and a tarnished reputation, prompting a reevaluation of AI integration strategies.

Given these contexts, the necessity for stringent regulations and ethical guidelines is evident. These should enforce transparency, accountability, and regular auditing of AI systems to ensure they align with both ethical norms and legal standards, thereby safeguarding patient welfare and rights.

**Effects of Societal Biases on AI Development**

Societal biases, ingrained in our cultural and social fabric, undeniably shape AI developments, potentially leading to systems that inadvertently perpetuate these prejudices. These biases originate from the collective values, experiences, and beliefs of those who contribute to AI's creation and training processes. Consequently, if the diversity of the development team or the data is limited, the AI system may mirror these limitations, failing to address or even identify needs outside this scope.

For instance, societal norms and biases toward medical treatments can influence which data sets are deemed relevant or prioritized. Traditional and indigenous healing practices might be undervalued or not captured at all, resulting in AI that is skewed towards Western medical paradigms. This oversight can alienate populations relying on alternative medicines, reducing the universality and utility of AI in health care.

Acknowledging these effects requires a concerted effort to incorporate a wide array of cultural contexts during the training of AI systems. This approach not only enhances the robustness and relevance of AI applications but also ensures a more equitable representation in healthcare innovations. Truly inclusive AI development is pivotal not just for ethical alignment but for advancing truly global healthcare solutions.

**AI Bias in Different Industries**

AI bias permeates beyond the healthcare sector, influencing outcomes in industries like finance, recruitment, and law enforcement. In finance, algorithms determine creditworthiness, yet often reflect existing socio-economic disparities, disadvantaging underrepresented groups. Similarly, in recruitment, AI-powered tools can perpetuate bias by favoring resumes from certain demographics based on historical hiring data, thus embedding institutional prejudices against certain candidates.

The consequences are just as profound in law enforcement, where predictive policing tools may disproportionately target specific communities, reinforcing racial profiling practices. These biases are not incidental but stem from the foundational data these industries employ to train AI systems. Without diverse and representative input, AI technologies inadvertently uphold the status quo, promoting inequality.

Addressing these widespread biases calls for a multifaceted approach involving regulatory oversight, industry-specific ethical guidelines, and a heightened commitment to data inclusivity. By employing more diverse datasets and implementing rigorous bias monitoring, industries can leverage AI's potential responsibly and ethically, promoting equity rather than perpetuating biases.

## Cultural Considerations in AI Bias

Acknowledging cultural considerations is pivotal when addressing AI bias, especially in medical contexts. Diverse cultures harbor unique medical knowledge and practice that AI tools may overlook if not properly integrated during the training phase. This oversight can skew AI's diagnostic and prognostic capabilities, potentially disadvantaging those who rely on non-Western medical traditions.

For instance, certain symptoms or health conditions recognized within indigenous practices might be completely absent from datasets predominantly composed of Western medical data. As a result, AI developed under such conditions may exhibit biases against these cultural practices, failing to recognize or misinterpreting crucial health information. Such exclusions not only compromise the effectiveness of medical AI but also perpetuate a form of cultural ignorance and insensitivity.

Therefore, it is essential to imbue AI systems with a rich diversity of cultural data. Collaborative efforts between technologists, cultural scholars, and practitioners from various medical systems should be intensified to ensure that AI recognizes and respects a wide spectrum of healing traditions. This will enhance medical AI's inclusiveness and accuracy, making it a truly global healthcare tool.

## Bias Transparency in AI Reporting

Transparency in AI reporting is pivotal for fostering an environment where biases are not only recognized but also addressed. It entails the explicit disclosure of the methodologies and data sources used in AI systems, helping stakeholders to understand how decisions are made and when biases may be influencing outcomes.

For instance, in the sphere of medicine, revealing that an AI system primarily analyzed Western medical literature might flag potential biases against traditional healing methods prevalent in other cultures. Consequently, medically underrepresented communities can advocate for more inclusive data practices. This transparency in reporting supports endeavors to ensure AI tools serve diverse global populations equitably.

Moreover, making these disclosures standard practice in AI development and deployment sets ground for fairer AI systems. Stakeholders, including regulators and the public, must critically assess AI transparency reports and demand thoroughness in documenting AI decision-making processes. This iterative scrutiny fosters an accountability loop, continuously sharpening AI fairness and usability across different medical and cultural contexts.

**Education and Bias Awareness in AI Practices**

Educational initiatives focusing on AI bias are crucial for cultivating a generation of technologists who prioritize fairness in AI development. By embedding courses on AI ethics and bias into curricula, academic institutions can prepare students to critically analyze AI systems, ensuring they recognize and mitigate bias. Such education should extend beyond technical skills, fostering an understanding of the sociocultural dimensions that influence AI.

Awareness programs play a critical role in ongoing professional development, equipping current AI practitioners with the tools needed to review and revise their work continually. Workshops, seminars, and online courses about bias in AI can help maintain high standards of practice, ensuring that awareness and corrective measures evolve with technological advancements.

Moreover, public education on AI bias is essential. By informing the broader community about how AI decisions are made and their potential biases, individuals can better advocate for systems that fairly represent diverse perspectives. This widespread awareness supports a transparent, inclusive approach to AI, essential for its ethical application in society.

**Intersectionality of Bias in AI Systems**

The concept of intersectionality is crucial when examining biases in AI systems. It refers to the complex, cumulative way different forms of discrimination overlap, intersect, and interact. In the context of AI, this means considering how biases related to race, gender, socio-economic status, and more can conflate to create unique disadvantages, particularly in medicine.

For instance, AI systems trained primarily on data from predominantly affluent, Western populations may fail to accurately diagnose diseases that are more prevalent in other socio-economic or ethnic groups. This could lead to misdiagnoses or lack of treatment options for individuals at the intersection of multiple marginalized identities, exacerbating health disparities and inequity.

Thus, addressing AI bias effectively requires a composite approach that accounts for these intersecting identities. AI developers must incorporate diverse datasets that reflect the wide range of human conditions and socio-cultural dynamics. Ensuring the representation of intersectional identities in AI training sets is essential for the development of fair and effective AI-driven medical solutions.

**Role of AI Ethics Committees**

AI Ethics Committees play a pivotal role in guiding and enforcing ethical practices in AI development, particularly in mitigating biases that can arise in AI systems. These multidisciplinary committees, comprising ethicists, technologists, legal experts, and representatives from impacted communities, review AI projects to ensure they adhere to established ethical standards and are sensitive to cultural and societal nuances.

Their responsibilities include scrutinizing AI development processes, from data collection to algorithm deployment, to identify and address potential biases. By evaluating the sources and impacts of bias, these committees help ensure that AI technologies are developed in ways that promote fairness and inclusivity. This oversight is crucial in medicine, where the stakes of biased AI can be life-altering.

Moreover, AI Ethics Committees advocate for transparency and accountability, demanding clear documentation and reporting on how AI systems make decisions. This initiative not only enhances public trust but also reinforces the commitment to ethical AI development across industries, fostering a culture where bias mitigation is a shared responsibility.

## Challenges in Correcting AI Bias

Correcting AI bias presents multifaceted challenges that span technical, ethical, and operational domains. Technically, the intricacy of AI algorithms and the vastness of data involved make identifying and rectifying biases a daunting task. Inaccuracies in primary data sources or inherent prejudices in data annotation can embed subtle biases deep within AI systems, often mirroring societal prejudices subtly integrated into algorithmic decisions.

Ethically, determining what constitutes fairness in AI systems is contentious and varies across cultures and contexts. This ethical ambiguity complicates the formulation of universally applicable correction strategies. Moreover, operational constraints such as cost, time, and the availability of diversified data further hinder the process of bias mitigation.

Engaging diverse groups in AI development is essential yet challenging. It demands extensive collaborations that traverse geographic and disciplinary boundaries, requiring significant resources and commitment. Despite these hurdles, overcoming these challenges is imperative to ensure AI technologies serve humanity equitably, enhancing their efficacy and trustworthiness across diverse populations.

## Bias in AI and Machine Learning Research

Research in artificial intelligence (AI) and machine learning (ML) harbors unique susceptibilities to ingrained biases, which can pervade the foundational stones of algorithmic development. This bias in research not only skews technological outcomes but also inevitably shapes the AI applications deployed in real-world scenarios, including medicine.

Primarily, the composition of research teams often reflects a narrow slice of global demographics, predominantly those from technologically advanced regions. This lack of diversity can lead to a homogenized perspective on problem-solving and technological development, sidelining traditional and indigenous knowledge systems that are crucial for comprehensive healthcare solutions. Additionally, research funding and publication bias towards high-impact problems pertinent to affluent societies amplify these skewed focuses, further marginalizing underrepresented groups and their healthcare practices.

To address these issues, integrating a broader range of cultural and academic perspectives in AI research is imperative. Cultivating inclusive research environments and promoting interdisciplinary studies could serve as vital steps toward mitigating bias. These efforts ensure that AI and ML technologies do not perpetuate existing disparities but instead foster equitable advancements in medicine.

## Future Trends in AI Bias Studies

The horizon of AI bias studies promises transformative shifts toward addressing and mitigating biases pragmatically and preemptively. Innovations are trending towards developing algorithms that are not only self-correcting but also capable of identifying and adapting to new biases as they emerge. This evolution of AI systems fosters a proactive rather than reactive stance on bias mitigation.

Furthermore, the focus is expanding to incorporate a broader spectrum of interdisciplinary research that includes ethicists, sociologists, and anthropologists. Their involvement ensures that AI systems are not viewed purely through a technological lens but are also assessed for their societal impacts. This holistic approach aims to enhance the cultural sensitivity of AI tools, allowing for a more inclusive representation of diverse populations.

In the realm of medicine, future studies will likely prioritize the integration of traditional, indigenous, and holistic medical knowledge into AI systems. This trend will address current gaps in training datasets and knowledge bases, potentially revolutionizing how AI understands and interacts with various health practices from around the world.

## Strategies for Inclusive AI Training Sets

Developing strategies for inclusive AI training sets requires a multifaceted approach to ensure representation across diverse populations. Initiatives must begin by expanding the scope of data collection to encompass a broad spectrum of demographic and environmental variables. It's crucial that these datasets not only include, but also emphasize, data from communities frequently underrepresented in technological developments, such as indigenous and remote populations.

To enforce inclusivity, adopting a framework that standardizes the incorporation of varied data sources can be instrumental. This includes establishing partnerships with organizations that hold insights into local health practices and norms. Moreover, transparent documentation of data provenance and processing methods helps in maintaining the integrity and accountability of the AI systems developed.

Moreover, periodic reviews and updates of datasets are essential to adapt to changing demographics and emerging health trends. Collaborative efforts involving interdisciplinary teams will further enhance the robustness of AI systems, ensuring they are attuned to the nuances of diverse medical traditions and practices.

## Public Trust and AI Bias Perceptions

Public trust in AI systems is deeply intertwined with how biases in these systems are perceived and addressed. For AI implementations in medicine, a field where decision accuracy can be a matter of life and death—the stakes are exceptionally high. Trust is not given freely; it must be earned through consistent demonstration of fairness and reliability.

The public's perception of AI bias is influenced significantly by transparency regarding how AI decisions are made. Documentation that clearly explains decision-making processes and the criteria used can help demystify AI operations, making them more accessible and understandable to a broader audience. However, when biases occur—whether due to flawed data sets or biased algorithmic design—the ripple effects on public trust can be profound, leading to skepticism and heightened scrutiny.

Efforts to educate the public on AI's role in medicine and the ongoing measures to mitigate biases are crucial. Initiatives that include open forums, educational campaigns, and detailed reporting on AI performance contribute significantly to trust-building. Such transparency not only clarifies how AI works but also highlights the commitment to ethical AI practices, reinforcing public confidence in the technology.

### Summary

The chapter explores various dimensions of bias within AI systems, particularly focusing on healthcare. Bias in AI refers to systematic errors in algorithms or data that lead to unfair outcomes, often reflecting societal inequalities. These biases manifest in numerous forms, including measurement, sampling, algorithmic, prejudice, and exclusion biases, which can originate from skewed training data, flawed algorithm design, or culturally narrow perspectives. The consequences are significant in healthcare, as they can lead to misdiagnoses or inappropriate treatments, particularly affecting minority groups or those practicing non-conventional medicine. Addressing these biases involves recognizing the sources and types of bias, measuring and detecting bias through statistical methods, implementing rigorous validation techniques, and continuously monitoring and updating AI systems. Mitigation strategies include diversifying training datasets, utilizing algorithmic fairness methods, and employing multidisciplinary teams to ensure ethical practices. Moreover, education about AI bias and the inclusion of diverse cultural and societal perspectives in AI training and development are pivotal for reducing biases. These efforts are essential not only for enhancing the accuracy and fairness of AI applications but also for maintaining public trust and ensuring ethical compliance in healthcare and other sectors affected by AI.

## References

[1] AI fairness 360: An extensible toolkit for detecting, understanding, and mitigating unwanted algorithmic bias. https://aif360.mybluemix.net/
[2] Gender Shades: Intersectional Accuracy Disparities in Commercial Gender Classification. https://proceedings.mlr.press/v81/buolamwini18a.html
[3] Fairness and Abstraction in Sociotechnical Systems. https://dl.acm.org/doi/10.1145/3287560.3287598

### Case Study: Mitigating Bias in AI-Driven Diabetic Retinopathy Screening

Diabetic retinopathy is a severe complication of diabetes that can lead to blindness if not detected and treated promptly. In Resolute Health Hospital, the endocrinology department partnered with a tech company to develop an artificial intelligence (AI) system aimed at early screening of diabetic retinopathy using retinal images. Initial outcomes were promising, showing high accuracy in detecting early signs of the condition. However, over time, the data revealed a concerning trend: the AI system was significantly less accurate in diagnosing patients from certain ethnic backgrounds, particularly those of Asian and Hispanic descent.

Further investigation into the AI model's training data showed a predominance of images from Caucasian patients, severely underrepresenting other ethnic groups. This lack of diversity in the data led to a biased model that did not perform equitably across all patient demographics. Resolute Health Hospital faced an ethical conundrum, as the uneven performance could potentially exacerbate health disparities.

To address this, the hospital initiated a multifaceted approach. First, they expanded the dataset by sourcing more inclusive image sets reflective of global demographics. They collaborated with international healthcare providers to access a diverse range of retinal images and incorporated expert feedback from ophthalmologists worldwide to annotate the images accurately. The model's algorithms were also reevaluated and adjusted to correct inherent bias, employing techniques like algorithmic fairness methods and regularization.

As a part of ongoing measures, Resolute Health Hospital established a continuous review system involving periodic audits of the AI system's performance. They also initiated community outreach programs to better understand and integrate patient feedback directly from influenced demographics. This comprehensive strategy not only aimed to enhance the AI system's accuracy but also its fairness, ensuring all patients benefited equally from the technology.

### Case Study: Enhancing Fairness in AI-Assisted Cardiovascular Risk Assessment

Cardiovascular diseases (CVDs) are the leading cause of death globally, prompting healthcare sectors to adopt advanced technologies like artificial intelligence (AI) to enhance early diagnosis and treatment strategies. HeartCare Clinics, a network specializing in cardiovascular health, integrated an AI system to predict patient risk levels based on historical data, physical examinations, and genetic information. Although the AI model initially displayed high efficiency in evaluating and predicting heart disease risks, discrepancies in its predictions across different racial groups became apparent over time.

A detailed analysis revealed that the AI system favored data patterns predominantly from White individuals, with considerable underrepresentation of African American, Hispanic, and South Asian populations. This imbalance mirrored societal and historical biases present in the healthcare system, inadvertently integrated into the training datasets by the predominance of existing studies focusing on White subjects. The skewed AI outcomes risked perpetuating existing health inequities, raising significant ethical concerns about the fairness and universal applicability of AI in medical diagnostics.

To address these critical issues, HeartCare Clinics initiated a comprehensive bias mitigation program. The first step involved collaborating with diverse healthcare institutions to gather a more balanced dataset that included a broader spectrum of racial and ethnic groups. They also partnered with AI ethics committees to reevaluate the data curation and algorithm development processes. By adjusting model parameters and implementing machine learning fairness techniques, such as equity constraints and bias correction algorithms, the clinic aimed to recalibrate the AI system's predictive accuracy and fairness.

Continuous monitoring was set up to track the AI system's performance, with periodic adjustments made based on real-time data and patient outcomes. Further, HeartCare Clinics engaged in community outreach initiatives to educate the public about AI's role in healthcare and gather broader feedback to continuously refine their approach. These steps were crucial in not only enhancing the technical accuracy of the AI system but also in building trust and ensuring equitable health service delivery across all patient demographics.

## Case Study: AI-Enhanced Mental Health Diagnosis and the Challenge of Cultural Bias

In the diverse metropolitan area of Sunfield, several mental health facilities began implementing an AI-augmented system to assist in diagnosing mental health disorders like depression and anxiety, drawing from patient interviews, historical health records, and ongoing behavioral data. This AI system was trained using vast datasets predominantly sourced from Western clinical studies and patient records. Initially, the system demonstrated an exceptional capability in identifying subtle patterns associated with mental health issues, promising a new era of precision in psychiatric care.

However, clinicians soon noticed troubling inconsistencies in diagnostic accuracy among patients from different cultural backgrounds. For instance, the AI system frequently misinterpreted expressions of distress that are culturally specific, such as certain verbal and non-verbal cues used by East Asian populations, which the system had not been adequately trained to recognize. This oversight led to lower diagnostic accuracy for these patient groups, inadvertently reinforcing the stigma and barriers to mental health services among minority communities.

The providers at these facilities, recognizing the potential for cultural bias embedded in the AI system, took proactive steps to correct these disparities. They formed a working group, including cultural psychologists, AI developers, and community representatives from various backgrounds, to audit the existing models and curate a more diverse training dataset. This group also implemented a continuous feedback loop with real-time data from patient interactions and community-based focus groups to dynamically refine the AI algorithms.

In addition to these technical adjustments, the health facilities launched educational initiatives aimed at healthcare providers. These programs focused on understanding cultural expressions of mental health and utilizing AI tools in a way that respects cultural diversity. With these comprehensive measures, the AI-augmented system saw improved diagnostic precision and user trust, creating a more inclusive approach that acknowledges the vital interplay between cultural context and mental health diagnosis.

## Case Study: Algorithm Bias Impact on AI-Assisted Oncology Treatments

In Globetrotter Oncology, a renowned cancer treatment center, a new AI system was implemented to optimize treatment plans for patients. The AI was programmed to analyze patient data including medical history, genetic information, and response to previous treatments, and suggest personalized treatment protocols. Initially, the system seemed revolutionary, offering precise treatment suggestions that often aligned closely with the latest research findings.

However, over time, discrepancies in treatment success rates began to emerge, particularly affecting racial minorities and economically disadvantaged groups. A deeper analysis revealed that the AI's training data predominantly consisted of information from middle to upper-class individuals, primarily of Caucasian ethnicity, who had easier access to newer treatment options. This data inadequacy resulted in the AI system proposing treatment options that were less effective for patients whose medical characteristics did not fit the main data demographic. The economic factors further complicated treatment accessibility, as the AI often recommended expensive treatment plans that were unaffordable for lower-income patients, inadvertently increasing healthcare disparities.

This bias revelation prompted Globetrotter Oncology to undertake a series of corrective measures. First, they collaborated with other medical institutions to diversify the data pool, incorporating more comprehensive data that included underrepresented groups. They also revised the AI algorithms to detect and correct biases by introducing fairness-aware machine learning techniques, such as re-weighting and calibration. Regular bias audits were set up to ensure ongoing compliance with equity standards.

As a long-term solution, Globetrotter Oncology initiated partnerships with public health organizations to better understand and integrate socio-economic factors into treatment planning. They also launched educational programs aimed at improving AI literacy among healthcare professionals, ensuring that practitioners understood the implications of AI suggestions and could make informed decisions when AI-recommended treatments seemed incongruent with patient-specific contexts.

### Case Study: Addressing AI Bias in Pediatric Asthma Treatment

In Lakeshore Medical, AI technology was introduced into pediatric care to better diagnose and manage childhood asthma, a prevalent chronic condition affecting millions worldwide. The AI system was programmed to analyze clinical data such as patient symptoms, environmental factors, and family medical history to recommend personalized management plans and predict potential exacerbations. Initial results showcased the system's potential in providing timely interventions, reducing the frequency of asthma attacks among treated children.

However, several months into deployment, pediatricians at Lakeshore Medical noticed a troubling pattern: the AI's recommendations were less effective for children living in lower-income urban areas, a demographic disproportionately affected by asthma. The AI tended to recommend standard treatments that did not account for environmental triggers prevalent in these areas, such as indoor allergens in poorly ventilated housing or high pollution levels. This oversight was traced back to the AI's training data, which predominantly included patient information from suburban areas with different environmental characteristics.

The discovery prompted Lakeshore Medical to revise its approach to AI in treating pediatric asthma. Acknowledging the biases present in the initial dataset, they partnered with urban public health departments to integrate more diverse environmental and socioeconomic data. This data enrichment aimed to provide the AI with a more comprehensive understanding of various living conditions and their impacts on asthma.

In addition to data diversification, Lakeshore Medical implemented a system for continuous learning, wherein the AI could update its models based on real-time patient outcomes and environmental changes. Pediatricians were also trained to critically assess AI recommendations, considering individual patient contexts to mitigate potential biases.

To ensure long-term effectiveness and fairness, Lakeshore Medical established a multidisciplinary oversight committee consisting of healthcare providers, AI ethics experts, and community representatives. This committee regularly reviews the AI system's outcomes by demographic segments, ensuring that asthma treatment recommendations are equitable and effective across all child populations.

**Case Study: Revamping AI Deployment in Cardiovascular Health Screening for Ethnic Diversity**

Crescent Medical Center, a renowned healthcare institution located in a diverse urban environment, implemented an advanced AI system designed to enhance early detection of cardiovascular diseases (CVD). Initially, the AI's integration boasted higher screening rates, helping in early intervention practices. However, disparities soon began to surface in its efficacy among the ethnically diverse clientele, particularly underdiagnosing individuals of African and South Asian descent.

An in-depth analysis revealed that the underlying issue was the AI system's training data, which predominantly consisted of biological and genetic markers from populations of European descent. This skewed data set failed to capture the variance in CVD manifestation across different ethnic groups, directly impacting the AI's predictive accuracy and subsequently, patient outcomes.

In response to these findings, Crescent Medical Center embarked on a complete overhaul of their AI system. First, they established partnerships with international health organizations to access a broader spectrum of data, encompassing a more comprehensive genetic and environmental array representing their diverse patient base. Additionally, the center initiated a unique community-based data collection campaign, directly engaging with different ethnic communities to contribute to the cultivation of an inclusive data set.

These efforts necessitated revisions in the AI algorithm to accommodate new data inputs and reconfiguration to adjust its predictive parameters more equitably. The center also integrated a continuous feedback mechanism, enabled by a dynamic data update system that assimilated real-time health outcomes to refine and recalibrate the AI algorithms consistently.

To sustain this initiative, Crescent implemented regular training sessions for their healthcare professionals, enhancing their proficiency in managing the AI system and raising awareness about potential biases. They also formed a community advisory board comprising representatives from various ethnic groups, who regularly reviewed the AI system's performance and reported findings directly influencing future AI updates. This multidimensional approach not only aimed to rectify the initial biases but also fostered an environment of trust and collaboration between the medical center and the communities it serves.

**Case Study: AI-Driven Diagnostic Tools in Rural Medical Practices: Addressing Bias and Enhancing Inclusivity**

In Emerald Valley, a rural healthcare center turned to AI to address the scarcity of specialized medical personnel and enhance diagnostic accuracy. The center initiated the deployment of an AI diagnostic tool designed to assist in the early detection and treatment of chronic illnesses such as diabetes and hypertension, which were prevalent in the local population. Initially, the implementation showcased promising results, providing rapid diagnostics that supported overburdened healthcare workers.

However, several months into its integration, the medical staff began observing unusual patterns in diagnostic outputs that appeared to favor patients with lifestyle and symptoms typical of urban demographics. For example, the AI system frequently misdiagnosed chronic conditions in farmers and other rural professions, attributing common occupational symptoms to non-related illnesses. This bias stemmed from the AI's training data, which primarily consisted of urban patient data and failed to represent the lifestyle and environmental factors typical of rural communities. The discrepancy in AI performance raised concerns about its reliability and fairness, risking patient trust and the effectiveness of treatments administered.

Emerald Valley's healthcare leadership, recognizing the potential for bias-induced disparities, launched an extensive review of the AI tool. They partnered with local universities to research rural health dynamics and gathered new, diverse datasets that included environmental factors and occupational health data peculiar to rural settings. These efforts aimed to retrain the AI with a balanced perspective on patient backgrounds.

In addition to technical adjustments, the center engaged with local community leaders to foster an understanding of AI's role in healthcare and gather direct feedback from the patients most affected by the technology. They implemented a continuous feedback system that incorporated patient outcomes into the AI learning process, ensuring that the tool evolved in alignment with the real-world health context of their community.

Such initiatives ensured that the AI system did not merely function as a technological solution but as an integrated tool that respects and adapts to the diverse needs of its users, aiming for equity in medical care across differing demographic landscapes.

### Case Study: AI in Neonatal Care: Addressing Ethnic Bias in Prematurity Risk Assessments

In MetroHealth Hospital's Neonatal Intensive Care Unit (NICU), an AI system was incorporated to improve the assessment and management of prematurity risks in newborns. This AI-driven tool utilized historical health data, genetic information, and real-time physiological signals to predict health complications and optimize care for premature infants. Initially, the technology showed substantial promise, reducing the time taken to intervene during critical situations.

However, several months into the application, clinicians noticed a pattern of inconsistent risk predictions particularly affecting infants from non-Caucasian ethnicities. A detailed examination of the AI model's training data exposure unearthed a significant overrepresentation of data from Caucasian infants, coupled with a severe underrepresentation from other ethnic groups such as African American, Hispanic, and South Asian origins.

This discovery led MetroHealth's NICU management to initiate a systematic overhaul of the AI system's dataset. The team broadened the scope of data collection efforts, prioritizing inclusivity and diversity. They collaborated with other hospitals across the state to form a consortium, sharing anonymized patient data to create a more balanced and representative dataset.

Despite expanding the dataset, the inherent challenge remained in recalibrating the AI system to handle the new diversity in data effectively. The NICU team worked with AI and neonatal specialists to revise the algorithms, integrating fairness-aware machine learning techniques designed to detect and minimize bias dynamically. These methods accounted for the range of ethnic-specific physiological factors influencing prematurity risks.

In addition to technical improvements, the NICU initiated a series of educational workshops for hospital staff. These workshops aimed to raise awareness about the potential biases in AI-driven tools and trained clinicians on culturally competent practices that complemented AI usage. The overall strategy not only aimed at refining the AI performance but also sought to build staff competency in understanding and countering biases inherent in their tools, fostering a culture of continuous learning and adaptation.

### Review Questions

**1. A 55-year-old woman with a history of knee osteoarthritis opts to visit an integrative health center after feeling wary of increasing her NSAIDs due to past stomach upset. During her visit, she receives a 30-minute session of Reiki and gentle yoga stretches that reportedly reduced her pain. Over the following weeks, she notes a decrease in her pain episodes and reduced use of painkillers. Given these outcomes, which of the following statements best reflects the principal benefits of integrating traditional and spiritual healing practices into modern healthcare?**

A) Traditional and spiritual healing practices often provide immediate and complete recovery from chronic conditions.

B) They can serve as complementary to conventional medicine, providing relief and reducing the need for medication through holistic care.

C) These practices can replace all forms of modern medicine as they are superior in managing chronic conditions.

D) Integrative approaches are generally met with skepticism and rarely provide measurable benefits to patients.

**Answer: B**

Explanation: This case highlights the benefits of incorporating integrative approaches alongside conventional treatments. The combination of Reiki and yoga provided relief that traditional NSAIDs alone could not achieve for the patient, illustrating how such therapies can complement conventional medical treatments to enhance patient outcomes. Integrative health practices like Reiki and yoga can address both physical and psychological aspects of health, offering relief from symptoms while reducing dependence on pharmacological treatments, which can sometimes have undesirable side effects like stomach upset experienced by the patient.

**2. Considering the case of a patient undergoing integrative therapy for knee osteoarthritis, which type of healthcare professional is typically NOT involved directly in the administration of Reiki therapy?**

A) Certified Reiki Practitioner

B) Orthopedic Surgeon

C) Holistic Health Coach

D) Yoga Instructor

**Answer: B**

Explanation: An Orthopedic Surgeon typically specializes in the surgical treatment of conditions involving the musculoskeletal system and is not trained in the administration of Reiki, a form of energy healing practiced by certified Reiki practitioners. While orthopedic surgeons may play a crucial role in the overall management of osteoarthritis, Reiki therapy is outside the scope of their professional practices. Integrative health settings might involve various specialists, but Reiki is specifically offered by practitioners trained in this unique modality.

**3. A patient with osteoarthritis experiences significant improvement in her symptoms after incorporating Reiki and yoga into her treatment regime. What is an appropriate next step in her healthcare management considering the positive response to integrative therapies?**

A) Discontinue all previous conventional treatments including medications.

B) Integrate these therapies consistently as part of a long-term management plan.

C) Only rely on Reiki and yoga, rejecting any new conventional treatments in the future.

D) Evaluate these therapies as placebos and not acknowledge their therapeutic value.

**Answer: B**

Explanation: Integrating effective therapies such as Reiki and yoga into a long-term management plan for osteoarthritis is a sensible approach following the patient's positive response. This strategy embraces the benefits of holistic treatments while maintaining the advantages of any necessary conventional medical interventions. Such an integrative approach helps in managing the condition comprehensively, potentially reducing the need for high dosages of pain-related medications and enhancing the overall quality of life. These therapies should not replace conventional medical treatments but rather complement them to maximize patient care outcomes.

## Historical Marginalization of Indigenous Healing Practices

### Colonial Impacts on Indigenous Health Practices

The colonial era ushered in profound disruptions to indigenous health practices which had evolved over centuries. As colonizers imposed their own medical systems, local traditions were often sidelined or outright discarded. Colonial medicine not only introduced new diseases but also undermined the efficacy of traditional healing methods by devaluing them as primitive or unscientific.

This assault was not merely biological but cultural, stripping indigenous peoples of their autonomy over health care. Traditional healers, who were custodians of both medicinal knowledge and spiritual wellness, faced persecution, marginalization, and loss of status within their communities. This erasure was facilitated by colonial policies that favored Western medical practices and institutions, relegating indigenous systems to the peripheries of health governance.

Moreover, the introduction of Western education systems further enshrined the supremacy of allopathic medicine, leaving little room for traditional teachings. Indigenous methods that survived did so in isolation, their integration into mainstream health systems stymied by ongoing biases and misunderstandings about their value and efficacy.

### Western Medicine's Dominance Over Traditional Methods

The ascendancy of Western medicine over traditional healing practices is a significant facet of medical history, often overshadowed by complex socio-political dynamics. As Western medical paradigms took root globally, traditional methods were frequently deemed inferior or unscientific. This dominance was not merely a reflection of advancements in medical science but also a strategic component of broader colonial agendas.

In areas where indigenous practices were once woven into the fabric of community life, the introduction of Western medicine created a dichotomy that marginalized native approaches. Traditional healers, who had maintained generational knowledge on natural remedies and holistic care, found their practices and roles diminished. Western medicine's systematic structures, backed by rigorous scientific validation, gradually usurped the credibility and utility perceived in traditional healing methods.

The imbalance fostered by this dominance resulted in a homogenized healthcare system where pharmaceutical solutions and surgical interventions became the norm, sidelining millennia-old practices that emphasized harmony with nature and preventative care. This shift has profound implications, influencing perceptions of health and healing across diverse cultures even today.

**Historical Exclusion from Formal Health Systems**

The exclusion of indigenous healing practices from formal health systems has deep historical roots, reflecting a larger narrative of neglect and marginalization. Traditional healing, rich in its reliance on natural remedies and ancestral wisdom, was systematically sidelined as Western medical practices became institutionalized. This institutionalization was not merely a transition in health care techniques; it was a cultural imposition that often dismissed the holistic and spiritual components integral to indigenous methodologies.

As formal medical education and licensing bodies emerged, they codified medical knowledge that adhered strictly to Western norms and scientific criteria, excluding non-Western practices by design. This codification process not only legitimized certain forms of knowledge but also delegitimized others, casting indigenous healing as unscientific and anecdotal. The result was a professional and public health narrative that largely ignored or trivialized indigenous medicine's contributions and efficacy.

This historical exclusion has lasting impacts today, manifesting as disparities in health outcomes and continued mistrust between indigenous communities and modern medical institutions. Efforts to reintegrate traditional healing into contemporary health systems often face bureaucratic and cultural barriers, further complicating the path to a truly inclusive health model.

**The Role of Legislation in Suppressing Indigenous Medicine**

The legislative framework historically served as a tool for the systematic suppression of indigenous healing practices. Laws often embodied colonial ideologies that prioritized Western medical approaches, categorizing traditional practices as unscientific or merely folkloric. This legal marginalization institutionalized the exclusion, severely limiting the practice and transmission of indigenous medical knowledge.

Restrictive laws frequently prohibited the practice of indigenous medicine, with healers facing penalties or even imprisonment. Such regulations were not limited to colonial times but persisted into modern legislations, reflecting deep-rooted biases. These policies not only hindered the development of indigenous practices but also eroded trust within communities that revered these traditions as integral to their identity and wellness.

Moreover, the legal system rarely recognized the intellectual property rights of indigenous communities over their medicinal knowledge, facilitating biopiracy and exploitation without compensation. Addressing these injustices requires a legal reformation aimed at acknowledging and integrating indigenous healing within the broader health care systems, respecting both its value and its rights to exist and evolve.

**Documentation and Loss of Indigenous Medical Knowledge**

The erosion of indigenous medical knowledge is not merely a result of neglect but also of inadequate documentation. Historically, oral transmission was the primary method of preserving and conveying medical wisdom within indigenous communities. This mode of knowledge sharing, inherently fluid and evolving, faced immense challenges with the onset of colonial influences that favored written documentation and formalized medical education systems.

As Western methods began to dominate, there was a significant decline in the systematic recording of indigenous medical practices. This oversight led to a considerable loss of valuable therapeutic knowledge, practices that had been refined over generations. Moreover, the few documented accounts by early ethnographers or missionaries often lacked depth and cultural context, sometimes misrepresenting the practices as mere folklore or superstition, further undermining their validity and scientific potential.

This loss has not only cultural implications but also affects biodiversity, as traditional knowledge often includes the use of local plants and minerals, which are overlooked in modern practices. Reviving and valuing this knowledge requires genuine documentation efforts that respect and understand the cultural significance behind the practices.

## Cultural Erosion and Healing Practices

The erosion of cultural identity is a significant repercussion of the marginalization of indigenous healing practices. As colonial and modern forces emphasized Western medical systems, the intrinsic connection between cultural traditions and health practices was weakened. Indigenous healing practices, deeply embedded in communal and spiritual life, began to fade, losing their prominence and functional relevance within their communities.

This cultural erosion went beyond the mere displacement of medical practices; it encompassed a profound disconnection from ancestral roots and wisdom. Traditional healers, once venerated as custodians of both health and spiritual wisdom, found their roles and societal respect diminishing. The homogenization of health care under Western practices not only sidelined these healers but also eroded the cultural tapestry that supported diverse healing traditions.

Efforts to reverse this erosion face numerous challenges. Reintegrating indigenous practices requires not just acknowledgment but a deep understanding and respect for their cultural significance. Addressing the psycho-social impacts of this cultural loss is equally crucial, as it involves restoring identity and healing integrity to communities stripped of their traditional practices.

## Impact of Modernization on Traditional Health Paradigms

Modernization, a process intertwined with industrialization and urbanization, has significantly altered traditional health paradigms. As societies shifted towards industrial economies, traditional healing, often rural and closely tied to nature, struggled to find its place in the rapidly urbanizing world. The infrastructure of modern healthcare, with its hospitals and clinics, centralized health services in urban centers, sidelining rural and indigenous practices that remained distant both physically and ideologically.

The advent of technology in health further exacerbated this divide. Advanced diagnostic tools and treatment methods became the benchmarks for effective healthcare, while traditional methods that emphasized prevention and holistic treatment were often dismissed as outdated. This technological disparity rendered traditional healing methodologies less visible and less accessible in the face of modern medical equipment and pharmaceutical innovations.

Despite these challenges, a resurgence in recognizing the value of holistic and natural remedies has begun to bridge the gap. Yet, the full integration of traditional paradigms within modern medical systems remains a nuanced and ongoing struggle, suggesting a complex interplay between cultural preservation and modern health advancements.

## Assimilation Policies and Their Impact on Health Sovereignty

Assimilation policies have historically played a profound role in undermining the health sovereignty of indigenous communities. Enforced predominantly through colonial regimes, these policies aimed to homogenize diverse cultural practices into a singular, dominant medical framework, often at the expense of indigenous methods. As traditional healing was stigmatized or outright banned, indigenous peoples were coerced into adopting Western medical practices, which frequently disregarded the holistic and spiritual components that were integral to indigenous health paradigms.

The impact on health sovereignty was dual-faceted. Firstly, these policies diluted the traditional knowledge base, as younger generations were alienated from their ancestral healing techniques. Secondly, they instilled a dependency on a health system that was often inaccessible or misaligned with indigenous needs and values, escalating health disparities.

Today, the legacies of these assimilation policies linger, evident in ongoing health inequities and the challenging process of reviving and legitimizing traditional practices within modern health systems. Recognizing and rectifying these historical injustices is crucial for restoring health sovereignty to indigenous communities.

## Economic Factors Contributing to the Displacement of Indigenous Healers

Economic shifts, often driven by rapid industrialization, have been significant in displacing indigenous healers. The replacement of localized economies with global trade systems fundamentally altered the economic landscape, in which indigenous healing practices had thrived. As a result, herbal medicines and traditional therapies were seen as less competitive against mass-produced pharmaceuticals that conformed to global market standards.

Moreover, land dispossession played a critical role. Commercial interests, supported by state policies favoring industrial agriculture or urban development, deprived indigenous communities of land. Land is not merely a source of income but the bedrock of many communities' herbal knowledge and healing practices. Displaced from these vital resources, indigenous healers found it increasingly difficult to practice their crafts under such economic pressures.

Project funding and financial aid typically allocated towards healthcare generally favor modern medical facilities over traditional healing. This disparity in funding not only marginalized indigenous healers economically but also diminished their visibility in the broader healthcare landscape, accelerating their exclusion and the decline of traditional medicine practices.

## Academic Dismissal of Non-Western Medicine

The dismissal of non-Western medicine within academic circles is a complex legacy of cultural imperialism intertwined with scientific bias. Historically, universities and research institutions, pillars of knowledge production, have predominantly endorsed Eurocentric paradigms. This endorsement systematically undermines indigenous healing practices, categorizing them as unscientific or backward without substantive evaluation of their efficacy or cultural significance.

In academic settings, this bias manifests through curriculum designs that privilege Western medical knowledge while excluding or misrepresenting traditional methods. Such educational practices not only marginalize non-Western medical traditions but also influence future healthcare professionals' perceptions, reinforcing a cycle of ignorance and prejudice. This skewed portrayal contributes to a hierarchical knowledge system where Western medicine is seen as inherently superior.

Efforts to integrate indigenous knowledge systems are often challenged by academic inertia and a lack of genuine interdisciplinary engagement. Overcoming these challenges requires not only curricular reform but also a profound shift in academic culture to embrace and respect the diversity of global medical knowledge systems.

## The Role of Religion in the Marginalization of Indigenous Practices

Religion played a pivotal yet complex role in the marginalization of indigenous healing practices globally. Historically, colonizing powers often imposed their own religious norms, which vilified and replaced traditional spiritual beliefs integral to indigenous medicine. The intrinsic linkage between indigenous spirituality and healing was strategically dismantled, with native rituals often branded as superstition or heresy, leading to a loss of their legitimacy and survival.

Missionaries and colonial doctors further solidified this rift. They frequently positioned Western medical practices as a component of 'civilizing' missions, where conversion to Western religions entailed adopting Western medical techniques. This merger of medicine and religion not only disenfranchised traditional healers but also disrupted the transmission of indigenous medical knowledge through generations.

Despite this historical suppression, modern initiatives aim to reconnect religious beliefs with traditional healing wisdom, advocating for a synthesis that respects and revitalizes indigenous practices. These efforts face significant challenges but highlight the ongoing struggle to restore cultural integrity and medical plurality.

## Historical Perceptions and Misinterpretation of Indigenous Healing

The misinterpretation of indigenous healing practices has deep historical roots, influenced heavily by colonial and ethnocentric perspectives. Often, these practices were dismissed as mere folklore or superstition, overshadowed by the empirical framework favored in Western medicine. This misunderstanding severed the holistic essence from the techniques, ignoring the cultural and spiritual depth that defines their efficacy.

Such misconceptions were not benign but carried severe implications for the preservation and respect of indigenous medical knowledge. As these practices were sidelined or misrepresented, crucial healing wisdom, passed through generations, began to fade, its integration into broader medical discourse stunted. This marginalization reflected broader patterns of cultural imperialism where indigenous life ways were systematically devalued.

The repercussions of this historical bias continue to echo today, as many health systems still grapple with fully integrating and valuing diverse medical paradigms. Overcoming these deep-rooted prejudices requires a re-examination of the historical narrative and a robust inclusion of indigenous voices in medical research and practice.

## Global Variations in the Recognition of Indigenous Medicine

The recognition of indigenous medicine exhibits profound global variations, influenced by historical, cultural, and political factors. In nations where colonial impacts have been most suppressive, the acknowledgment and integration of these traditional practices into mainstream health systems remain minimal. Conversely, countries with a strong resurgence of indigenous identity often witness more substantial institutional recognition and incorporation of these healing arts.

Countries like New Zealand and Canada have begun to integrate Maori and First Nations' healing practices respectively into public health strategies, recognizing their value through legislative support and funding. However, in many parts of Africa and Asia, traditional medicine often operates informally, acknowledged more by the community than by the state. This informal status limits research opportunities and formal development of these practices within national health systems.

The global health community, influenced by WHO's traditional medicine strategy, is beginning to foster greater inclusivity. Acknowledging the disparities and embracing a more holistic approach to health could pave the way for a globally integrated medical paradigm that respects and utilizes the full spectrum of indigenous knowledge.

## The Erasure of Shamanic Practices in Western Scholarship

The erasure of shamanic practices in Western scholarship is a stark example of the broader marginalization indigenous healing has faced historically. Academia, primarily dominated by Western methodologies, has often dismissed shamanic traditions as pseudoscientific or primitive. This dismissal is not only a loss of cultural heritage but also a significant gap in the understanding of holistic healing methods that have benefited communities for centuries.

In many scholarly texts, shamanic practices were often misrepresented or reduced to exotic curiosities, stripping them of their therapeutic value and depth. This reductionist view fails to capture the complex interplay of spirituality, community, and environment in shamanic healing, aspects that are now recognized as integral to effective therapeutic practices in modern psychology and medical anthropology.

Efforts to revive and reintegrate shamanic wisdom into academic discourse face substantial hurdles. Institutional biases, coupled with a lack of comprehensive documentation, continue to sideline these practices in scholarly research and discussions. Overcoming these challenges requires not only academic openness but also a collaborative approach to preserve and learn from shamanic traditions.

## Colonial Medical Campaigns and Their Legacy

Colonial medical campaigns were often justified under the guise of humanitarian aid, but they carried a deeper agenda: the diminishment and replacement of indigenous healing practices with Western medicine. These campaigns, rooted in a colonial mindset that viewed Western science as superior, systematically devalued and undermined traditional knowledge, leaving a legacy of mistrust and health disparities.

As Western medicine was introduced into colonized regions, it often clashed with, and sought to suppress, existing medicinal practices that were deeply intertwined with the cultural and spiritual life of the communities. The introduction of hospitals and Western-trained doctors eroded the role of traditional healers, not just as healthcare providers but as essential cultural stewards, accelerating the decline of holistic health paradigms.

Today, the impact of these campaigns is still evident as many indigenous communities struggle with healthcare systems that do not accommodate their cultural perspectives or practices. Rebuilding these bridges requires recognizing the historical damages and actively involving indigenous knowledge in contemporary health practices.

## Historical Biases in Medical Research and Funding

Through history, the allocation of medical research funding has starkly favored Western methodologies, sidelining indigenous healing systems. This bias is not merely a reflection of scientific preference but is deeply rooted in colonial legacies and ethnocentric perspectives that valorize Western medical paradigms as more legible and legitimate. As a result, traditional practices have been under-researched and underfunded, perpetuating a cycle of marginalization and delegitimization.

The implications of these biases are profound, as they influence which health interventions are developed, scaled, and accepted in mainstream medicine. This has systematically constrained the integration of holistic and indigenous healing methods that are often preventive, less invasive, and harmoniously aligned with the cultural contexts of their communities.

Efforts to address these disparities have been emerging, with calls for inclusive funding strategies that recognize the value of diverse medical traditions. Yet, the journey towards equitable research investment is fraught with challenges, requiring rigorous advocacy and a restructuring of funding priorities to embrace a pluralistic approach to health science.

## Effects of Industrialization and Urbanization

The rapid rise of industrialization and urbanization has significantly impacted indigenous healing practices. As cities expanded, they drew populations away from rural areas, where many traditional healing practices were rooted. The migration not only dispersed communities but also diluted the transfer of knowledge as younger generations sought modern professions over traditional healer roles.

Urban environments, characterized by their technological and infrastructural focus, often lack the natural resources crucial for many traditional remedies, pushing indigenous medicine into obscurity. Furthermore, urban health systems are predominantly designed around Western medical practices, which are better funded and globally recognized, further marginalizing indigenous methodologies.

The pace of industrial growth frequently overlooks the sustainability of cultural practices, leading to a diminished practice of, and respect for, traditional medicine. This exacerbates the loss of biodiversity, which is essential not only for physical health but for the cultural identity that supports holistic well-being in indigenous communities.

## Anthropological Perspectives on Indigenous Health Practices

Anthropologists have long been fascinated by the depth and diversity of indigenous health practices, which encapsulate more than just medical treatment; they embody a holistic view integrating the social, spiritual, and environmental realms. Investigating these practices offers insights into how health and well-being are perceived and managed within different cultures, contrasting markedly with the biomedical approaches that dominate Western medicine.

Through ethnographic studies, anthropologists observe the roles of community, ritual, and tradition in healing processes, highlighting how these elements foster a sense of collective identity and support. Such studies also reveal the adaptive nature of traditional practices, which evolve in response to both internal cultural shifts and external pressures, including those from modern medical practices.

Critically, anthropological research challenges the marginalization of indigenous wisdom by providing a platform for these voices in the global health dialogue. This inclusion not only enriches our understanding of health and healing but also promotes a more inclusive approach to global health challenges, advocating for the integration of indigenous knowledge systems alongside conventional medical science.

## Psycho-social Effects of Losing Traditional Healing Practices

The loss of traditional healing practices carries profound psycho-social effects for indigenous communities. These practices are not merely medical interventions but are integral to the cultural and spiritual identity of the people. Their erosion often leads to a sense of loss and alienation, which can manifest as psychological distress or communal disintegration.

As traditional healing practices diminish, replaced by often inaccessible Western medicine, communities lose more than just healthcare—they lose a common thread that binds them. This disruption in continuity can lead to a breakdown in community cohesion and weaken the transmission of ancestral knowledge, which is pivotal not only for health but for the survival of cultural heritage.

Furthermore, the marginalization of these practices contributes to systemic biases in health care that disregard the holistic aspects of indigenous health, leading to inadequate treatment and increased stigmatization of cultural practices. Addressing these psycho-social impacts requires a concerted effort to preserve traditional knowledge and integrate it respectfully into broader health systems.

## Nationalist Agendas and the Suppression of Local Medicine

Nationalist agendas have historically played a pivotal role in the suppression of local medicine, often favoring a homogenized medical approach that sidelines indigenous practices. Nationalistic policies, driven by the desire to unify diverse populations under a single cultural and medical standard, frequently marginalized traditional healing methods deemed 'unscientific' or 'backwards'.

In many instances, these policies were implemented through healthcare reforms that established Western medicine as the superior and only legitimate form of healthcare, with government support funneled exclusively into modern medical facilities and education. Traditional healers were either restricted by licensing requirements that were biased against their practices or outright banned.

The consequences of such suppression extended beyond healthcare, affecting the cultural identity and self-perception of indigenous communities. The undermining of local medicine under nationalist policies not only eroded health sovereignty but also stripped communities of a vital component of their heritage and knowledge systems.

## Case Studies in Cultural Preservation and Loss

The exploration of case studies in cultural preservation and loss uncovers the complex layers of how indigenous healing practices have been preserved or lost over time. In regions like the Amazon, efforts to document traditional knowledge before it vanishes have seen mixed results. While some tribes have successfully archived their medicinal practices through collaboration with researchers, others have witnessed a near-total erosion due to external pressures such as deforestation and cultural assimilation.

Contrastingly, in places like New Zealand, the formal recognition of Maori healing techniques through government-supported initiatives illustrates a proactive approach to cultural preservation. These programs not only safeguard medical knowledge but also integrate it into the public health system, providing a model for other nations.

However, the loss of native American healing traditions in the United States serves as a stark reminder of the challenges. Urbanization and strict regulations have marginalized these practices, often relegating them to historical anecdotes rather than living, evolving forms of medicine.

## Cultural Revival Movements in Indigenous Medicine

In recent years, indigenous communities have initiated cultural revival movements to reclaim and restore traditional healing practices marginalized by centuries of colonial dominance and modernization. These movements emerge as powerful rebuttals to historical suppression, utilizing both knowledge preservation and contemporary platforms to reinforce the validity and value of indigenous medicine.

Engagement with digital media, coupled with academic collaborations, has allowed for a wider dissemination of traditional knowledge that was once on the brink of extinction. Such efforts are not merely archival but are active restorations, often integrating traditional wisdom with modern health practices to create innovative, culturally sensitive healthcare solutions. This blend addresses both community-specific and global health challenges, recognizing the profound benefits of holistic and nature-based treatments that have been refined over generations.

Furthermore, these movements also foster stronger community identity and resilience by reinforcing cultural heritage as a source of healing power. They challenge the ongoing narratives that have historically undermined these practices and inspire a new generation to rediscover and respect their ancestral knowledge.

## Role of UNESCO and Other Agencies in Protecting Indigenous Health Knowledge

UNESCO, among other global agencies, plays a pivotal role in preserving traditional healing knowledge, particularly in contexts where such practices face erasure by dominant medical paradigms. Through initiatives like the Intangible Cultural Heritage list, UNESCO fosters recognition and respect for indigenous medicinal practices, which are often closely tied to the cultural identity of communities. These efforts provide a platform for indigenous voices in the global health landscape, ensuring these practices are not only remembered but integrated into current health systems.

Such protection is crucial, as it empowers communities to maintain and control the use of their indigenous knowledge. Agencies like the World Health Organization have begun to collaborate with UNESCO to develop policies that incorporate traditional healing within national health frameworks, enhancing the diversity of healthcare options available to populations worldwide.

Beyond preservation, these initiatives also aim to revive knowledge systems that have dwindled under the weight of globalization and industrialization. By providing resources and facilitating dialogue between traditional healers and modern medical practitioners, these organizations pave the way for a more inclusive understanding of health and wellness that respects and utilizes centuries-old knowledge alongside contemporary science.

## The Historical Impact of Missionaries and Colonial Doctors on Indigenous Cultures

The introduction of missionary and colonial medical practices profoundly impacted indigenous cultures, often undermining traditional healing methods. Missionaries, while primarily focused on spiritual conversions, also introduced Western health practices that conflicted with and frequently dismissed indigenous medicine. This led to a decline in the use and transmission of native healing knowledge, prioritizing Western methods as more 'civilized' or scientifically valid.

Colonial doctors frequently accompanied these missions; their approach to medicine not only displaced traditional practices but also ignored the holistic integration of spiritual, environmental, and physical health that characterizes indigenous healing. As these foreign practitioners established institutional health systems, they systematically marginalized local healers by labeling them as primitive or ineffective, significantly eroding cultural confidence in traditional medicine.

This historical trend resulted in a lasting skepticism towards indigenous practices and contributed to their gradual disappearance. Even today, the remnants of this impact linger, affecting how indigenous communities view their own cultural practices in the sphere of global health.

## Summary

The chapter 'Historical Marginalization of Indigenous Healing Practices' provides an in-depth analysis of the systematic suppression and displacement of indigenous health practices through colonial, legislative, and economic impacts. It starts by discussing how the colonial era brought significant disruptions to indigenous health practices, which were often sidelined or discarded in favor of Western medical practices. This not only introduced new diseases but also undermined the efficacy and cultural value of traditional healing methods. The introduction of Western education systems further entrenched the dominance of allopathic medicine, systematically marginalizing indigenous methods. Moreover, the legislative frameworks in colonial times and beyond restricted the practice and evolution of indigenous healing, often dismissing it as unscientific or primitive. The assimilation policies and economic factors, such as industrialization and land dispossession, further displaced indigenous healers, eroding the infrastructure of traditional healing practices. Additionally, the academic and scientific dismissal of non-Western medicine perpetuated a hierarchy where Western methodologies were deemed superior. The chapter discusses the psychological and social impacts of these losses, emphasizing the disconnection from spiritual and communal roots which were centrally integrated with traditional health paradigms. Modernization and urbanization further widened the gap, diluting the efficacy and presence of indigenous practices in the face of technological advances in healthcare. Despite such historical marginalization, there's a growing recognition of the value of traditional methods, with movements aimed at reviving and integrating indigenous wisdom into modern healthcare systems gaining ground. Agencies like UNESCO and the WHO are starting to foster greater inclusivity, acknowledging the vast potential of these time-tested practices not just for indigenous populations but for global health paradigms. This chapter highlights the need for a more equitable and respectful inclusion of indigenous healing practices in contemporary health discourse to bridge the cultural and knowledge gaps created over centuries.

## References

[1] Montenegro, R. A., & Stephens, C. (2006). Indigenous health in Latin America and the Caribbean.. https://www.ncbi.nlm.nih.gov/pmc/articles/PMC2080455/

[2] Waldram, J. B. (2000). The Efficacy of Traditional Medicine: Current Theoretical and Methodological Issues.. https://journals.uvic.ca/index.php/IC/article/view/12368

[3] Cohen, K. (1998). Native American Medicine, Alternative Therapies.. https://www.nejm.org/doi/full/10.1056/NEJM199812033392206

[4] World Health Organization (WHO). Traditional Medicine Strategy 2014-2023.. https://www.who.int/publications/i/item/9789241506097

[5] Gracey, M., & King, M. (2009). Indigenous health part 1: determinants and disease patterns.. https://www.thelancet.com/journals/lancet/article/PIIS0140-6736(09)60914-4/fulltext

[6] Kirmayer, L. J. & Valaskakis, G. G. (2009). Healing Traditions: The Mental Health of Aboriginal Peoples in Canada.. https://www.ubcpress.ca/healing-traditions

## Case Study: Integrating Maori Healing Practices in New Zealand's Health System

In recent years, New Zealand has emerged as a model for the integration of indigenous healing practices within its national health system, specifically through the incorporation of Maori traditional medicine. The Maori, the indigenous people of New Zealand, have a rich history of using native herbs, bodywork, and spiritual healing to maintain health. This case study examines the challenges and successes of integrating these practices into the modern healthcare framework.

The initiative began as a response to the persistent health disparities faced by the Maori population, who often reported feeling marginalized by the predominantly Western-oriented New Zealand health services. In an innovative approach, the government, in collaboration with Maori health practitioners, began to actively incorporate Maori healing techniques, known as Rongoā Maori, into the public healthcare system. This was facilitated through legislative support that recognized the value of these traditions and provided funding for their development and dissemination.

However, integration presented multiple challenges. One prominent issue was the credentialing of traditional Maori healers, who typically transmitted knowledge orally and did not adhere to formal educational frameworks common in Western medicine. Moreover, skepticism among medical professionals, who were trained in evidence-based practices, posed significant barriers. Additionally, logistical issues arose in attempting to blend these disparate health services in a way that maintained the integrity of each approach.

Despite these challenges, the integration has seen significant success. Pilot programs have demonstrated improved health outcomes for Maori patients, reflecting the efficacy and cultural relevance of their traditional practices. Additionally, this move has fostered a greater sense of cultural identity and empowerment within the Maori community, paving the way for a more inclusive and holistic approach to health in New Zealand.

### Case Study: Revival of Native American Healing Practices in the U.S. Healthcare System

The case study focuses on the efforts and challenges in reviving and integrating Native American healing practices within the broad framework of the U.S. healthcare system. Native American healing practices, steeped in centuries-old traditions and spiritual beliefs, have faced significant erosion due to historical suppression and marginalization. However, recent decades have seen a concerted effort to revive these practices, recognizing their value in providing culturally sensitive and holistic care to Native American populations.

Initiatives have been undertaken by various tribal leaders and health advocates, backed by federal support, aiming to incorporate traditional healing within health services provided to Native American communities. Key steps included the establishment of health facilities that operate under the principles of both Western and traditional medicine, as well as the development of training programs for healers and health workers on the cultural nuances and methodologies of Native American medicinal practices.

This integration, however, has not been without challenges. One significant barrier has been the clash between the structured, evidence-based approach of Western medicine and the more spiritual and holistic approach of traditional practices. Issues of credentialing and standardizing practices that are inherently diverse and often orally transmitted have also posed substantial hurdles. Moreover, there remains a degree of skepticism and resistance among some healthcare professionals and even within some segments of Native American communities, where trust in the federal health system remains low due to historical grievances.

Despite these challenges, there have been notable successes. Health programs that combine traditional healing with Western medical practices have reported higher levels of patient satisfaction and improved health outcomes among Native American patients. These programs have also played a critical role in preserving and revitalizing cultural heritage, boosting community health sovereignty by allowing Native Americans to take greater control over their health needs and solutions. Such initiatives mark essential steps toward a more inclusive and culturally attuned healthcare system in the United States.

### Case Study: Reclaiming Ancestral Wisdom: The Integration of Shamanic Practices in Modern Mental Health Therapies

The rise of mental health awareness has opened new avenues for exploring various healing methodologies, including the integration of traditional shamanic practices into contemporary treatment models. Shamanic practices, deeply rooted in the spiritual and communal life of indigenous cultures worldwide, have historically been marginalized or misunderstood in the context of modern psychology. This case study explores the potential benefits and challenges associated with integrating these ancestral wisdoms into modern mental health therapies, particularly for treating conditions like depression, anxiety, and post-traumatic stress disorder (PTSD).

One notable initiative has been the adaptation of shamanic techniques such as guided imagery, drumming sessions, and ritualistic healing into therapeutic settings. For instance, a mental health clinic in the United States has collaborated with a group of indigenous shamans to create a culturally sensitive therapeutic program that blends cognitive-behavioral therapy with shamanic rituals. The program aims to provide patients with a more holistic treatment, addressing not just the mind but also the spiritual and emotional dimensions of well-being.

However, the integration of shamanic practices into mainstream therapy presents numerous challenges. Firstly, there is significant resistance from practitioners trained exclusively in Western medical traditions, who may view these methods as unscientific or anecdotal. Secondly, ethical considerations arise regarding cultural appropriation and the authenticity of the shamanic elements being integrated. Ensuring that these practices are represented and administered respectfully and accurately requires careful collaboration with authentic practitioners from indigenous communities.

Despite these challenges, preliminary results from the integrated therapy programs have been promising. Patients have reported deeper emotional resolutions and improved mental health outcomes, suggesting that these ancient practices may offer valuable insights and techniques for contemporary health challenges. As mental health professionals continue to explore these integrations, the potential for a more diversified and culturally enriched therapeutic landscape becomes increasingly apparent.

**Case Study: Revitalizing Indigenous Health Systems in South America: The Ayahuasca Renaissance**

The resurgence of interest in traditional South American healing practices, notably those involving the psychoactive brew Ayahuasca, encompasses a broad spectrum of cultural, medical, and ethical dimensions. Originating from the Amazon basin, Ayahuasca is a concoction traditionally used by indigenous tribes for spiritual and healing purposes. This case study delves into the recent movements aimed at integrating Ayahuasca-based therapies into contemporary health systems, analyzing the interplay between traditional knowledge and modern medical practice.

Recently, countries like Brazil and Peru have witnessed a revival in the use of Ayahuasca, not only within indigenous communities but also among urban populations seeking alternative mental health therapies. The brew, composed of Banisteriopsis caapi vine and other indigenous plants, has been the center of both anthropological interest and biomedical research due to its potent psychoactive properties, which some studies suggest can be beneficial in treating depression and PTSD.

The renaissance of Ayahuasca has prompted both indigenous and non-indigenous healers to advocate for its integration into national health systems. This movement poses unique challenges, including the standardization of dosing and administration, the clinical training of practitioners, and legal issues surrounding its use due to its psychoactive components. Additionally, there is a robust debate regarding the ethical implications of utilizing indigenous knowledge and practices within a Western medical framework without proper cultural sensitivity and compensation.

Despite the challenges, the integration efforts have seen significant advancements. Research initiatives and pilot healthcare programs aimed at safely and respectfully incorporating Ayahuasca have been launched, with preliminary findings indicating positive therapeutic impacts. These efforts also aim to bolster the recognition and preservation of indigenous medical knowledge, fostering a more inclusive approach to health care. However, the path forward requires careful navigation of cultural rights, scientific validation, and legal frameworks to ensure that these traditional practices are respected and preserved, avoiding exploitation while enhancing global health diversity.

**Case Study: The Erosion and Revitalization of Gwich'in Healing Practices in Canada**

The case study focuses on the Gwich'in communities in Canada, particularly examining the erosion and subsequent revitalization efforts of their traditional healing practices. The Gwich'in are a group of First Nation peoples, primarily located in the Northwest Territories, who have historically relied on a rich array of medicinal practices rooted in deep ecological knowledge and spiritual beliefs.

During the 19th and 20th centuries, the introduction of Western medical systems alongside missionary activities resulted in a significant decline of these indigenous practices. Government policies not only promoted Western medicine but often actively suppressed traditional Gwich'in healing methods, which were labeled as superstitious or unscientific. This suppression was further compounded by the residential school system, which sought to assimilate indigenous youths into Western norms, thereby severing their cultural ties and knowledge of ancestral healing techniques.

In recent decades, there has been a noticeable shift towards reclaiming and revitalizing these indigenous practices. Initiated by community elders and supported by cultural preservation groups, these efforts have led to the establishment of programs aimed at educating younger generations about traditional Gwich'in healing practices. These programs incorporate elder teachings, hands-on experience with medicinal plants, and the revitalization of spiritual healing ceremonies.

However, the path to revitalization is fraught with challenges. One significant hindrance is the intergenerational trauma inflicted by past oppressive policies, which affects both community health and cultural continuity. Additionally, there exists a skepticism about the efficacy of traditional methods within the broader medical community, making integration into modern healthcare systems difficult. Despite these challenges, preliminary outcomes from these initiatives have shown improvements in community health metrics and an increased sense of cultural identity among the Gwich'in. This resurgence not only bolsters health sovereignty but also plays a crucial role in the cultural and spiritual reclamation for the community.

**Case Study: Restoration of Traditional Healing Practices in Aboriginal Australia**

The case study examines the concerted efforts to restore and integrate traditional Aboriginal healing practices in Australia, a country with a rich history of Indigenous medicinal knowledge that suffered suppression under colonial rule. Aboriginal Australians have utilized natural remedies and spiritual healing, deeply rooted in their connection to the land and ancestral wisdom, to maintain health for centuries. This investigation highlights the complexity of reintegrating such practices into a predominantly Western-aligned health system while addressing the nuances of cultural sensitivity and medical efficacy.

The initiative to revive these traditional practices began in response to health inequalities faced by Aboriginal communities, marked by higher rates of non-communicable diseases and reduced access to healthcare services in remote areas. Australian health authorities, in collaboration with Aboriginal health councils, initiated programs to document, sustain, and integrate these traditional healing techniques—which include herbal medicines, physical therapies, and spiritual healing—into the public health service. This integration was supported by government funding and policies that recognized the cultural and therapeutic value of these practices.

However, this process presented numerous challenges. One primary concern was the systemic bias within the healthcare system, which historically undervalued non-Western medicine as unscientific. This bias was evident in the reluctance of healthcare professionals to adopt practices that lacked stringent empirical validation. Another significant hurdle was ensuring that the traditional knowledge was passed down and maintained authentically, combating the erosion of knowledge caused by generations of cultural assimilation and suppression.

Despite these obstacles, the project has shown promising results. Collaborative health programs that combine traditional Aboriginal healing with Western medical science have been reported to increase engagement and satisfaction among Aboriginal patients, indicating a respectful integration of health services. In addition, these initiatives have empowered Aboriginal communities, fostered a sense of agency and cultural pride while contributing to the broader aims of reconciliation and cultural preservation.

### Case Study: Addressing Health Disparities through Community-Based Indigenous Healing in Rural India

The Indian subcontinent hosts a rich tapestry of indigenous cultures, each with its own set of traditional healing practices that have been honed over millennia. This case study explores the efforts to integrate these indigenous practices into the broader healthcare system in rural India, highlighting the socio-cultural dynamics at play and the implications for improving health outcomes in these communities.

In the heart of rural Rajasthan, a pilot program was initiated by local NGOs in collaboration with the Indian Ministry of Health to harness the capabilities of traditional healers, known locally as 'Vaidyas,' in addressing prevalent health issues such as malnutrition, maternal health, and infectious diseases. The program aimed to blend Ayurvedic medicine, one of India's traditional systems of medicine, with contemporary allopathic treatments, creating a comprehensive, culturally sensitive healthcare model.

However, integrating these diverse medical systems presented considerable challenges. First, there was significant resistance from the allopathically trained medical community, who often viewed traditional practices as empirically weak and unstandardized. Furthermore, the logistical challenges of training and standardizing practices among Vaidyas, who largely pass their knowledge orally and rely heavily on local herbs and personal experience, were immense.

Despite these challenges, the initiative saw pockets of success attributable to community engagement strategies that emphasized respect and cooperation between different medical practitioners. Activities such as joint medical camps, cross-training workshops, and community health education sessions facilitated a mutual understanding of various health paradigms. These efforts culminated in increased acceptance and usage of combined health services, leading to improved healthcare delivery in remote areas.

This case study underscores the vast potential of integrating indigenous healing practices into formal health systems, particularly in rural settings where conventional medical resources are scarce. By leveraging local knowledge and cultural beliefs, health programs can enhance their effectiveness and reach, significantly improving public health outcomes. This integration not only promotes a pluralistic approach to health but also aids in preserving invaluable cultural heritage.

### Case Study: The Preservation and Integration of Ainu Medicinal Practices in Modern Japan

The Ainu people, the indigenous population of northern Japan, have long relied on a comprehensive system of medicinal practices derived from their deep connection with nature. However, the gradual dominance of Western medicine brought by the Meiji Restoration and subsequent modernization efforts in Japan has severely threatened these ancient practices. Aimed at examining the multifaceted approach taken to preserve and reintegrate Ainu healing traditions within Japan's health system, this case study delves into the recent policies, community efforts, and educational programs fostering this integration.

Historically, the Ainu's extensive herbal knowledge and rituals were undermined during Japan's rapid industrialization, with many Ainu forcibly assimilated into mainstream Japanese society, leading to the severe decline of their cultural practices. Recognizing this erosion, recent governmental and non-governmental initiatives have sought to preserve Ainu culture by documenting medicinal knowledge and facilitating its practice. For example, the establishment of the Ainu Culture Promotion Act and the subsequent creation of the Symbolic Space for Ethnic Harmony in Hokkaido represent significant steps towards cultural preservation.

Challenges in this integrative process include the skepticism of the medical community trained in allopathic methods, regulatory hurdles for the recognition of Ainu herbal remedies, and the generational gaps within the Ainu community, often resulting from historical disruptions to the transmission of knowledge. Efforts to overcome these barriers have included partnerships between national health institutes and Ainu cultural organizations, aiming to validate the efficacy of Ainu remedies through scientific research and to introduce educational modules on Ainu medicine in medical schools.

Despite such efforts, the road to full integration is fraught with complexity. The case underscores a critical tension between preserving the authenticity of traditional practices and adapting them within a modern regulatory and scientific framework. The way forward, as suggested by this study, involves a collaborative approach that respects cultural sensitivities while rigorously evaluating and incorporating traditional knowledge into public health practices, offering a model that could inspire similar initiatives worldwide.

## Review Questions

**1. A 62-year-old male suffering from chronic back pain after noticing that traditional medical treatments were not effectively alleviating his discomfort, he decided to try court-type traditional Thai massage, based on suggestions from friends who had positive outcomes. After several weeks of treatment, he reports significant improvement in pain management and mobility. Given this case, what is a potential reason for the success of Thai massage in treating his chronic back pain?**

A) Thai massage incorrectly diagnosed the underlying condition.

B) The physical manipulation involved in Thai massage improved blood circulation and reduced muscle tension.

C) The placebo effect solely contributed to the reported improvements.

D) Thai massage treatments typically include pharmaceutical interventions.

**Answer: B**

Explanation: Thai massage involves various techniques, including deep pressure and stretching, which helps improve blood circulation and reduce muscle tension, often addressing underlying causes of back pain such as tight muscles and poor circulation. The man's improvements are likely due to these physiological changes, which are common benefits associated with Thai massage, rather than a placebo effect or pharmaceutical interventions, which are not typically part of Thai massage treatments.

**2. A patient suffering from diabetic neuropathy and lower back pain opts to try Traditional Thai Massage based on its reputed benefits in similar cases. After a treatment period, the patient notices a significant reduction in pain levels, improved mobility, and better blood sugar level management. What could explain the multifactorial benefits experienced by this patient from Thai massage?**

A) Thai massage only masks the pain but does not address underlying causes.

B) Thai massage provides temporary psychological relief without physical health benefits.

C) Thai massage includes secret medicinal ingredients that treat diabetes.

D) Thai massage can help improve circulation, reduce stress, and enhance lymphatic drainage, contributing to overall health improvements.

**Answer: D**

Explanation: Thai massage is known to enhance circulation and reduce stress, which are beneficial for managing diabetic neuropathy and back pain. By improving circulation, Thai massage helps in effective nutrient delivery and waste removal at the cellular level, which can alleviate symptoms of neuropathy. Stress reduction from massage can improve overall endocrine function, potentially stabilizing blood sugar levels. There are no secret ingredients in Thai massage; its benefits are primarily due to mechanical and reflexological effects.

## Case Studies of AI Bias in Medicine

### Analysis of Misdiagnosis Due to Training Data Limitations

Artificial intelligence in medicine often mirrors the biases present in its training data. Predominantly sourced from homogeneous populations, these datasets frequently neglect the nuances of genetic, environmental, and lifestyle variations across different ethnicities and regions. This oversight leads to AI systems that are less adept at diagnosing and treating diseases in non-represented groups, potentially resulting in harmful misdiagnoses.

Furthermore, the reliance on data from mainstream medical research disregards traditional, indigenous, and holistic health practices, which differ fundamentally from Western medicine. Consequently, AI systems may misinterpret symptoms that are commonly understood and treated within these traditional frameworks. This not only compromises patient care but also diminishes the credibility of valuable alternative medicinal practices.

Correcting these flaws requires integrating diverse data sources that encompass a wide range of human conditions and healing practices. By acknowledging and incorporating these varied perspectives into AI training datasets, the technology can achieve a truly inclusive, accurate, and culturally sensitive application in healthcare.

### Racial Disparities in Healthcare AI Outcomes

The promise of AI in healthcare often clashes with the reality of racial disparities, which manifest significantly in AI-driven medical practices. Data used to train AI models generally reflects the majority population's health profiles, inadvertently neglecting the specific health markers and outcomes pertinent to racial minorities. Consequently, this skew leads to AI systems that are less accurate and potentially harmful when used in racially diverse settings.

For instance, AI tools developed for diagnosing skin cancer have shown lower accuracy rates for darker skin tones, leading to delays in diagnosis and appropriate care. Similarly, predictive algorithms in cardiology have been critiqued for overestimating the risk of cardiovascular diseases in certain racial groups based on biased historical data.

Efforts to recalibrate and audit these AI systems are crucial. Incorporating a broader spectrum of data that accurately represents all racial groups can mitigate these disparities. Moreover, continuous monitoring and transparent reporting on AI performance across different demographics must be instated to ensure equitable AI-driven healthcare outcomes.

## Economic Bias in AI Treatment Recommendations

Artificial intelligence systems in healthcare often unknowingly perpetuate economic biases, tilting treatment recommendations toward more lucrative options rather than most effective or necessary ones. This scenario disproportionately affects lower-income individuals who may be nudged towards less optimal or affordable care due to the profit-oriented training models of these AI systems.

Additionally, economic bias manifests in the accessibility of cutting-edge treatments. AI algorithms, trained primarily on data from wealthier demographics, skew towards solutions that those groups are more likely to afford, further marginalizing economically disadvantaged patients by not providing equally effective alternatives within their financial reach.

In these contexts, AI's decision-making processes mirror the inequities found in broader society, emphasizing the need for a recalibration of these technologies to consider economic diversity. Mechanisms must be integrated to recognize and adjust for socio-economic factors, ensuring equitable treatment recommendations across all economic strata.

## AI's Failure in Recognizing Non-Standard Symptoms

Artificial intelligence in medicine often remains tethered to normative datasets, predominantly reflecting common symptoms exhibited by the majority. However, these databases occasionally overlook non-standard symptoms, which are atypical yet crucial indicators of underlying health issues. This model limitation poses a significant challenge in recognizing and responding to unusual symptom presentations, leading to instances where AI-based diagnostic tools fail to identify rare or less typical conditions effectively.

One pertinent example is the dismissal of atypical cardiac symptoms in women, which often differ from the classic 'chest pain' generally reported in men. AI systems, having been trained primarily on male-centric data, struggle to recognize these variations, contributing to misdiagnoses and delays in critical intervention. Similarly, mental health conditions exhibiting non-conventional symptoms might be overlooked by AI models rigid in their symptom recognition patterns.

Addressing these failures requires enhancing the diversity in training datasets and incorporating comprehensive symptomatology. Medical AI developers must prioritize updating algorithms with broader clinical inputs to reduce the risk of oversight. Only through such integrative measures can AI truly support all patients, recognizing the spectrum of human health variability.

## Gender Bias in AI Health Screening Tools

Gender bias in AI health screening tools conspicuously undermines the accuracy and effectiveness of medical diagnostics and treatment recommendations. Historically, much of the health data used to train AI models has been male-centric, often overlooking key physiological and symptomatic differences unique to women. For example, heart attack indicators are well-documented in men, but women may exhibit less typical symptoms, leading AI diagnostics to undervalue or misinterpret critical signs in female patients.

This bias is not just a technical oversight; it reflects deeper societal and institutional disparities that AI technologies inadvertently perpetuate. The repercussions are profound, affecting not only diagnostic precision but also the long-term health outcomes for women. In conditions like osteoporosis or autoimmune diseases, which predominantly affect women, biased AI tools can delay crucial interventions, exacerbating health issues.

Efforts to recalibrate these systems must prioritize gender-diverse data integration and continuous algorithm auditing to ensure equitable health care. By confronting these biases head-on, developers and healthcare providers can craft AI tools that promote justice and accuracy in medical assessments across all genders.

## Impact of AI Bias in Mental Health Assessments

The infusion of AI in mental health assessment processes brings to light significant biases that can exacerbate disparities in mental healthcare delivery. Often, AI algorithms are formulated based on datasets that fail to consider the full spectrum of psychological symptoms across different cultures and ethnic backgrounds. This oversight can lead to inappropriate treatment recommendations or overlook critical, culturally specific mental health issues.

For instance, depression and anxiety manifest differently across cultural contexts; symptoms that are prominent in one cultural group may be subtler or entirely different in another. If AI algorithms are trained predominantly on data from Western populations, they may not accurately identify or interpret symptoms expressed by individuals from diverse backgrounds. This can lead to misdiagnoses or underdiagnosis, affecting the quality of care and outcomes for patients from non-Western cultures.

Addressing these challenges requires an inclusive approach to training AI systems in mental health. By incorporating a diverse range of mental health profiles and understanding different cultural expressions of psychological distress, AI can be calibrated to provide more accurate assessments. Continuous monitoring and adaptation of these systems are critical to ensure fairness and effectiveness in AI-driven mental health services.

## Cross-Cultural Issues in AI-Derived Therapeutic Plans

Artificial Intelligence (AI) in healthcare reveals profound cross-cultural issues in therapeutic plan generation, often leading to non-optimal treatment outcomes for patients from diverse backgrounds. While AI aims to streamline and personalize healthcare, its reliance on dominant culture datasets significantly restricts its efficacy across different cultural spectrums. For example, therapeutic plans derived from AI models primarily trained with Western medical practices may not align well with the traditional healing approaches used in other regions like Asia or Africa.

This misalignment can result in the overlooking of effective indigenous treatments or the misapprehension of patient compliance and receptivity to prescribed interventions. Cultural nuances in symptom expression and health management practices are frequently underrepresented in AI datasets, leading to generalized and sometimes ineffective healthcare strategies.

To address these shortcomings, it is critical for AI development in healthcare to integrate culturally diverse data and expertise. Engaging with medical professionals from varied cultures and incorporating patient feedback on a global scale can help refine AI algorithms, making them more inclusive and representative of the global population they serve.

## Age-Related Bias in AI-Predictive Health Models

The age-related bias in AI-predictive health models emerges as a critical challenge, exacerbating discrepancies in healthcare delivery to different age groups. Training on data skewed toward middle-aged populations, these models may inadequately assess risks or misdiagnose illnesses in the elderly or the young. For instance, AI systems often underpredict cardiovascular risks in younger demographics because their training data is predominantly derived from older individuals.

Moreover, symptoms of diseases like Alzheimer's or diabetes manifest differently across ages, yet AI models frequently fail to adjust their algorithms accordingly. This one-size-fits-all approach can lead to over or under-treatment, significantly affecting health outcomes and increasing healthcare costs due to unnecessary procedures or delayed interventions.

To overcome these biases, it's imperative to diversify AI training sets to include wider age ranges and continuously update the models as new age-specific medical research becomes available. Incorporating clinical input from geriatric and pediatric care specialists might also recalibrate predictive models, making them more equitable across all ages.

## AI Misinterpretations Affecting Chronic Disease Management

Chronic disease management relies heavily on consistent and accurate data interpretation, yet AI systems often falter by adhering too rigidly to narrow data models derived from less diverse patient histories. When AI interprets chronic disease data, it may inadvertently apply biases that ignore less common disease manifestations or variations in progression across different populations. For instance, diabetes management AI tools frequently misinterpret the nuances of disease management in ethnic minorities, leading to less personalized and effective care plans.

These AI misinterpretations can result in suboptimal drug dosage recommendations or flawed monitoring schedules that fail to consider individualized metabolic differences or culturally influenced dietary patterns among patients. The implications are profound, directly impacting patient outcomes by potentially exacerbating conditions or not fully addressing disease progression factors.

To correct these AI deficiencies, there is an urgent need to integrate more comprehensive datasets that include a wide array of chronic disease scenarios and patient backgrounds. This approach not only enhances the accuracy of chronic disease management but also ensures fairness and inclusivity in healthcare AI applications.

## Misaligned AI Algorithms and Emergency Medical Responses

Emergency medical responses require swift and accurate decision-making, a task increasingly delegated to AI systems. However, misaligned AI algorithms can have catastrophic consequences, particularly when they fail to accommodate diverse emergency scenarios. For example, AI systems programmed primarily with data from urban settings may perform poorly in rural emergency situations due to differing environmental factors and available resources.

Moreover, these algorithms sometimes prioritize efficiency over nuanced patient care. In cases of cardiac arrest or stroke, where every second counts, AI-driven protocols that misinterpret symptoms or delay appropriate responses can exacerbate patient outcomes. The urgency and variability of emergencies make it crucial for AI systems to be robust and adaptable, traits often compromised by current training paradigms based on limited datasets.

To rectify these critical issues, it is essential to incorporate a broader spectrum of emergency scenarios in AI training processes, ensuring algorithms are tested across varied and unpredictable conditions. Constant feedback loops between on-ground emergency personnel and AI developers must be established to keep these systems relevant and reliable.

**Neurodiversity and AI's Standardization Challenges**

AI's integration in healthcare, while innovative, poses unique challenges when addressing neurodiversity. Standard AI models often fail to adequately capture the wide spectrum of neurodevelopmental conditions, such as autism and ADHD, where symptoms and behaviors can vary vastly among individuals. These models, typically trained on data reflecting neurotypical patterns, struggle to interpret atypical neural behaviors, leading to misdiagnosis or inappropriate treatment strategies.

For instance, an AI system might misclassify the hyperfocus associated with certain forms of autism as an obsessive-compulsive trait, missing the broader context of the individual's neurodiverse condition. Such oversights can significantly affect treatment paths, emphasizing the need for AI systems to be educated on the nuances of neurodiversity.

Addressing these challenges requires a concerted effort to diversify AI training datasets and involve experts in neurodiversity during the development phase. Only through an inclusive approach can AI truly enhance healthcare delivery for all, accommodating the rich variety of human cognitive experiences.

**Inequities in AI Drug Prescription Practices**

Artificial Intelligence (AI) systems in drug prescription practices reveal significant inequities, often stemming from biases in their training datasets. These AI models, primarily trained on data from largely homogeneous population samples, inadvertently perpetuate disparities in treatment outcomes. For instance, the underrepresentation of minority ethnic groups in these datasets can lead to less effective or inappropriate drug recommendations for these populations.

Moreover, socioeconomic biases coded into these systems can further skew prescriptions. AI might favor more expensive treatments accessible to wealthier demographics, ignoring equally effective but more affordable alternatives crucial for lower-income patients. This not only exacerbates healthcare inequalities but also limits patient access to necessary medications based on economic status rather than medical need.

To rectify these issues, there's an urgent need for inclusivity in the data used for training AI in healthcare. Integrating a diverse array of health profiles and socio-economic backgrounds can help create more balanced and equitable drug prescription practices. Continuous monitoring and updating of these AI systems are also essential to prevent the perpetuation of existing biases.

**Biased AI in Oncological Treatment and Patient Outcomes**

In the realm of oncology, AI has promised precision yet often delivers bias. Oncological treatment recommendations and prognosis determinations generated by AI systems tend to reflect the racial, gender, and socioeconomic biases embedded in their training data. For instance, algorithms can oversimplify complex cancer markers that vary significantly across ethnic groups, potentially leading to suboptimal treatment strategies for non-majority populations.

Moreover, gender disparities in outcome predictions further complicate the efficacy of AI in cancer care. Studies highlight that certain AI models underpredict survival rates for women with lung cancer compared to men, despite clinical evidence suggesting otherwise. This skewed output arises not from clinical reality but from historical data biases that overlooked gender differences in symptomatology and response to treatment.

Addressing these biases requires a multifaceted approach. Integrating diverse datasets that encompass a broad spectrum of patient demographics is critical. Collaboration between oncologists, data scientists, and ethicists can ensure AI tools in oncology not only advance treatment but also uphold fairness, ultimately improving outcomes across all patient groups.

## Evaluating AI's Impact on Pediatric Medicine

Pediatric medicine faces unique challenges when integrating AI, primarily due to the diverse developmental stages and variable symptom presentations in children. AI systems often struggle to accurately interpret pediatric data, partly because most algorithms are designed and trained using adult-centric databases. This can lead to misdiagnoses or oversights, particularly in early childhood diseases that manifest differently than in adults.

For instance, AI tools that analyze speech patterns to diagnose conditions such as autism might miss subtleties in younger children who are naturally at varied stages of language development. Additionally, pediatric AI dosing tools might default to simplified adult-equivalent formulas, disregarding critical weight and growth variations among children, leading to either underdosing or overdosing scenarios.

To address these shortcomings, it is crucial to refine AI models with pediatric-specific datasets, involving clinical pediatricians in the training process to tailor AI systems to the nuances of child health care. Continual monitoring and adaptation, with a strong emphasis on pediatric guidelines, will enhance AI's reliability and efficacy in treating younger patients.

## The Consequences of AI Bias in Remote Patient Monitoring

The integration of AI into remote patient monitoring aims to enhance healthcare efficiency and reach; however, biases inherent in AI systems introduce significant risks, particularly for underrepresented groups. Predominantly homogeneous data used for training AI can fail to detect conditions unique or more prevalent in minority populations, potentially leading to delayed or incorrect diagnoses and treatments.

Furthermore, socioeconomic bias in AI algorithms can restrict access to remote monitoring technologies for lower-income patients. This not only perpetuates healthcare disparities but also weakens the potential for early intervention strategies that could reduce hospitalizations and improve patient outcomes. As such, the less affluent patients, who could benefit most from remote monitoring due to geographic and economic constraints, often receive the least benefit.

Corrective measures must involve diversifying training datasets and developing rigorous testing standards to ensure AI systems perform equitably across all demographics. Collaborative efforts between technologists, clinicians, and ethicists are essential to mitigate the risks and maximize the benefits of AI in remote healthcare.

## AI in Dermatology: Model Failures Due to Skin Tone Variations

AI applications in dermatology showcase significant biases, particularly in diagnosing conditions across different skin tones. These systems are often trained on datasets that predominantly consist of lighter skin tones, resulting in less accurate diagnoses for individuals with darker skin tones. This disproportionality not only undermines the effectiveness of AI but also exacerbates existing healthcare disparities.

For example, melanoma detection AI tools demonstrate higher error rates when evaluating darker skin, potentially delaying life-saving diagnoses and treatments for patients of color. This stark bias prompts the need for a more inclusive approach in training AI models to recognize a diverse range of skin conditions across all skin tones.

Corrective steps must include the collection and integration of balanced data, encompassing a comprehensive spectrum of skin tones. Only through such enriched datasets can AI tools in dermatology become truly universal in their application and utility, ensuring equitable healthcare outcomes for every demographic.

**Bias in Cardiac Care Algorithms Affecting Patient Treatments**

In the realm of cardiac care, AI algorithms harbor the risk of replicating and amplifying existing biases, which can directly impact patient treatments and outcomes. Predominantly trained on data from specific population subsets, these algorithms can miss critical nuances in cardiac conditions across different demographics. For example, certain heart diseases manifest differently in women compared to men, yet AI systems often reflect the male-dominated clinical data more prominently.

Racial and ethnic disparities further complicate the efficacy of AI in cardiology. Studies have shown that algorithms might not accurately assess risk or recommend appropriate treatments for non-white patients, due to a lack of diverse data inputs. This can lead to underdiagnosis or inadequate treatment strategies, exacerbating health disparities.

Addressing these biases requires a multidimensional approach, including the diversification of training datasets and the involvement of a broader range of cardiologists in AI development. Continuous oversight and validation processes are critical to ensure these tools perform fairly and effectively across all patient groups.

**Algorithmic Errors in AI-Assisted Surgical Procedures**

AI-assisted surgical procedures denote a monumental shift in operative care, promising enhanced precision and reduced human error. However, this frontier technology is fraught with algorithmic errors that could have dire consequences. Notably, the reliance on historical surgical data to train these algorithms may inadvertently perpetuate outdated practices or amplify existing biases in surgical approaches. For instance, certain surgical techniques favored in these datasets may not be universally optimal across different patient demographics, such as varying anatomical differences or co-morbidities more prevalent in specific populations.

Moreover, the intricacies of real-time surgical decision-making are sometimes oversimplified by AI models, which can lead to errors that may affect the outcome. The absence of nuanced data input results in a lack of adaptability in AI systems, making them less effective in handling unanticipated complications or unique surgical scenarios.

Therefore, continuous oversight, rigorous validation against contemporary surgical standards, and inclusive data enrichment are essential. Engaging multidisciplinary teams in the AI training process could address these issues, paving the way for safer, more effective AI-assisted surgeries.

**Privacy Concerns with AI in Healthcare Personalization**

The integration of AI into personalized healthcare raises substantial privacy concerns, particularly regarding the management and protection of sensitive patient data. AI systems, designed to tailor healthcare solutions by analyzing personal health records, risk unauthorized data exposure if not properly safeguarded.

Notably, the complexity of AI algorithms can make it difficult for patients to understand how their data is being used. This lack of transparency can erode trust, as patients may fear their health information could be used for purposes beyond their direct care, such as commercial profiling or insurance evaluations.

Comprehensive regulations and clear communication are essential in ensuring that patients are informed and consenting participants in these AI-driven processes.

Moreover, the potential for security breaches poses a significant risk. As AI systems become more interlinked with cloud-based data storage, the vulnerability to cyberattacks increases, necessitating advanced cybersecurity measures to protect patient information from malicious intent. Prioritizing robust encryption methods and continuous monitoring of data access are crucial steps in mitigating privacy risks associated with healthcare AI.

## Legal Implications of AI's Misdiagnosis and Treatment Failures

The integration of AI in healthcare, while propelling advancements, also brings forth serious legal challenges, particularly in the realms of misdiagnosis and treatment failures. These AI-driven errors can have severe consequences for patient health, potentially leading to incorrect treatments or overlooked conditions, thereby increasing the liability of healthcare providers.

Legal frameworks are currently wrestling with assigning responsibility for AI errors. Traditional medical malpractice law typically focuses on human error; however, with the advent of AI, the question of liability extends to software developers and the algorithms themselves. This raises complex issues around the standard of care and who is ultimately accountable – the healthcare provider using the AI, or the developers of the AI technology?

These issues necessitate clear regulatory guidelines and robust legal protections for patients. Ensuring that AI systems are transparent and their decisions are understandable is crucial for accountability. Legislation must evolve to address these unique challenges, safeguarding patient rights while fostering the responsible use of AI in medicine.

## Geographical Bias in AI Healthcare Services Distribution

The distribution of AI-driven healthcare services reveals significant geographical biases that can exacerbate disparities in medical access and outcomes. Urban areas, which are often the focal points for technological advancements, tend to have a higher concentration of AI-enabled healthcare facilities. This disparity leaves rural and remote communities at a significant disadvantage, as they lack similar access to innovative AI tools that facilitate early diagnosis and personalized treatment plans.

For instance, AI systems designed to manage chronic illnesses or provide remote monitoring are less likely to be implemented in underdeveloped regions where technological infrastructure is lacking. Without reliable internet access or adequate healthcare databases, these areas remain underrepresented in algorithm training processes, leading to a lack of representation in AI-driven healthcare benefits.

The need for equitable AI distribution is critical, necessitating intentional programming that incorporates diverse geographical data. Strategies to counteract this bias include enhancing data collection from underrepresented areas and adjusting algorithms to ensure they serve a broader demographic spectrum. Without such measures, geographical biases will continue to marginalize already underserved populations.

## Cultural Insensitivity in End-of-Life Care AI Systems

Artificial intelligence systems involved in end-of-life care face critical challenges related to cultural sensitivity. These systems are often programmed with a narrow set of cultural norms, primarily reflecting Western biomedical ethics and practices. This limitation fundamentally undermines the quality of care for patients from diverse backgrounds, whose end-of-life customs and preferences may differ significantly.

For instance, some cultures emphasize holistic and family-centered decision-making in end-of-life situations, a nuance that generic AI systems might not recognize or prioritize. The lack of cultural competence in AI programming can result in recommendations that clash with patient and family expectations, leading to increased distress during already challenging times.

Addressing this form of AI bias demands a thoughtful integration of cultural diversity in algorithm development. This includes engaging with cultural experts and ethicists during the design and training phases of AI systems to ensure they can competently navigate the complex landscape of global end-of-life care practices.

**Correction Measures for Identified AI Bias in Clinical Trials**

Addressing AI bias in clinical trials requires a multifaceted approach, beginning with the diversification of data sources. By integrating a broader array of demographic and geographical datasets, developers can enhance the robustness and representativeness of AI models. This includes actively seeking out and incorporating data from traditionally underrepresented groups, ensuring that trial outcomes are applicable across diverse populations.

Additionally, implementing stringent regulation and oversight mechanisms is crucial. Establishing guidelines that mandate routine bias audits, alongside transparent reporting practices, can help identify and mitigate bias effectively. Independent review boards specializing in AI ethics could oversee these procedures, providing an added layer of accountability.

Enhancing stakeholder involvement, particularly from communities affected by AI decisions, further strengthens the effectiveness of correction measures. Engaging these groups in the dialogue around algorithm design and result interpretation fosters a more inclusive AI system. Feedback loops from end-users and continuous adaptation of the AI systems based on real-world outcomes ensure persistent alignment with ethical standards and practical efficacy in clinical applications.

**Education and Retraining Strategies for AI Healthcare Systems**

To address AI bias in healthcare, ongoing education and retraining strategies for AI systems are crucial. This involves continuous learning from diverse datasets and regular updates to AI algorithms to accommodate new medical insights and demographic changes. Educative measures must emphasize the importance of inclusivity in training data to prevent biases against certain patient groups.

Programs designed for AI retraining should include modules on recognizing and integrating traditional, indigenous, and holistic healing practices. By broadening the scope of AI's learning, we can enhance its applicability and sensitivity to varied medical philosophies and practices. These initiatives demand collaboration between technologists, traditional healers, and medical professionals to ensure comprehensive knowledge transfer.

Moreover, educational frameworks should encourage the ethical use of AI, focusing on transparency and accountability within these systems. Implementing regular ethical audits and stakeholder feedback mechanisms will further align AI operations with human rights and equity in healthcare services.

Ultimately, these strategies foster a resilient healthcare ecosystem where AI complements diverse therapeutic approaches, reducing bias and improving patient care outcomes across all populations.

## Summary

Artificial Intelligence (AI) holds transformative potential for healthcare; however, its deployment raises critical concerns regarding bias, which reflects the limited and homogeneous nature of training datasets. These datasets often primarily include data from the majority populations, disregarding the diverse genetic, environmental, and lifestyle nuances across various ethnicities and regions. Such oversights can lead to AI systems that are less effective, potentially resulting in misdiagnosis and inappropriate treatment for under-represented groups. Predominant use of mainstream medicine data often excludes traditional, indigenous, and holistic health practices, leading to misinterpretations of symptoms well-understood within these traditional frameworks. Furthermore, racial disparities emerge prominently, with AI in healthcare often perpetuating inequities, misdiagnosing diseases like skin cancer, or misinterpreting cardiovascular risk in minorities due to skewed training data. AI systems also exhibit economic bias by favoring treatments aligned with more profitable or standard practices among affluent demographics, thereby disadvantaging patients from economically disadvantaged backgrounds. The problem extends to gender biases where AI fails to recognize symptoms unique to women, and age-related biases where AI does not adequately cater to the needs of the very young or elderly. AI's challenges are not just in diagnosis but also extend to treatment recommendations and management, particularly in chronic diseases, where it fails to accommodate variations in progression and manifestation across different populations. These deficiencies necessitate integrating broader and more diverse datasets, continuous monitoring of AI performance, and genuine collaboration between developers, clinicians, and ethicists to recalibrate technologies to serve the full spectrum of the global population inclusively and equitably. This recalibration should also consider legal, privacy, and ethical implications, ensuring AI systems in healthcare not only advance treatment but also promote fairness and accountability.

## References

[1] Rajkomar, A., Dean, J., & Kohane, I. (2019). Machine Learning in Medicine. New England Journal of Medicine. https://www.nejm.org/doi/full/10.1056/NEJMra1814259

[2] Obermeyer, Z., Powers, B., Vogeli, C., & Mullainathan, S. (2019). Dissecting racial bias in an algorithm used to manage the health of populations. Science. https://science.sciencemag.org/content/366/6464/447

[3] Vyas, D.A., Eisenstein, L.G., & Jones, D.S. (2020). Hidden in Plain Sight — Reconsidering the Use of Race Correction in Clinical Algorithms. New England Journal of Medicine. https://www.nejm.org/doi/full/10.1056/NEJMms2004740

[4] Buolamwini, J., & Gebru, T. (2018). Gender Shades: Intersectional Accuracy Disparities in Commercial Gender Classification. Conference on Fairness, Accountability and Transparency. https://proceedings.mlr.press/v81/buolamwini18a.html

[5] Char, D.S., Shah, N.H., & Magnus, D. (2018). Implementing Machine Learning in Health Care — Addressing Ethical Challenges. New England Journal of Medicine. https://www.nejm.org/doi/full/10.1056/NEJMsb1710591

## Case Study: Bias and Misdiagnosis in Dermatological AI Applications

In the realm of dermatology, the application of Artificial Intelligence (AI) has been viewed as a transformative breakthrough, particularly in the diagnosis of skin cancer. However, a comprehensive case study reveals significant challenges, particularly concerning bias towards patients with darker skin tones. A notable instance involves an AI-powered diagnostic tool used in a multi-center dermatology clinic network, which is primarily trained on datasets consisting of lighter skin examples. Due to this skewed training, the tool demonstrated a significantly higher error rate when diagnosing conditions like melanoma in individuals with darker skin, leading to delayed treatments and increased patient anxiety.

The scenario escalated when a patient, referred to here as John Doe, visited his dermatologist with a concerning lesion. The AI tool, which had been integrated into the clinic's diagnosis process, initially assessed the lesion as benign. This misdiagnosis was partly due to the underrepresentation of individuals with dark skin in the training data. John's condition worsened over time, which eventually required more aggressive treatment than would have been necessary had the melanoma been correctly identified at the first visit.

This case underscores the dire need for inclusivity in AI training datasets. To address this challenge, dermatologists, alongside AI specialists, initiated an overhaul of the AI system's training protocol. This involved gathering a more balanced dataset that included a diverse range of skin tones and collaborating with international dermatological databases to expand the range of examples.

Furthermore, to combat the ongoing bias, the clinic network implemented routine reviews and updates to the AI's algorithm, aiming to adapt to new research and demographic changes continually. This proactive approach aimed not only to enhance diagnostic accuracy but also to restore patient trust in AI-driven medical processes, thereby ensuring fairness and effectiveness in healthcare outcomes across diverse populations.

### Case Study: AI-Based Cardiovascular Risk Assessment and the Challenge of Ethnic Diversification

A major hospital in an urban setting has recently implemented an AI system designed to assess cardiovascular risk using machine learning models. These models were primarily trained using health data from the majority population, which is predominantly Caucasian, accounting for approximately 70% of the dataset used. This model was used to streamline the diagnosis process and offer proactive treatments. Soon, however, clear gaps began to emerge in the AI system's performance, especially regarding patients from minority ethnic backgrounds.

For example, Mr. Adebayo, a 45-year-old African American patient, exhibited multiple risk factors for cardiovascular disease, including high blood pressure and a family history of heart disease. Despite these factors, the AI system initially classified his cardiovascular risk as moderate, rather than high. The system's underestimation of Mr. Adebayo's condition was later attributed to the lack of diverse ethnic data in the training dataset, as cardiovascular disease manifests differently across ethnicities. This misclassification could have led to insufficient monitoring and preventive treatment, potentially worsening his health condition.

Upon reviewing several similar cases, the healthcare provider recognized a pattern of misdiagnoses that disproportionately affected ethnic minorities. This sparked an initiative to re-evaluate and diversify the AI system's training dataset. The hospital partnered with international health organizations to gather a broader spectrum of health data representing a variety of ethnic groups. They also instituted a continuous feedback mechanism, allowing clinicians to provide direct input into the AI system's development based on observed discrepancies in patient outcomes.

This adaptive response not only improved the AI system's diagnostic accuracy but also underscored the critical need for incorporating diverse data in training AI for healthcare applications. It emphasized the importance of continuous oversight and modification of AI systems, ensuring they evolve in line with new medical insights and population diversity, thereby mitigating risk and enhancing patient care equity across all demographic groups.

### Case Study: Disparities in AI-Driven Mental Health Diagnostics

The integration of Artificial Intelligence (AI) in mental health services has been touted as a potential game-changer for diagnosing and managing psychiatric conditions. However, a detailed case study underscores significant challenges, particularly the failure to capture diverse cultural expressions of mental health symptoms. This issue was highlighted in the experience of a mental health facility implementing an AI diagnosis tool trained primarily on data from Western populations.

A 38-year-old Hispanic woman, referred to as Maria, presented symptoms that were inconsistent with typical Western psychological diagnostic criteria. Maria reported feelings of 'nervousness' (nerves), a culturally specific syndrome involving symptoms akin to anxiety and depression but recognized primarily in Latin American communities. The AI system, lacking data on such culturally nuanced symptoms, categorized her symptoms as general anxiety disorder. This misclassification led to a treatment plan that was not fully effective for her specific cultural needs.

The facility's reliance on a one-size-fits-all AI diagnostic tool not only resulted in inadequate care for Maria but also highlighted broader issues in the application of AI in mental health diagnostics. Other patients from diverse backgrounds shared similar experiences where their culturally unique mental health expressions were either misunderstood or overlooked by the AI system.

In response, the mental health facility undertook several corrective measures. They partnered with cultural psychiatrists to integrate a broader spectrum of cultural expressions and symptoms into the AI's training data. They also implemented continuous learning protocols for the AI system to adapt to new and emerging cultural expressions of mental health in their patient population.

Efforts were made to audit and continuously update the AI system with feedback from both patients and clinicians. This proactive approach aimed to transform the AI tool into a truly inclusive system, capable of accurately diagnosing and treating mental health conditions across diverse cultural landscapes, ensuring equitable and effective mental health care for all patients.

### Case Study: AI and Gender Disparities in Pulmonary Disease Diagnostics

The use of Artificial Intelligence (AI) in pulmonary disease diagnostics presents several unresolved challenges, notably those related to gender-specific biases in diagnosis accuracy. A recent examination explored a significant healthcare facility that integrated AI systems to identify and predict patterns in pulmonary conditions such as chronic obstructive pulmonary disease (COPD). Predominantly trained on clinical data captured from male patients, the AI system provided high accuracy in diagnosing male patients but faltered with female patients, indicating underlying gender disparities in medical AI applications.

Consider the case of Elizabeth, a 53-year-old woman having trouble breathing and recurring bronchitis. Her initial digital consultation through the AI-assisted platform concluded a mild respiratory infection, advising minimal treatment, belying the underlying severity of her situation. As her condition gradually deteriorated, a subsequent physical examination by a pulmonologist and a thorough review of her imaging and health history beyond the AI's preliminary analysis revealed stage II COPD, a diagnosis the AI system failed to predict.

This incident not only shed light on the gaps in AI's diagnostic capabilities across genders but also prompted a more exhaustive institutional review. Analysis showed that the AI model's decision-making algorithms favored symptom manifestations typically observed in males, such as prolonged exposure to pulmonary irritants commonly cataloged in occupational health data and underplayed 'atypical' female-presenting COPD symptoms, including frequent bronchitis that tends to be less connected to occupational factors.

To mitigate these discrepancies, the healthcare institution implemented several corrective strategies. They initiated the expansion of the AI training dataset to include more balanced gender representation and a wider range of clinical manifestations of pulmonary diseases. Health practitioners were also involved in a continuous feedback loop to provide real-time insights into the system's accuracy and biases, aiding much-needed model recalibrations based on wide-ranging patient interactions. This proactive adjustment aims not just to refine diagnostic accuracy but also galvanize broader efforts toward ensuring gender equity in medical AI diagnostic systems and patient care overall.

### Case Study: AI and Socioeconomic Bias in Predictive Healthcare Models

In an ongoing effort to personalize healthcare and improve predictive outcomes through advanced technology, a prominent hospital network has implemented an AI-driven predictive analytics platform designed to enhance treatment plans across its patient base. This initiative, however, inadvertently illuminated profound socioeconomic biases, impacting low-income patient groups disproportionately due to training datasets skewed towards higher-income populations.

A critical case involved Sarah, a single mother with two children, who was part of a lower economic segment and suffering from Type 2 diabetes. The AI system, relying primarily on data from economically advantaged patients, recommended a treatment regimen that included expensive medications and frequent monitoring through wearable technology, which Sarah could not afford. Consequently, this led to a lack of adherence to the recommended plan, resulting in poor disease management and repeated hospital admissions.

It became evident that while the AI system was technically advanced, it did not account for the financial limitations of a sizeable segment of the patient community. This oversight not only risked patient health but also strained the hospital resources with frequent, preventable readmissions. The healthcare provider began to recognize the critical need for a recalibrated AI system that could adapt to the realities of all patients' demographic groups, particularly those in lower socioeconomic strata.

To address this issue, the hospital initiated a comprehensive review and restructuring of the AI system's training module. They partnered with social workers and community health programs to gather broader socioeconomic data. These data inputs were integrated into the system to refine its predictive algorithms, ensuring they align more accurately with the resources available to all patient categories.

Moreover, the hospital network implemented a feedback system that allowed patients to report on their ability to follow through with AI-recommended treatment regimens, enabling ongoing recalibration of the system based on real-world outcomes. This proactive and inclusive approach was instrumental not only in mitigating socioeconomic biases but also in enhancing the overall effectiveness and equity of AI-driven healthcare services.

### Case Study: Geographical Disparities in AI Enhanced Stroke Diagnosis

A regional hospital in a rural area recently incorporated an AI-based system designed to enhance early stroke detection and improve patient outcomes. This new technology, trained primarily on datasets obtained from urban healthcare settings, promised to streamline the diagnostic process and provide rapid intervention options. However, the implementation phase revealed significant geographical biases that reduced its efficacy in less urbanized settings.

For instance, the case of Susan, a 63-year-old woman living in the rural outskirts, underlines the impact of these regional discrepancies. Susan experienced early signs of a stroke, characterized by sudden dizziness and an abnormal gait, symptoms that the AI model should readily identify for immediate care. However, the AI system was slow to flag her symptoms as critical because most of the training data involved cases from urban settings with slightly different symptomatology and younger patient profiles.

In response to Susan's scenario and several similar cases, the hospital staff recognized the AI system's inability to fully adapt to the dynamics of rural healthcare, where patient demographics and prevalent health conditions differ from those in urban-centric databases. Consequently, Susan received the correct diagnosis and necessary treatment, but only after critical delays that could have been minimized with a more responsive AI system.

To address these geographical disparities, the hospital initiated a series of modifications to its AI system. This involved integrating health data from rural communities into the training set and adjusting the AI algorithms to represent the regional patient demographics better. Additionally, the hospital established a collaboration with nearby medical facilities and local health workers to update the dataset and improve AI predictions continually.

Furthermore, to ensure the effectiveness of the AI system, continuous monitoring and real-time data analysis were implemented to enable swift adaptation to any emerging trends or nuances specific to rural medical care. In doing so, the hospital aims to enhance the AI system's responsiveness and reliability, ensuring that all patients, regardless of geographical location, receive timely and accurate medical assessments.

## Case Study: Cultural Bias and Misinterpretation in AI-Driven Pain Assessment Tools

In a recent comprehensive case study, a major metropolitan hospital faced significant challenges when deploying an Artificial Intelligence (AI) system designed to assess and manage patient pain levels. The case involved an AI model that was primarily trained on datasets derived from a population that did not adequately represent the hospital's diverse patient base, particularly overlooking the cultural differences in pain expression and tolerance.

One notable instance involved a patient, 58-year-old Mrs. Nguyen, a Vietnamese woman who reported chronic back pain. The AI tool, which had been set up to standardize and streamline pain management protocols, initially assessed her pain as minor based on the verbal and non-verbal cues interpreted through its algorithms. However, cultural nuances in pain expression, particularly the stoic demeanor often maintained by patients from Asian backgrounds — led to a significant underestimation of her pain levels. The AI's failure to assess her pain accurately resulted in inadequate pain management and prolonged discomfort, ultimately necessitating her family's intervention to secure appropriate care.

This incident highlighted the broader systemic issue of cultural insensitivity within AI healthcare applications. The hospital recognized the need to enhance the AI's training data to include a broader range of cultural pain expression patterns, which led to several initiatives aimed at collecting more inclusive data directly from their diverse patient demographics.

To address these challenges, the hospital enlisted the help of cultural competence experts to provide insights into nonverbal and verbal pain indicators specific to different cultural groups. They integrated these findings into the AI training protocols and continuously updated the algorithms based on real-world feedback and outcomes. Additionally, a layered assessment strategy was implemented, wherein AI assessments were supplemented by human evaluations, especially in cases involving patients from culturally diverse backgrounds.

These responses were critical in transforming the AI tool into a more effective and sensitive instrument for pain assessment, paving the way not only for better patient outcomes but also for the establishment of AI as a truly supportive healthcare technology across culturally diverse patient populations.

## Case Study: Ethical Concerns in AI-Assisted End-of-Life Care Decisions

The integration of Artificial Intelligence (AI) into healthcare extends to sensitive areas, including end-of-life care decisions, which pose profound ethical challenges and underscore the necessity for culturally and personally sensitive implementations. In a recent case, a well-established metropolitan hospital implemented an AI system intended to support clinical decisions by predicting patient outcomes based on historical health data. This system, however, was primarily trained on datasets from a predominantly Western patient population.

The challenges became evident with the treatment of Mr. Hassan, a 72-year-old patient with a Middle Eastern background suffering from terminal cancer. The AI system recommended a highly aggressive treatment path, typically preferred in Western medical practices but contrary to Mr. Hassan's cultural values and personal wishes, which favored a dignified and less invasive end-of-life experience, reflecting a common preference in his culture for minimal medical intervention when facing terminal conditions.

Upon recognizing this, the care team faced the complex task of aligning AI-driven recommendations with culturally sensitive care. This discord highlighted a profound need to adjust the AI system to acknowledge the diverse cultural and individual preferences surrounding end-of-life care, which are often overlooked in AI's empirical, data-driven logic.

To address this, the hospital initiated several corrective measures. The first step involved incorporating a broader, more culturally diverse dataset, including patients' cultural backgrounds and their treatment preferences, into the AI's learning algorithms. This was supplemented by training sessions for clinical staff on the potential biases of AI tools and the development of protocols for manual overrides when AI recommendations conflict with patient values or clinical judgments.

Continuous feedback loops were established, incorporating insights from ongoing patient care experiences to improve the AI model's accuracy and sensitivity. By integrating these layers of cultural and ethical consideration, the hospital aimed not only to enhance the AI system's functionality but also ensure that it aligns closely with the ethical standards and diverse needs of all patients.

## Review Questions

**1. In a non-profit medical center treating patients with traditional Thai Yoga therapy and acupuncture, a 55-year-old patient diagnosed with idiopathic osteoarthritis of the knees reports improved mobility and reduced pain levels after 3 months of consistent treatment. Which of the following aspects of the treatment contributed most to the patient's improvement?**

A) Regular deep tissue massage is applied during sessions

B) Integration of spiritual healing practices within the therapy sessions

C) Consistent application of heat treatments during sessions

D) Use of Western pharmacological interventions alongside therapy

**Answer: B**

Explanation: Although multiple factors might contribute to the patient's improvement, the integration of spiritual healing practices within traditional Thai Yoga therapy sessions is known to significantly enhance the therapeutic effects by addressing the holistic aspects of patient care. This approach fosters a deeper connection between the mind, body, and spirit, which is particularly effective in managing pain and improving mobility in conditions such as osteoarthritis. Traditional Thai Yoga therapy emphasizes holistic healing that combines physical, mental, and spiritual therapies, often resulting in improved outcomes compared to purely physical treatments.

**2. During a clinical trial evaluating the efficacy of a new AI-driven health monitoring system, it was found that the system failed to integrate feedback from patients utilizing indigenous herbal remedies for managing hypertension. This oversight affected the treatment recommendations provided to a significant portion of the patient population. What might be the primary cause of this AI system's failure in this context?**

A) Lack of adequate training data that includes information about indigenous herbal remedies

B) Technical glitches within the AI system's software

C) The AI system's algorithms are designed to prioritize pharmaceutical treatments over herbal remedies

D) Patients' refusal to share information about their use of herbal remedies

**Answer: A**

Explanation: The most likely cause of the AI system's failure to account for indigenous herbal remedies in its treatment recommendations is the lack of adequate training data that includes this type of information. AI systems rely heavily on the data provided to them during the training phase. If indigenous herbal remedies were not included or were underrepresented in the dataset used to train the AI, it would not be equipped to recognize or consider these treatments when making treatment recommendations. This illustrates a significant challenge in AI development for healthcare: ensuring that the training data is comprehensive and accurately represents diverse treatment modalities to effectively cater to all patient needs.

## AI's Impact on Holistic and Indigenous Medicine Practices

### Understanding Holistic Medicine: Definitions and Principles

Holistic medicine, a healing approach that seeks to address the individual, integrates various elements of physical, emotional, spiritual, and social health. Unlike conventional medicine, which often focuses on treating specific symptoms or illnesses, holistic practices emphasize the interconnectedness of the body and mind, advocating for balance and harmony as the foundations of health.

The principles of holistic medicine revolve around the belief that healing occurs naturally when the body is in a state of equilibrium. It encourages the use of diverse therapies, some derived from age-old traditions, to facilitate the body's innate healing response. This approach not only aims to alleviate symptoms but also to identify and treat the root causes of illness, emphasizing preventive care and maintaining optimal health.

Integrating these practices into modern medical settings requires a deep respect for and understanding of these principles. As AI technology advances, it becomes vital to ensure that these holistic health paradigms are recognized and preserved in digital health platforms, maintaining the essence of traditional healing in the era of technological medicine.

### Defining Indigenous Medicine: Cultural and Historical Context

Indigenous medicine encompasses a rich tapestry of healing practices rooted in the cultural traditions and historical experiences of indigenous peoples. These practices are deeply interwoven with spiritual beliefs, herbal knowledge, and rituals that have been passed down through generations, often orally and within specific community contexts.

Historically, indigenous medicine has served not only as a means of health care but also as a central element of cultural identity and spiritual life. These healing modalities can vary significantly from one community to another, influenced by local environments and cultural histories. While some use herbs and natural pharmacopeias, others might incorporate spiritual healing or physical therapies unique to their culture.

The understanding of these practices confronts considerable challenges in the era of digital health advancements, particularly with the advent of AI. The risk lies in oversimplifying or misinterpreting these culturally grounded practices through a technological lens, which often aligns poorly with non-materialistic and community-focused healing approaches.

**Surveying AI's Current Role in Holistic Medical Practices**

The integration of Artificial Intelligence (AI) into holistic medical practices marks a pivotal evolution in healthcare. AI is actively being incorporated to enhance diagnostic processes, tailor treatment plans, and analyze health data through a broader, more integrative lens. However, its penetration into holistic medicine also raises significant questions about the depth and appropriateness of its application.

One significant role of AI in this domain has been in analyzing large, complex datasets to identify patterns that might not be apparent through traditional methods. This capability is used to track wellness trends and predict potential health issues before they manifest, thereby supporting the preventive ethos of holistic medicine. Yet, the challenge remains to ensure these AI systems capture the nuanced philosophies and practices that define holistic healing, without reducing them to mere data points.

Moreover, while AI can offer substantial support in managing patient records and personalizing care plans, its role in understanding and integrating non-conventional healing practices—like energy healing or spiritual counseling—remains minimal. Bridging this gap necessitates a cohesive effort among AI developers, practitioners, and patients themselves, aiming to foster a technology that truly complements holistic health perspectives rather than overshadowing them.

**Impact of AI on Traditional Herbal Medicine**

The intersection of AI and traditional herbal medicine presents a fascinating convergence of ancient wisdom and modern technology. AI's analytical prowess offers unprecedented opportunities to explore the vast pharmacopeia of herbs through bioinformatics and molecular chemistry, potentially accelerating the discovery of new therapeutic compounds. Yet, this integration is not without its perils. The risk of cultural appropriation and the commodification of sacred knowledge looms large, as AI systems, primarily designed within Western scientific frameworks, may fail to capture the holistic essence embedded in herbal practices adequately.

Moreover, AI's role in patenting processes raises ethical concerns. The ability to rapidly identify active compounds can lead to patents that may restrict access to traditional medicines for the very cultures that discovered and nurtured these remedies. Such actions undermine the communal and open nature of indigenous medical knowledge, turning healing practices into monopolized commodities.

Despite these challenges, AI could foster a more profound respect for herbal wisdom by documenting efficacy and safety, validating traditional uses in global contexts. If aligned with ethical considerations and developed collaboratively with indigenous communities, AI could help preserve heritage while enhancing the efficacy of traditional herbal medicine.

**AI's Role in Enhancing Personalized Medicine Approaches**

Artificial Intelligence (AI) holds promise for a revolution in personalized medicine, particularly within holistic and indigenous healthcare settings. By leveraging AI, practitioners can personalize treatments more effectively, considering not just the biological aspects of a patient's health but their emotional, spiritual, and environmental influences as well. This nuanced approach to healthcare delivery respects the individual preferences and cultural significances that define holistic medicine.

Integrating AI facilitates the analysis of vast amounts of data from diverse sources, including traditional medical records, patient genetic information, and environmental factors. This capability enables the crafting of tailored healthcare plans that consider unique personal health narratives and cultural backgrounds. However, the challenge is to ensure that AI systems are trained on sufficiently diverse datasets to understand and appropriately apply these ancient and culturally rich healing practices.

To truly benefit personalized medicine, AI must be developed in collaboration with traditional healers and patients. This ensures that technology is not merely imposed on indigenous practices, but woven into them, enhancing both their efficacy and respect for traditional knowledge. This coalition supports a bridge where AI technology respects and amplifies the principles of holistic health care.

## Case Study: AI in Traditional Chinese Medicine

Exploring the intersection of Artificial Intelligence (AI) and Traditional Chinese Medicine (TCM) unveils a compelling case study. AI's analytical capabilities are being employed to decode complex TCM formulations, which typically involve an intricate balance of various herbs and elements. This synergy aims at enhancing the understanding and application of these ancient remedies in a contemporary setting.

However, the integration of AI into TCM has also sparked debates concerning the potential loss of the deeply embedded philosophical and spiritual nuances of TCM practices. While AI can efficiently analyze patterns and predictions in herbal efficacy, there is a looming concern about its ability to fully grasp the qi (energy flow) and yin-yang principles that are central to TCM. The challenge lies in programming AI to respect these non-materialistic dimensions that are crucial for holistic treatment approaches.

Despite these challenges, there have been successes. AI-driven projects have helped identify new applications for traditional herbs and improve diagnostic precision through pattern recognition in patient data. Medical practitioners are gradually recognizing the potential benefits of this technology, advocating for a more nuanced integration that respects the essence of TCM while leveraging AI's power to enhance patient outcomes.

### Effects of AI on Spiritual Healing Practices

The integration of Artificial Intelligence (AI) into spiritual healing practices poses profound implications, navigating a realm traditionally guided by intangible, sacred elements. Spiritual healing, which relies on the metaphysical energies and deep-rooted beliefs of various cultures, finds an ambiguous ally in AI. The primary challenge for AI in this domain is its inherent design to interpret quantifiable data, which starkly contrasts with the qualitative essence of spiritual practices.

The deployment of AI in spiritual healing has led to innovative approaches, such as analyzing emotional and psychological data to enhance the healing process. However, this technological intrusion raises concerns about the dilution of traditional authenticity, as AI may not fully comprehend the subjective experiences and spiritual nuances that are crucial to these practices.

Despite this, there are potential benefits. AI can assist in cataloging vast amounts of undocumented spiritual healing techniques, potentially preserving them for future generations. Yet, ensuring these technologies are developed in respectful collaboration with spiritual healers is vital to maintain the sanctity and effectiveness of these age-old practices.

### AI's Interpretation of Indigenous Healing Data

The process of Artificial Intelligence (AI) interpreting indigenous healing data presents a complex landscape fraught with challenges and potential misinterpretations. AI's capabilities, primarily structured around Western scientific paradigms, may struggle to appreciate the deeply cultural and spiritual nuances embedded in indigenous medicinal practices. This issue is not merely technical but deeply cultural, potentially leading to a superficial understanding of healing techniques that have been refined over centuries.

For example, many indigenous healing traditions rely on an intimate understanding of local environments, spiritual beliefs, and community relationships, and aspects that are often intangible and poorly translated into digital data forms. When AI systems attempt to digest such holistic information, they can inadvertently strip away these essential contexts, reducing rich, nuanced practices to crude data points.

Nevertheless, with careful design and input from indigenous knowledge holders, AI has the potential to become a supportive tool rather than an invasive technology. Collaborative efforts are necessary to develop AI systems that are truly inclusive and culturally sensitive. This involves programming AI to consider non-quantifiable factors and incorporating ethics that respect and preserve the integrity of indigenous knowledge.

**Technological Advancements and Their Impact on Native Healing Techniques**

The integration of technological advancements, particularly artificial intelligence (AI), into native healing techniques presents both exciting opportunities and complex challenges. By incorporating AI, researchers can analyze historical usage and outcomes of traditional remedies more efficiently, offering potential improvements in their application and broader acceptance in global healthcare systems.

However, the mechanization and data-driven approach of AI often clash with the fundamentally spiritual and experiential nature of native healing practices. There is a significant risk that AI could oversimplify or misinterpret the nuanced traditions that are deeply rooted in cultural identity and heritage. This can lead to a form of cultural disenfranchisement, where invaluable indigenous knowledge is reduced to mere data points, devoid of context and community significance.

Despite these hurdles, if handled with care and respect, AI can aid in the preservation and revitalization of traditional healing techniques. Collaborations between technologists and indigenous communities are crucial, ensuring technologies are developed that honor and preserve the integrity and intentions of traditional practices.

**Criticisms of AI in Handling Non-Western Medicine**

The criticisms surrounding AI's role in non-Western medicine stem from the technology's failure to appreciate the profound cultural and metaphysical dimensions inherent in indigenous health practices. While AI has facilitated notable advances in data processing and pattern recognition, its reliance on quantifiable metrics can starkly misrepresent holistic healing traditions that emphasize spiritual and environmental interconnectedness.

Another critical issue is the potential imposition of a Western scientific framework onto non-Western practices, which can undermine their intrinsic values and lead to inappropriate cultural generalizations. This misalignment distorts the nuanced understandings necessary for effective indigenous therapies and risks transforming deeply personal and community-centric practices into standardized, commodified medical solutions.

Despite AI's promise to revolutionize various sectors, its integration into traditional medicine requires cautious and culturally sensitive approaches. It is imperative that this integration does not prioritize technological prowess over respect for heritage and the depth of ancestral knowledge. Engaging with traditional healers and communities in the development of AI applications can help bridge these gaps, ensuring technology supports rather than erodes non-Western medicinal wisdom.

**AI Integration Challenges with Animistic Cultures**

Integrating Artificial Intelligence (AI) with animistic cultures introduces complexities that echo broader concerns about cultural sensitivity in technology. Animistic beliefs, which see spirits as integral to both living beings and inanimate objects, pose a particular challenge for AI, which relies on empirical data and algorithms. This grounding in materialism starkly contrasts with the spiritual and relational foundations of animistic traditions.

For AI to function effectively in these contexts, it must navigate the non-quantifiable nature of spiritual relations and the interconnectedness perceived in animistic environments. However, AI systems designed within a predominantly materialistic framework may inadvertently overlook or misinterpret these non-material dimensions, risking cultural insensitivity or even harm by imposing inappropriate technological structures on deeply spiritual practices.

Despite these challenges, opportunities for respectful and beneficial integration exist. This requires a concerted effort to design AI that can 'understand' and incorporate the nuances of animistic beliefs, potentially through the inclusion of cultural experts in the development process to ensure that AI respects and preserves the integrity of these traditions.

**Data Collection Biases Affecting Indigenous Medicinal Knowledge**

The collection and interpretation of data on indigenous medicinal practices by AI systems embed significant biases, largely due to the overriding use of Western scientific methodologies. These methodologies often fail to capture the essence of indigenous knowledge, which is deeply rooted in oral traditions, spiritual beliefs, and environmental interactions. Consequently, the data collected can be inherently skewed, misrepresenting or even omitting the holistic and interconnected nature of these practices.

Moreover, the data collection process frequently overlooks the subtle nuances that characterize indigenous medicine, such as the timing of herbal collection, specific local rituals, or the spiritual states induced during healing practices. These elements are crucial but typically defy quantification and standard data-collection protocols, leading to a partial or distorted database.

This challenge requires a reevaluation of data collection methodologies in AI processes to adopt a more inclusive and culturally sensitive approach. Engaging directly with indigenous communities and healers to co-design data collection frameworks can help ensure that AI systems are informed by a comprehensive understanding of indigenous medicinal knowledge, thereby reducing biases and enhancing the applicability and respectfulness of AI in these contexts.

**The Role of AI in Preserving Endangered Indigenous Practices**

The potential of Artificial Intelligence (AI) to preserve endangered indigenous practices opens a vital discourse on integrating modern technology with ancient wisdom. By analyzing patterns in traditional methods, AI can help document and safeguard the intricate details of these practices, which are often passed down orally and are at risk of being lost. This technological intervention could facilitate the cataloging of rare medicinal plants, traditional healing techniques, and ritual practices, thereby creating digital repositories that ensure their preservation for future generations.

However, the implementation must be handled with sensitivity and respect for cultural nuances. Collaboration with indigenous communities is crucial for creating AI systems that accurately reflect their knowledge without stripping it of its cultural essence. Indigenous experts can provide insights that guide AI programming to capture not only data, but also the context and cultural significance of these practices.

Critically, AI has the capability to actively engage in the cultural preservation process, but this must align with ethical considerations, avoiding exploitation and ensuring data sovereignty remains with the indigenous communities. Through respectful collaboration, AI could become a powerful ally in the fight against the erosion of invaluable cultural heritage.

**AI and the Standardization of Holistic Health Metrics**

The aspiration to standardize holistic health metrics through AI harbors profound implications for both the preservation and transformation and possible confusion-misinterpretation of traditional healing wisdom. AI's approach, fundamentally data-driven and quantitative, risks simplifying the rich and often subjective experiences intrinsic to holistic practices into numerical data points. This translation from a deeply personal to a universally standardized format might dilute the essence of therapies that are heavily tailored to individual experiences and cultural contexts.

Conversely, such standardization offers potential for broader acceptance and integration of holistic methods into global healthcare systems, potentially increasing their credibility and reach. Establishing standard metrics could facilitate comparative studies and the blending of holistic practices with conventional medicine, driving innovation in integrative health approaches.

However, the ethical landscape of AI-driven standardization raises critical concerns. Preserving cultural sovereignty and ensuring that these metrics do not overshadow or trivialize the inherent value of traditional wisdom is paramount. Collaborative efforts, involving both AI technologists and traditional healing practitioners, are essential to address these challenges, striving for a balance that respects and uplifts the diverse healing practices worldwide.

**Ethical Implications of AI in Integrative Healthcare Settings**

The integration of Artificial Intelligence (AI) into integrative healthcare settings, which often includes holistic and indigenous practices, raises significant ethical considerations. Firstly, the potential for AI to inadvertently impose Western medical paradigms on diverse cultural health practices can lead to ethical conflicts. This imposition risks marginalizing traditional knowledge systems and undermining the autonomy of indigenous communities, prioritizing data-driven approaches over culturally embedded wisdom.

Moreover, the ethical use of AI in these settings involves navigating the privacy and data sovereignty of individuals whose health data may be particularly sensitive or sacred. Mismanagement of such data can breach trust and violate ethical norms established in medical practice. Therefore, safeguarding these elements is crucial when designing AI systems that merge with integrative health practices.

Finally, engaging with local communities to co-develop AI solutions ensures that these technologies are implemented in ways that respect and enhance indigenous practices, rather than diluting or replacing them. This collaborative approach supports ethical integrity, aligning AI advancements with the preservation and respect for traditional healing approaches.

**Privacy and Data Sovereignty Concerns for Indigenous Populations**

The intersection of AI with indigenous medicinal practices necessitates serious considerations regarding privacy and data sovereignty. Indigenous populations often rely on traditional knowledge that has been passed down through generations, often through oral traditions and ceremonial practices. This knowledge encompasses healing techniques, herbal medicines, and spiritual therapies, deeply intertwined with cultural identity and communal values.

However, the advent of AI in medicine brings challenges to maintaining this privacy and data sovereignty. Digitizing such information risks exposure to unauthorized entities, possibly leading to cultural appropriation or exploitation (Misappropriation). Furthermore, traditional knowledge is collective rather than individual, which complicates consent processes typically structured by Western norms that may not necessarily translate across cultures.

To address these concerns, AI development must incorporate mechanisms that prioritize these communities' control over their own medicinal knowledge. This includes tools for enforcing data encryption, secure sharing protocols, and agreements that acknowledge and respect data sovereignty. Engaging with tribal elders and healers in AI projects not only ensures ethical practices but also enriches the technology's sensitivity to these invaluable cultural insights.

## Community Reactions to AI's Involvement in Traditional Practices

Community reactions to AI's integration into traditional practices vary widely, reflecting a spectrum of acceptance and skepticism. In many indigenous communities, there is a cautious curiosity about how AI might bolster the preservation and dissemination of ancestral knowledge. Elders and healers, often gatekeepers of these traditions, express a conditional interest, predicated on assurances that their intellectual and cultural property rights are prioritized and safeguarded.

Conversely, there is tangible and very realistic apprehension concerning AI's capability to genuinely comprehend and respect the depth of holistic and spiritual components inherent in traditional practices. The fear that AI might oversimplify or misinterpret these complex systems leads to resistance among practitioners. They advocate for an AI that is not just a tool of technology but one that learns under the guidance of those who live these traditions.

Amid these divergent views, a common thread emerges: the demand for collaborative development of AI tools. Communities seek active involvement in shaping AI applications to ensure they are not only culturally sensitive but also beneficial in enhancing the effectiveness and reach of traditional medicine.

## Potential Benefits of AI in Global Herbal Research

The integration of Artificial Intelligence (AI) into global herbal research heralds unprecedented opportunities for advancing our understanding and utilization of herbal medicine. By leveraging machine learning algorithms, AI can analyze vast datasets of plant properties and uses, identifying potential new medicinal applications and efficacies that might otherwise remain undiscovered due to the limitations of human capacity.

Furthermore, AI can streamline the process of drug discovery and development from herbal sources. Predictive modeling can forecast interactions between herbal compounds and human biology, speeding up the development of effective, natural medications. This functionality not only catalyzes the research phase but also enhances safety profiles by predicting adverse effects before clinical trials.

Lastly, AI's role in global herbal research can bridge the gap between traditional and modern medical practices. By validating the effectiveness of herbal remedies through robust, data-driven analyses, AI fosters a deeper integration of these age-old practices into contemporary healthcare paradigms, potentially leading to wider acceptance and utilization worldwide.

**Navigating AI's Limitations in Understanding Non-Material Healing**

Artificial Intelligence (AI) has significantly advanced medical science, yet it grapples with understanding the non-material aspects of healing inherent in holistic and indigenous practices. The crux of AI's struggle lies in its inherent mechanical nature, which renders it ill-equipped to interpret the subtleties of spiritual, emotional, and energy-based healing modalities that emphasize balance and harmony beyond the physical body.

Such healing traditions often rely on intuitive knowledge and subjective experiences that cannot be easily quantified or reproduced in datasets, which are fundamental to AI operations. The challenge extends to AI's ability to respect and integrate these non-material perspectives adequately without distorting their essence. This incompatibility prompts critical questions about the application of AI in settings where healing is deeply intertwined with cultural and spiritual dimensions.

Efforts to bridge this gap must involve collaborative engagements between AI developers and traditional healers. This partnership could foster innovations in AI programming, enabling the development of new algorithms that respect and incorporate non-material aspects of healing, thereby enhancing AI's applicability in diverse medical contexts.

**Prospective Technologies Enhancing Shamanic and Energy Healing**

The realm of shamanic and energy healing, rooted deeply in spiritual and holistic traditions, presents a fertile ground for nurturing through advanced technologies. Innovators are exploring how augmented and virtual reality can create immersive healing environments that replicate sacred spaces and rituals, enhancing the spiritual connection vital for these practices. This technological infusion also aims to extend the healer's reach, enabling practices that were previously confined to physical interaction.

Moreover, wearable technology is being tailored to track and influence energy fields, attempting to quantify and optimize the flow of energy. These devices, which combine traditional knowledge with modern sensor technology, propose a novel method for monitoring spiritual well-being, introducing an interesting blend of age-old wisdom and contemporary precision.

The integration of AI and machine learning offers predictive insights that could revolutionize energy healing. Algorithms that learn from vast amounts of holistic health data can suggest refinements and personalize healing protocols, potentially enhancing the efficacy of these ancient practices within a modern healthcare framework.

**Collaborative Efforts Towards Culturally Sensitive AI Models**

The push for culturally sensitive AI models in holistic and indigenous medicine necessitates a collaborative approach that includes diverse stakeholders from medicine, technology, and indigenous communities. As AI becomes more prevalent in healthcare, the need to integrate it respectfully with traditional practices has become more critical. Developers must engage with healers and community leaders to understand the nuances of traditional knowledge and ensure AI tools are developed responsibly.

Ensuring cultural sensitivity in AI involves rigorous training phases, where AI systems are exposed to diverse datasets under the guidance of cultural experts. This collaborative training helps AI to interpret and respect the cultural context of the data it processes. Moreover, the involvement of indigenous practitioners can provide valuable feedback that guides the adaptation of AI technologies in a culturally congruent manner.

These joint efforts also address ethical concerns, ensuring AI does not misappropriate or misinterpret sacred knowledge. With structured and transparent collaborations, AI has the potential to support a wide range of benefits in global healthcare settings, enriching both traditional and modern practices.

## Training AI to Respect Holistic Health Paradigms

The integration of AI in holistic health paradigms necessitates a profound respect for the nuances of these systems. Essential to this process is training AI to recognize and value the breadth of holistic practices, from herbal remedies to energy healing. Achieving this requires encoding AI with an understanding that goes beyond empirical data, delving into the philosophical and spiritual underpinnings of holistic methods.

Developers must collaborate closely with holistic health practitioners to imbue AI with a genuine comprehension of these paradigms. This involves not only input from practitioners during the algorithm design phase but also iterative feedback to refine AI behavior. Such partnerships ensure AI technologies are aligned with the intent and ethics of holistic practices, fostering mutual respect and trust.

Moreover, the adaptability of AI must be enhanced to accommodate the diverse expressions of holistic health. This flexibility is crucial for AI to interact effectively with traditional knowledge systems, adapting to various healing environments without imposing rigid scientific frameworks. Through these dedicated efforts, AI can become a valuable ally in the global practice of holistic medicine.

## Predictive Analytics in Indigenous Medicine: Opportunities and Pitfalls

Predictive analytics in indigenous medicine harnesses AI to forecast health outcomes based on traditional knowledge. This integration offers significant opportunities, such as enhancing diagnostic precision and personalizing treatment plans, which may potentially increase the efficacy of indigenous practices in modern medical settings.

However, the pitfalls are substantial. Key among them is the risk of cultural misinterpretation, where AI systems may oversimplify or misrepresent complex cultural practices that are integral to indigenous healing. Moreover, the reliance on data that may not accurately capture the holistic and spiritual dimensions of indigenous medicine can lead to inappropriate medical recommendations, potentially harming patients rather than helping them.

Further, issues of data sovereignty pose critical concerns. Indigenous communities might become vulnerable to exploitation, as their medicinal knowledge is highly valuable. Ensuring that communities retain control over their traditional knowledge is crucial for preventing ethical breaches and maintaining trust.

## The Future of AI in Supporting Holistic and Indigenous Health Systems

As we gaze into the horizon of healthcare, the fusion of AI with holistic and indigenous medicine holds unparalleled promise. Harnessing AI's power to integrate vast data pools could significantly amplify the reach and impact of ancestral healing wisdom, tailored to modern ailments and personalized health needs.

Imagine AI systems that intricately map the effects of herbal combinations used for centuries, predicting outcomes and suggesting enhancements with precision. Such advanced systems could facilitate a resurgence of indigenous practices, respected and integrated within global health networks. Moreover, deploying AI to document and preserve disappearing healing traditions could serve as a bridge between generations, securing a legacy of healthcare knowledge.

Yet, the journey towards this future must be navigated with care and profound respect for cultural nuances. Collaborative frameworks involving AI developers, indigenous healers, and global healthcare professionals could ensure that technological advancements enrich rather than overwrite the deeply rooted values of holistic and indigenous health paradigms.

## Summary

The exploration of Artificial Intelligence (AI) in holistic and indigenous medicine practices underscores a transformative yet complex intersection. Holistic medicine, known for its integrative approach that considers emotional, spiritual, and social aspects of health, faces both challenges and opportunities in integrating AI. This technology aids in diagnostics and data analysis, enhancing the personalization of healthcare, but struggles to fully grasp the non-material aspects crucial to these traditions. Indigenous medicine, deeply rooted in cultural heritage and natural environments, risks cultural appropriation and misinterpretation through AI, which typically operates within Western scientific frameworks. The potential benefits of AI include accelerated discovery of therapeutic compounds in traditional herbal medicine, supported by AI's capability in bioinformatics. However, this raises ethical questions about intellectual property and access to these resources by the originating cultures. In enhancing personalized medicine, AI can help tailor treatments by analyzing diverse datasets that encompass genetic information, environmental factors, and traditional remedies. This allows for healthcare that respects patients' cultural backgrounds and personal health narratives. Yet, the risk of oversimplifying complex traditional practices into quantifiable data underscores the need for culturally sensitive AI applications. The chapter also highlights the specific case of Traditional Chinese Medicine (TCM), where AI assists in understanding herb combinations but may neglect the philosophical and spiritual nuances of TCM practices. Likewise, the implementation of AI in spiritual healing practices and the interpretation of indigenous healing data present significant challenges, requiring careful consideration to avoid reducing rich traditional knowledge to simplistic algorithms. Efforts to build culturally sensitive AI models involve collaboration with indigenous healers and communities, ensuring that AI respects and preserves traditional wisdom while advancing healthcare.

## References

[1] Atanasov, A. G., Waltenberger, B., Pferschy-Wenzig, E. M., Linder, T., Wawrosch, C., Uhrin, P., ... & Stuppner, H. (2015). Discovery and resupply of pharmacologically active plant-derived natural products: A review.. https://www.ncbi.nlm.nih.gov/pmc/articles/PMC4762214/

[2] James, P. B., Wardle, J., Steel, A., & Adams, J. (2018). Traditional, complementary and alternative medicine use in Sub-Saharan Africa: a systematic review.. https://www.ncbi.nlm.nih.gov/pmc/articles/PMC6195014/

[3] Luxton, D. D. (Ed.). (2016). Artificial intelligence in behavioral and mental health care.. https://www.sciencedirect.com/book/9780128007938/artificial-intelligence-in-behavioral-and-mental-health-care

[4] Ventola, C. L. (2014). Current issues regarding complementary and alternative medicine (CAM) in the United States: Part 1: The widespread use of CAM and the need for better-informed health care professionals to provide patient counseling.. https://www.ncbi.nlm.nih.gov/pmc/articles/PMC4104560/

[5] Horrigan, B. (2020). Integrative Approaches to Pain Management: How to Get the Best of Both Worlds.. https://www.ncbi.nlm.nih.gov/books/NBK553141/

[6] Sharma, A., Minh Duc, N. T., Luu Lam Thang, T., Nam, N. H., Ngoc Quyen, T., Rajendran, P., ... & Gathergood, N. (2019). Herbal Medicine for Anxiety, Depression and Insomnia.. https://www.sciencedirect.com/science/article/pii/S0753332219310315

## Case Study: Integrating AI in Native American Healing Practices

The integration of Artificial Intelligence (AI) into Native American healing practices provides a compelling case study on blending traditional wisdom with contemporary technology. The Navajo Nation, spanning parts of Arizona, Utah, and New Mexico, has a rich heritage of medicinal practices deeply interwoven with spiritual beliefs, rituals, and a profound connection to nature. These practices, passed down through generations, include the use of herbal remedies, spiritual healing techniques, and community-based ceremonies.

In an initiative to preserve these traditions and enhance healthcare accessibility, a collaborative project involving AI developers, local healers, and cultural experts was launched. The project's goal was to develop an AI system capable of documenting and analyzing vast amounts of indigenous medicinal knowledge, identifying patterns, and suggesting integrative health approaches that preserve cultural significance. For instance, AI was used to analyze the effectiveness of various traditional herbs, which are often harvested based on lunar cycles and specific spiritual ceremonies.

However, the project encountered significant challenges. One major issue was ensuring that the AI systems respected and accurately represented the non-materialistic and spiritual dimensions of Navajo healing practices. Traditional healers expressed concerns that the AI, based primarily on data-driven logic and algorithms, might fail to capture the essence of healing practices that rely on spiritual and environmental connectivity. To address these concerns, ongoing workshops and feedback sessions were conducted, where healers guided AI developers on the subtle nuances of their practices.

The case study provided valuable insights into how AI can be used not only to preserve indigenous knowledge but also to integrate it into modern healthcare frameworks, provided it's developed under the guidance of the indigenous communities it serves. Such integrations could potentially enhance diagnosis and treatment while maintaining the integrity and cultural relevance of traditional practices.

### Case Study: AI and the Revitalization of Traditional Chinese Medicine

Advancements in Artificial Intelligence (AI) have begun to play a transformative role in revitalizing Traditional Chinese Medicine (TCM), a practice rooted in a holistic view of the human body and its connection to the natural world. The Essence of Nature Clinic in Shanghai presents a lengthy and detailed case study on the intersection of modern technology and traditional health practices. This clinic has integrated AI to enhance the diagnostic accuracy and treatment efficiency of TCM, leveraging the power of big data to analyze the complex interactions between natural elements and their impact on health.

The clinic utilizes AI systems that process information from a vast database containing centuries-old Traditional Chinese Medicine (TCM) insights, as well as contemporary health data. These systems assess patient symptoms and cross-reference them against historical cases and traditional Chinese medicine (TCM) texts. For instance, using predictive analytics, the AI can suggest customized treatment plans that incorporate a combination of acupuncture, herbal remedies, and dietary modifications tailored to individual patient profiles.

This integration faced numerous challenges, especially regarding the accuracy and cultural faithfulness of AI interpretations. AI developers and TCM practitioners underwent extensive training and adaptation to ensure that the AI algorithms were sensitive to the subtleties of TCM theory, including concepts such as Qi, Yin-Yang balance, and the five elements. Ensuring that AI properly understood and suggested treatments in line with these ancient principles necessitated a collaborative environment where TCM experts played a crucial role in the iteration and validation processes of the tools being developed.

From these extensive collaborative efforts emerge critical lessons about the potential and pitfalls of integrating AI with holistic and indigenous medical practices. While AI technology offers unprecedented potential for enhancing treatment personalization and predictive accuracy in Traditional Chinese Medicine (TCM), the inherent risks of misinterpretation and cultural dilution are substantial. Effective communication and ongoing partnership between AI developers and traditional medicine practitioners have proven essential in addressing these challenges, highlighting a model of integration that respects and leverages the strengths of both worlds.

### Case Study: AI-Enhanced Predictive Analytics in Ayurvedic Medicine

A significant step into the fusion of Artificial Intelligence (AI) with traditional Ayurvedic medicine practices forms an intriguing case study highlighting both the challenges and opportunities of technological integration. Ayurveda, an ancient Indian system of medicine, is based on balancing bodily systems and uses herbal compounds, dietary guidelines, and yogic breathing techniques. The AyurGenomics Clinic in Mumbai undertook an ambitious project to integrate AI-driven predictive analytics, enhancing the diagnostic precision and effectiveness of treatments offered in Ayurveda.

The AI system was designed to analyze a large set of both historical Ayurvedic texts and modern genetic data to uncover patterns that could predict susceptibility to certain diseases based on genetic markers and lifestyle choices. By integrating traditional Ayurvedic knowledge with cutting-edge genomics, the clinic aimed to offer personalized healthcare that anticipates potential health issues and recommends preventive Ayurvedic treatments.

However, several challenges arose during the project's implementation. The primary issue was the AI's ability to understand and interpret the deep philosophical and holistic concepts central to Ayurveda, such as the theories of 'Prakriti' (the individual constitution) and 'Dosha' (the bioenergy that governs body functions). There was also a significant cultural barrier in training AI systems to recognize the nuanced interactions between different herbs and their effects on various body types.

To mitigate these issues, a continuous collaboration was established between AI data scientists and seasoned Ayurvedic practitioners. Workshops and joint sessions were held to translate the traditional knowledge into a form that could be effectively utilized by AI algorithms. This process was pivotal in ensuring that the AI system not only collated data but also respected and incorporated the holistic and individual-focused philosophy of Ayurveda.

This case provides a profound insight into how AI can be tailored to support traditional medicinal systems in a manner that respects their unique cultural paradigms and philosophical foundations. The successful integration of AI into Ayurveda not only has the potential to transform health diagnostics and predictions but also ensures the preservation and modern interpretation of ancient wisdom.

### Case Study: Enhancing African Traditional Medicine with AI Integration

The integration of Artificial Intelligence (AI) into African traditional medicine presents a unique case study, particularly examining the collaborative efforts in the Zola Herbal Solutions initiative in Nigeria. This project was designed to modernize and enhance the accessibility and efficacy of traditional herbal remedies that have been used generationally across various African cultures. African traditional medicine is characterized by its reliance on herbal remedies, spiritual healing, and community-based practices, all of which are deeply embedded within the cultural and historical context of different tribes.

The Zola Herbal Solutions initiative leveraged AI to catalog and analyze the healing properties of local herbs, drawing on historical data and contemporary research findings. AI-powered tools were developed to predict the efficacy of herbal combinations for specific ailments and to personalize treatments for individuals based on their unique health profiles. This was achieved by combining local herbal knowledge with global biomedical data, leveraging AI's sophisticated pattern recognition capabilities.

However, several cultural and technical challenges emerged during the initiative. One significant issue was the translation of qualitative, experience-based knowledge into quantitative data that can be effectively utilized by AI. This necessitated a meticulous process of data capture and analysis, often requiring direct input from traditional healers who possessed intricate knowledge passed down orally for generations. Furthermore, the project faced ethical considerations regarding the ownership and commercial use of traditional knowledge, leading to comprehensive engagement with local communities to strike a balance between modernization and cultural preservation.

Through painstaking efforts and continuous adaptations, the project successfully enhanced the diagnostic and treatment capabilities of African traditional medicine while respecting its cultural roots. The case study highlights both the potential and limitations of applying AI to indigenous medicinal knowledge, underscoring the need for deeply collaborative approaches that honor and integrate traditional wisdom with modern technology.

### Case Study: AI's Role in Supporting Shamanic Practices in the Peruvian Amazon

In the heart of the Peruvian Amazon, shamanic practices have been a cornerstone of indigenous culture, emphasizing profound spiritual connections and the utilization of natural resources to promote healing. These traditions, heavily reliant on ancestral knowledge and spiritual interactions, are being explored through the innovative lens of Artificial Intelligence (AI) to enhance their preservation and effectiveness.

The case study revolves around the partnership between AI researchers and the Shipibo-Conibo community, which is renowned for its intricate knowledge of plant medicine and spiritual healing. The initiative aimed to document and analyze traditional practices using AI, creating a database that could aid in diagnosing illnesses based on symptoms described in spiritual terms and suggest potential herbal remedies. The AI system was trained to recognize patterns in herbal efficacy and spiritual diagnoses, employing natural language processing to interpret the community's dialect and codify their knowledge.

However, integrating AI into such a spiritually oriented context presented considerable challenges. The primary concern was the AI's capacity to understand and translate non-materialistic, spiritual healing practices into quantifiable data. Another challenge was ensuring the respectful capture and use of sacred knowledge, closely tied to the identity and spiritual life of the community. To address these issues, the project included extensive collaborative workshops where AI developers spent time with shamans to learn about the spiritual and communal significance of their practices. This hands-on engagement allowed for the development of AI algorithms that were more sensitive to the cultural and spiritual nuances of the practices.

Throughout the project, direct, personal feedback from the shamans was crucial in refining the AI models. This ongoing interaction ensured that the AI system not only collected data but also respected and reflected the depth of shamanic knowledge. The outcome was a sophisticated tool that supported the community in preserving their heritage and enhancing the accessibility of their medicinal knowledge for younger generations, potentially enriching global health perspectives with its unique insights.

### Case Study: AI-driven Analysis and Preservation of Indigenous Amazonian Botanical Knowledge

The Amazon rainforest, a biodiversity hotspot, is home to thousands of species of plants and herbs, many of which have established uses in local indigenous medicine. These plants are utilized according to traditional knowledge passed down through generations, often only within specific tribes. The potential for this botanical knowledge to contribute to global health is immense, provided it can be accurately understood, preserved, and shared. An intriguing initiative in this context is the Amazonian Ethnobotanical AI Project (AEAP), a collaborative effort involving AI researchers, environmental scientists, and indigenous communities that aims to catalog and analyze this vast pharmacopeia using advanced AI technologies.

The AEAP utilizes machine learning algorithms to aid in the identification and classification of unknown plant species, as well as to predict their potential medicinal properties based on their genetic markers and historical usage by indigenous communities. This digital catalog aims not only to preserve this precious knowledge but also to make it accessible for potential pharmaceutical applications, ensuring equitable benefits for the native communities.

However, this ambition encounters profound challenges. The primary concern is ensuring the fidelity of digital representations to the complex, often spiritual narratives that accompany traditional plant use. The AI's capability to manage and interpret non-quantitative data, such as tribal lore and ceremonial contexts, is inherently limited. To mitigate this, the project has developed a unique participatory model in which indigenous healers work alongside data scientists to input traditional knowledge into the AI system, thereby guiding the context and interpretation of the data.

The case study further explores ethical considerations, including intellectual property rights and benefit-sharing. Continuous dialogue and legal frameworks ensure that any commercialization of discoveries provides reciprocal benefits to the indigenous peoples who hold this traditional knowledge. The project serves as a profound case of how AI can be leveraged to bridge ancient wisdom with modern scientific inquiry, fostering a sustainable and respectful use of endemic natural resources while potentially unlocking new avenues in global healthcare solutions.

### Case Study: The Integration of AI in Maori Healing Practices in New Zealand

The integration of Artificial Intelligence (AI) into Māori healing practices in New Zealand presents a pioneering case study in the fusion of technological innovation with indigenous healthcare. Māori healing, known as Rongoā Māori, encompasses a range of practices including the use of medicinal plants, physical therapies, and spiritual healing, deeply rooted in the traditional knowledge and cultural values of the Māori people.

A collaborative project was initiated by a tech consortium in partnership with local Māori health practitioners to explore how AI could support the preservation and application of Rongoā Māori. The goal was to develop an AI system that could catalog extensive historical and cultural knowledge of healing practices and potentially suggest personalized treatment plans based on traditional Maori approaches to health and well-being.

The AI system employed machine learning algorithms to analyze data from various sources, including historical records, patient medical histories, and documented outcomes of traditional treatments. However, integrating these diverse data types posed significant challenges, particularly in capturing the nuances and complexities of spiritual and cultural dimensions in Maori healing. Another challenge was ensuring that the algorithms were trained on culturally relevant datasets without perpetuating any biases or misinterpretations.

To address these concerns, ongoing workshops and knowledge-sharing sessions were established where Maori healers could directly interact with AI developers. These interactions were crucial for providing insights into the culturally specific aspects of Rongoā Māori and ensuring that the AI system respected and accurately reflected Māori healing philosophies. The project also included stringent ethical guidelines to govern data use and sharing, ensuring that Maori intellectual and cultural property rights were protected.

Despite the hurdles, the project demonstrated promising results. The AI system effectively identified patterns in traditional treatment efficacy, suggesting optimized combinations of medicinal plants that were previously undocumented. More importantly, the technology reinforced the intergenerational transmission of Maori healing knowledge, making it accessible to younger Maori populations and healthcare professionals interested in integrative medical practices.

### Case Study: Utilizing AI to Revitalize South American Quechua Healing Practices

In the heart of Ecuador's dense rainforest, Quechua healers have long utilized a vast array of plants, spiritual ceremonies, and ancestral wisdom for healthcare, grounded deeply in their connection to their environment and cultural beliefs. A groundbreaking project aimed to integrate Artificial Intelligence (AI) into these traditional healing practices, presenting a unique intersection of ancient heritage with modern technology. Conducted in collaboration with a local university and an international tech firm, the project sought to digitize and analyze historical and contemporary Quichua medicinal knowledge.

The objective was twofold: to preserve endangered knowledge as elder healers pass away and to identify potential new applications for traditional remedies in broader healthcare practices. AI algorithms were trained to categorize plant properties and their reported healing effects, using both structured data entry by healers and unstructured data from community-shared oral histories. Additionally, natural language processing tools have been developed to interpret the Quechua language, which is rich in nuances crucial for understanding the context of use in traditional medicine.

Despite the technological promise, several significant challenges surfaced. First was the deep skepticism among some community members about the potential for AI to 'westernize' their traditional practices, fearing loss of spiritual significance that could not be quantified and captured by data algorithms. To mitigate these concerns, project leaders established ongoing dialogue sessions that allowed healers to express their concerns and actively influence the development process.

Moreover, ethical issues concerning data sovereignty and consent were prominent. The project navigated these challenges by developing a framework that ensured all digitalized knowledge remained the intellectual property of the Quechua community, with strict controls on external access and use.

This case study highlights the complexities and potential of integrating AI with indigenous healing practices. It encapsulates the necessity for a respectful, collaborative approach in melding technology with ancient wisdom, ensuring that AI serves as a tool to enhance and preserve cultural practices rather than diminish or exploit them.

## Review Questions

**3. A health policy maker is reviewing AI models for adoption in public hospitals and comes across a model that predicts treatment outcomes based on clinical data. However, the model does not involve any traditional healing practices widely used among the local indigenous population. What should be the policymaker's approach to address this limitation?**

A) Reject the AI model and seek alternative solutions that include traditional healing practices

B) Approve the AI model as is, considering the clinical accuracy of its predictions

C) Work with AI developers and local traditional healers to integrate traditional healing practices into the model's dataset

D) Conduct further research on the efficacy of traditional healing practices before deciding

**Answer: C**

Explanation: The best course of action for the health policy maker would be to work with AI developers and local traditional healers to integrate traditional healing practices into the model's training dataset. This collaboration would enhance the model's ability to better serve the entire population, including those who utilize traditional healing methods. Such AI health systems need to reflect the diversity of medical practices within the community they serve, thereby providing equitable and effective care. By incorporating traditional healing practices, the AI model could become more inclusive and holistic, potentially increasing its acceptance and effectiveness.

**Techniques for Decolonizing Medical AI**

**Understanding Decolonization in Medical AI Contexts**

Decolonization in the context of medical AI involves dismantling the traditional hierarchies and biases that are inherently tied to colonial pasts, which often overshadow global health perspectives. It involves acknowledging the respective Native communities healing and medical history and practices, giving credit where credit is due and avoiding any cultural misappropriation while doing so. This crucial step forward requires redefining the frameworks of medical knowledge to include and elevate indigenous, traditional, and holistic health practices that have been historically marginalized.

By critically analyzing how medical AI technologies are currently designed, we can identify embedded biases that perpetuate a predominantly Western medical paradigm. This awareness enables the integration of diverse healing practices into AI systems, ensuring they are equitable and representative of various cultural approaches. The goal is to create AI tools that recognize and adapt to a wide range of medical systems and beliefs, thereby broadening their applicability and effectiveness.

Implementing such changes also involves scrutinizing and altering the AI development process, from data collection to algorithm training and implementation stages. It's essential that these processes inclusively reflect the cultural, spiritual, and empirical wisdom of non-Western medical systems, fostering a truly global medical AI that respects cultural sovereignty.

**Revisiting Historical Contexts: The Colonization of Medicine**

The history of medicine is deeply intertwined with the forces of colonization, where Western medical practices often supplanted indigenous health systems. This historical context is crucial in understanding the pervasive biases present in contemporary medical AI. By examining the past, we observe a pattern in which medical practices have been used as tools for control and assimilation, sidelining traditional healing wisdom that has sustained communities for generations.

In many regions, colonial powers introduced Western medical systems that marginalized and delegitimized local health practices and knowledge bases, thereby creating a hierarchy that persists in medical education and practices to this day. This legacy of dominant institutional Western medicine systems dominates how medical data is collected, interpreted, and valued, often overlooking the nuanced approaches of traditional medicine.

Decolonizing medical AI demands addressing these historical imbalances. It requires an intentional dismantling of the lingering colonial frameworks within AI algorithms and databases to revalidate and integrate diverse, culturally specific knowledge. Only then can AI in healthcare truly become inclusive, delivering solutions that respect and incorporate the full spectrum of global medical wisdom.

**Challenging Western Dominance in Medical Practice**

The domination of Western medical practices often eclipses diverse healing traditions, including those rooted in indigenous cultures. Challenging this dominance means reassessing the biases entrenched within AI technology, promoting a broader view of health. By acknowledging the validity and effectiveness of non-Western medical practices, AI can benefit from an enriched dataset that brings traditional wisdom to the forefront of medical innovation.

Integrating these diverse healing methods involves more than just data inclusion; it demands a fundamental redesign where AI systems are developed by teams reflecting global diversity. This change requires a shift in mindsets and educational systems that perpetuate Western medical superiority, ensuring that future AI developers are equipped to consider and respect a wide range of healing traditions.

Ultimately, confronting Western dominance is not merely about adding diversity for show. It's about rectifying historical inequities in healthcare, providing equal validity to all health sciences. This move towards decolonization can usher in a new era of truly comprehensive and equitable healthcare solutions powered by AI.

## Promoting Diversity in AI Development Teams

Promoting diversity within AI development teams serves as a cornerstone in decolonizing medical AI. Diverse teams bring a wide range of cultural perspectives and experiences, which are crucial for incorporating a multitude of traditional and indigenous healing practices into AI technologies. This diversity extends beyond ethnic backgrounds to encompass a range of professional domains, genders, economic backgrounds, and geographical locations, ensuring a holistic approach to AI development.

Integration of diverse perspectives can dramatically reduce the risk of biased algorithms that typically arise from homogeneous development environments. Representing multiple demographics within AI teams fosters an environment where cultural insights are acknowledged and valued, not only enriching the development process but also enhancing the effectiveness of AI applications in real-world, diverse medical settings.

Moreover, the inclusion of team members from different cultural and traditional backgrounds enables the critique and redesign of AI systems that respect and incorporate local healing practices and knowledge. It is a step towards building AI that is not only technically sound but also culturally sensitive and inclusive, leading to better healthcare outcomes globally.

## Incorporating Indigenous Knowledge Systems into AI

The incorporation of indigenous knowledge systems into AI is a transformative step towards decolonizing medical AI. This involves recognizing and validating the empirical nature of non-Western healing practices, rather than merely relying on anecdotal evidence. AI systems can be adapted to consider local plant-based remedies, spiritual rituals, and community-wide health practices, once considered peripheral by mainstream medicine.

For instance, algorithms could be enhanced to analyze patterns from centuries-old herbal medicine databases, integrating these insights with contemporary medical protocols. This approach not only diversifies the AI's knowledge base but also offers a holistic view of patient care that respects cultural heritage and community wisdom. In practicing this integration, AI developers must collaborate closely with indigenous healers and scholars to ensure accuracy and cultural sensitivity.

Furthermore, this integration promotes the sustainability of indigenous knowledge by digitizing and digitally preserving sacred wisdom for future generations. Such collaborative efforts can lead to innovative health solutions that are culturally tailored and technologically advanced, thereby redefining health equity and inclusiveness in the global medical landscape.

## Ensuring Equitable Participation in AI Data Collection

Ensuring equitable participation in AI data collection is vital for the democratization of medical AI. Historically, data pools have predominantly been sourced from non-diverse demographics, skewing AI's understanding and outputs toward these populations. To truly decolonize medical AI, the scope of data collection must widen to include underrepresented groups, capturing the richness of global, particularly indigenous and traditional, medical knowledge.

Broadening data collection entails targeted outreach and education, ensuring communities understand the benefits and implications of their participation. This process should be built on trust, with clear communication strategies that are culturally sensitive and accessible to all parties involved. By actively engaging these communities, we not only enrich the data sets but also empower these groups by valuing their contributions to global health insights.

Additionally, implementing strict ethical guidelines to protect participants' data ensures that the collection process respects individuals' privacy and the cultural significance attached to their medical information. Such measures foster a more inclusive AI that is representative of the true diversity in health practices worldwide.

**Addressing Power Imbalances in Health AI Technologies**

Addressing power imbalances in health AI technologies is crucial for creating equitable healthcare solutions. Existing AI models often reinforce existing disparities by primarily being developed and tested in high-resource settings, neglecting the diverse needs and conditions of marginalized communities. To rectify this, diverse stakeholder involvement in AI development is paramount, ensuring voices from varied socio-economic and cultural backgrounds shape the technologies that affect their health outcomes.

Moreover, power dynamics can be rebalanced by democratizing AI development tools and resources, allowing broader access and innovation from previously underserved communities. This includes open-source frameworks and collaborative platforms where traditional and indigenous knowledge can influence foundational AI models. Such inclusivity enhances AI's ability to address diverse global health challenges comprehensively.

Lastly, continuous monitoring and regulation of AI applications in healthcare must be implemented to ensure compliance with equitable practices. This involves setting standards that require AI to be transparent, accountable, and continuously evaluated for bias and fairness across all user demographics. Only through such comprehensive measures can AI genuinely support global health equity and justice.

**Building AI Systems that Acknowledge Cultural Sovereignty**

Building AI systems that acknowledge cultural sovereignty is essential in fostering a globally inclusive medical field. This requires the integration of diverse cultural norms and values directly into the AI's decision-making processes, ensuring these systems adhere to the cultural rights and customs of the populations they serve.

Firstly, the development of culturally aware AI demands collaboration with leaders and experts within indigenous and underrepresented communities. This engagement allows for an in-depth understanding of cultural nuances, which can guide the AI modeling. Such participatory approaches empower communities by giving them a role in shaping technologies that impact their healthcare outcomes.

Moreover, AI systems must be designed with mechanisms that allow them to adapt to evolving cultural norms and ethical standards. This dynamic adjustment ensures that AI technologies remain relevant and respectful to cultural sovereignty over time.

Ultimately, recognizing and integrating cultural sovereignty in AI systems sets a precedent for technology that not only heals but deeply respects the diverse world it serves.

**Designing AI with Sensitivity to Traditional Healing Practices**

To genuinely advance the mission of decolonizing medical AI, designing AI with sensitivity to traditional healing methods is paramount. This facet of AI design goes beyond mere inclusion; it entails a profound understanding and respect for healing traditions that have been nurtured over generations. By integrating these practices, AI can offer more comprehensive and personalized healthcare solutions.

Collaborative engagements with practitioners of traditional medicine can help in mapping out the vast landscape of indigenous healing. AI systems designed in these collaborative settings benefit from the nuanced insights of traditional healers, ensuring the technology is not only adaptive but also respectful and efficacious. The insights derived from traditional practices, such as herbal medicine, spiritual healing, and community-based therapies, provide AI with a richer, more diverse data set to draw from.

To effectively implement this sensitivity, AI developers must undergo cultural sensitivity training and establish ethical guidelines that protect and honor traditional knowledge. The development process should aim for inclusivity, allowing AI to serve as a bridge between modern medical practices and traditional healing arts, thereby fostering an environment where technology and tradition coalesce for improved health outcomes.

**Redefining Success Metrics in AI Health Solutions**

Redefining success metrics in AI health solutions involves a fundamental shift towards valuing cultural inclusivity and holistic outcomes. Traditionally, AI metrics focused on clinical accuracy and cost-effectiveness, often overlooking the nuanced benefits of integrating indigenous and traditional healing methods. By broadening these metrics to encompass patient satisfaction across diverse cultural contexts and the preservation of cultural heritage, AI can more effectively reflect the varied health needs and values of different populations.

Such metrics might include the ability of AI to adapt recommendations to include traditional remedies acknowledged by local communities, or the extent to which AI supports patient-centered care that aligns with their cultural practices. Additionally, success could be assessed by community impact, gauging how well AI technologies help sustain and rejuvenate indigenous medical knowledge rather than merely extracting data.

Implementing these revised metrics requires ongoing collaboration with indigenous communities and health practitioners, ensuring that AI development aligns with both modern medical standards and the deep-seated cultural traditions of these communities. Through these endeavors, AI can truly become a tool for equitable and culturally respectful healthcare.

**Legal Frameworks to Protect Indigenous Data Rights**

In the realm of medical AI, robust legal frameworks must be instituted to safeguard indigenous data rights, prioritizing confidentiality, consent, and the cultural significance of data. This initiative requires crafting laws that not only recognize but also enshrine the ownership rights of indigenous communities over their data, ensuring they have absolute control over how their information is used.

Implementing such legal provisions involves clear regulations that govern data access and the purposes for which it is utilized, preventing misuse and unauthorized sharing. Collaboration with indigenous representatives is vital to ensure that these laws resonate with the unique ethical standards and privacy concerns of each community.

Moreover, these legal frameworks should facilitate the ability of indigenous peoples to benefit equitably from the advancements in AI, including sharing in the economic gains derived from data-driven innovations. Ensuring legal protection for indigenous data rights is not just a regulatory necessity but a moral obligation to respect and preserve the integrity of diverse cultures in the digital age.

## Community-Based Approaches to AI Development

Community-based approaches to AI development harness the collective wisdom of local communities to create inclusive and effective health technologies. Engaging with community members throughout the AI lifecycle not only promotes understanding and acceptance of AI solutions but also ensures these technologies are tailored to meet the specific needs of those they serve.

By involving communities early in the design process, developers can gain valuable insights into cultural practices and local health challenges. This collaboration enables the development of AI systems that are culturally competent and more likely to be accepted by the communities they aim to support. Moreover, it supports the sustainability of AI initiatives by fostering a sense of ownership and accountability among local stakeholders.

Furthermore, community-based development encourages the use of local data sources, which can enhance the accuracy and relevance of AI applications in healthcare. Incorporating these diverse data inputs helps prevent biases that typically arise from homogeneous data sets, making AI tools more equitable and effective.

## Strategies for Authentic Representation in AI Datasets

Authentic representation in AI datasets is crucial for decolonizing medical AI, particularly in accurately representing minority and Indigenous health perspectives. This process begins with systematically identifying gaps in existing datasets, which are frequently compounded by historical neglect and ongoing disparities. Developers must engage with indigenous and traditional communities to incorporate diverse health data that reflects different healing practices, epidemiological patterns, and health outcomes.

Strategies include involving community liaisons and cultural consultants in the data collection phase to ensure that data gathering respects cultural norms and values. This collaboration can also help in decoding complex traditional knowledge systems into data formats suitable for AI applications, bridging a crucial gap between ancient wisdom and contemporary technology.

Furthermore, data anonymization processes must be adapted to protect personal and community identities without compromising the contextual richness necessary for meaningful AI analysis. Finally, continually iterating on data collection and analysis methods to proactively handle biases is essential. Such rigorous, culturally informed methodologies cultivate datasets that uplift authentic voices and foster trust in AI-driven medical applications.

## Creating Inclusive AI Training Environments

Creating inclusive AI training environments is vital for decolonizing medical AI. This requires a foundational change in how training settings are structured and who is involved in these processes. Bringing together a diverse mix of developers, ethicists, and practitioners from various cultural backgrounds significantly enhances the development of AI tools that are culturally sensitive and broadly effective.

Inclusion extends beyond mere representation; it requires the active participation and empowerment of traditionally marginalized voices in AI development. Training environments must not only be welcoming but also equip participants with the ability to influence the core functionalities of AI technologies. This means training sessions should cover cultural competence and the ethical dimensions of AI, ensuring all involved have a robust understanding of the diverse contexts in which AI will operate.

Furthermore, creating spaces that promote open dialogue and shared learning can foster innovations that respect and integrate traditional, indigenous, and holistic healing practices into AI solutions. These environments must continuously evolve to reflect new understandings and challenges as AI technology progresses.

## Re-examining AI algorithms through a Decolonized Lens

Re-examining AI algorithms through a decolonized lens necessitates a profound reevaluation of the foundational principles underlying algorithm design and their application in health contexts. It requires confronting the biases rooted in historical data, which are traditionally used to train these systems, often marginalizing non-Western medical knowledge and practices. This process should begin with critical scrutiny of the datasets and decision frameworks that underpin AI, ensuring they represent a globally diverse perspective.

The inclusion of indigenous health practices and holistic healing traditions in AI development can enrich algorithmic diversity, fostering models that appreciate the full spectrum of human health and wellness practices. Such an approach would enable AI to support a broader array of patient needs and cultural contexts, making it a more inclusive tool in global health systems.

Ultimately, re-examining algorithms means actively dismantling the colonialist residues that persist in AI. It involves continuous dialogue with indigenous and traditional communities, integrating their insights and values into AI systems. This transformative approach will yield AI technologies that are not only culturally sensitive but also ethically responsible and widely applicable across different cultural landscapes.

## Transparency and Accountability in AI Deployment

In the pursuit of decolonizing medical AI, the principles of transparency and accountability stand central. Transparent AI deployment involves clear communication of how AI systems operate, the data they use, and the rationale behind their decisions. This openness is crucial for building trust, especially among indigenous and traditional communities who may be skeptical of technologies that have historically overlooked their medical frameworks.

Accountability in AI extends beyond technical accuracy; it encompasses ethical obligations and the social impact of AI applications. Developers must ensure AI systems do not perpetuate existing disparities or introduce new forms of bias. Establishing robust oversight mechanisms can help monitor AI operations, ensuring they align with ethical standards and contribute positively to health outcomes across all cultural spectrums.

Engagement with community representatives in auditing AI systems enhances transparency and enforces accountability. Such collaborations should aim to assess the impact of AI solutions, adjusting them based on feedback to serve the community's needs better. Ultimately, maintaining a transparent and accountable AI deployment reassures all stakeholders of the technology's integrity and fairness.

## Partnerships between AI Developers and Indigenous Communities

Forging partnerships between AI developers and indigenous communities is crucial in developing medical AI systems that respect and incorporate traditional healing knowledge. Such collaborative ventures aim to co-create technologies that are culturally attuned and technically proficient. These partnerships often begin with establishing trust, necessitating transparency in intentions and mutual respect for both technological expertise and ancestral wisdom.

The engagement process involves regular and meaningful dialogues where community input directly influences the development of AI. Workshops, joint research initiatives, and shared projects ensure that AI solutions are not only informed by indigenous knowledge but also support local health needs and priorities. This collaborative model also facilitates capacity building within indigenous communities, empowering them with new skills and knowledge related to AI and technology.

A sustained commitment to and adaptability in response to feedback from community stakeholders characterizes successful partnerships. This approach ensures that AI systems remain relevant and beneficial to indigenous health outcomes, thus supporting a model of continued collaboration and mutual growth. Ultimately, these partnerships can serve as a blueprint for integrating diverse cultural knowledge into global health technologies.

**Feedback Mechanisms from Community to AI Developers**

Establishing robust feedback mechanisms from the community to AI developers is a cornerstone in decolonizing medical AI. These systems empower indigenous and traditional communities by giving them a direct voice in the development of AI. Ensuring that feedback is not only heard but actively incorporated is vital for the relevance and acceptance of AI technologies in diverse cultural contexts.

Mechanisms for feedback should involve multiple platforms and methodologies, such as digital forums, community meetings, and dedicated liaison officers who translate community concerns into actionable insights for developers. These platforms must be accessible and tailored to meet the linguistic and cultural nuances of the communities involved. Regular and structured feedback sessions facilitate an iterative process where AI systems are continually refined to meet community health needs.

Moreover, incorporating community feedback directly impacts the utility of AI, enhancing the system's responsiveness to cultural specifics in medical practices. It also fosters a sense of ownership and trust among indigenous populations, which is crucial for the successful integration of AI into local healthcare frameworks. Ultimately, these feedback mechanisms foster a dynamic dialogue where AI development is a collaborative and culturally informed journey.

**AI and the Reinforcement of Stereotypes in Healthcare**

Artificial Intelligence (AI) in healthcare can inadvertently reinforce existing stereotypes, particularly when the underlying data reflects historical biases. Traditional and indigenous healing practices, often sidelined in medical datasets, are thus at risk of further marginalization. This perpetuates a cycle in which these valuable knowledge systems are underrepresented in AI outcomes, reinforcing the dominance of Western medical paradigms and potentially harming those who rely on other forms of healing.

Addressing this requires a conscious effort to diversify data and include a broader spectrum of health practices. It is crucial to continuously audit AI systems for biases that may skew AI decision-making against non-Western medical traditions. These audits should involve experts from diverse medical systems and should strive to identify and correct disparities in AI recommendations.

Ultimately, the goal is to create AI that is as inclusive as it is innovative. Developing guidelines for equitable AI representation can help ensure that all healing practices are respected and integrated, providing a more holistic approach to health that reflects global diversity.

**Ethical Guidelines for Decolonizing AI Practices**

Establishing ethical guidelines for decolonizing AI in medicine is crucial to ensure the technology supports and respects diverse medical traditions. These guidelines start by clearly defining ethical use, particularly in the exploitation of data related to indigenous and traditional healing practices. Ethical AI must prioritize consent, ensuring that communities understand how their data and knowledge are being used.

Moreover, it's imperative to involve indigenous representatives in the creation of these guidelines. Their input guarantees that AI systems uphold dignity, respect, and fairness in handling culturally sensitive data. Ethical guidelines should enforce the validation of AI outcomes by culturally knowledgeable individuals to maintain relevance and accuracy.

Lastly, the guidelines must advocate for transparency about AI failures and successes in a culturally sensitive manner and provide mechanisms for grievance redressal. Compliance with these ethical standards should be monitored and enforced rigorously to cultivate trust and truly decolonize AI practices in healthcare.

**Addressing Language and Communication Barriers in AI**

Addressing language and communication barriers in AI is essential for decolonizing medical AI. Implementing multilingual support across AI platforms can significantly enhance accessibility for indigenous communities, supporting a more inclusive health ecosystem. This adaptability not only breaks through the language barrier but also respects the linguistic diversity of these communities, facilitating more equitable access to healthcare technologies.

Language sensitivity in AI goes beyond mere translation; it involves the contextual understanding of cultural nuances that affect health communication. AI systems must be designed to interpret and respond effectively in diverse cultural contexts, ensuring that all patients receive care that is not only medically competent but also culturally sensitive and coherent. This approach requires deep learning algorithms to be trained on a diverse corpus of linguistic data, representing various dialects and colloquial terms.

Moreover, communication in healthcare AI should consider non-verbal cues prevalent in many cultures, adapting interfaces to accommodate such nuances. This dedication to overcoming communication barriers can bridge the gap between technology and traditional healthcare practices, making AI tools more effective and respectful of cultural identities.

**Educational Initiatives to Foster Alignment in AI Practices**

Educational initiatives play a crucial role in aligning AI practices with the diverse needs of both indigenous and global communities. By focusing on inclusive education, we can bridge the knowledge gap that often exists between AI developers and the communities they serve. Initiatives such as specialized courses on cultural competency and the development of ethical AI are essential. These courses should not only teach technical skills but also emphasize the importance of understanding and respecting diverse healing traditions.

Workshops and seminars that bring together AI professionals and indigenous healers can foster mutual learning and appreciation. These interactions encourage the exchange of ideas and knowledge, ensuring that AI technologies are developed with a comprehensive understanding of different medical paradigms. This collaborative educational approach helps in creating AI systems that are culturally sensitive and medically inclusive.

Moreover, online platforms can provide continuous learning opportunities that are accessible to a wide audience. These platforms can host a variety of resources, including case studies, guidelines, and expert talks that delve into the nuances of decolonizing AI in the medical field. Ensuring that such educational resources are widely available and regularly updated is key to maintaining an ongoing dialogue about the best practices for AI development in healthcare.

## Re-evaluating the Tools and Methods Used in AI Training

Re-evaluating the tools and methods used in AI training is pivotal for decolonizing medical AI. Current AI training methodologies still heavily rely on datasets and algorithms that mirror Western-centric medical perspectives, which often marginalize traditional healing methods. To address this, it is essential to incorporate a broader range of data sources that reflect the diversity and richness of global medical practices.

This re-evaluation must also consider the design and functionality of AI tools. Tools should be adaptable to various medical systems and capable of handling diverse health concepts and terminologies. Techniques such as cross-cultural semantic understanding and context-aware computing could play crucial roles. By diversifying the tools utilized in AI training, we ensure that the technology is relevant and respectful to all health paradigms.

Furthermore, adopting new methods might involve leveraging insights from ethnomedical research and participatory design approaches. This ensures the AI not only comprehends but also appreciates the value of indigenous knowledge systems, providing a balanced and inclusive healthcare solution.

## Future Challenges and Prospects in Decolonizing Medical AI

The future of decolonizing medical AI presents a complex landscape of challenges and opportunities. As technology evolves, continually adapting AI systems to respect and integrate diverse medical traditions will be essential. This includes constant updates to ensure AI algorithms are free from biases that exclude or misinterpret non-Western medical knowledge. The expansion of AI into global medical practices demands robust frameworks to manage these updates effectively and ethically.

Looking ahead, the engagement of indigenous communities in AI development processes remains crucial. Creating ongoing partnerships will facilitate the exchange of knowledge and ensure that AI systems are culturally sensitive and medically comprehensive. However, sustaining such collaborations poses logistical and financial challenges that must be addressed to maintain momentum in decolonizing efforts.

Moreover, the legal and ethical implications of AI in medicine are continuously evolving. Policymakers must collaborate closely with technologists and cultural experts to develop laws that safeguard indigenous data rights and foster equity in AI-driven healthcare. The journey towards a decolonized medical AI is ongoing, requiring unwavering commitment to inclusivity and justice.

### Summary

The chapter 'Techniques for Decolonizing Medical AI' delves into crucial strategies necessary for reforming medical artificial intelligence (AI) systems by integrating culturally diverse, traditional, and indigenous medical knowledge, combating the dominance of Western medical practices. Decolonization within medical AI necessitates the dismantling of existing biases derived from colonial influences and the inclusive redesign of AI systems to respect and integrate a diverse range of medical perspectives. This transformation involves revisiting historical contexts to uncover how colonization has shaped contemporary medical practices, thereby influencing the data and algorithms used in current AI technologies. The chapter emphasizes the importance of challenging and redefining these historical biases through a concerted effort between data scientists, medical professionals, and communities that have been historically underrepresented in medical data. By embedding indigenous healing practices and acknowledging diverse health paradigms from the outset of AI development, these systems can deliver more equitable and culturally sensitive health solutions. Key techniques discussed include promoting diversity within AI development teams, ensuring equitable participation in AI data collection, addressing power imbalances, and ensuring AI applications are sensitive to cultural sovereignty and traditional healing practices. Furthermore, the establishment of legal frameworks to protect indigenous data rights and community-based approaches to AI development are underscored as essential for fostering a reciprocal relationship between AI developers and indigenous communities. This ensures that AI technologies not only advance technically but are also rich in cultural empathy and ethical practice. By redefining success metrics to include cultural inclusivity and implementing continuous feedback mechanisms from diverse communities, medical AI can evolve into an equitable tool that respects and preserves the integrity and value of global medicinal diversity. This change is envisioned not only as a technical overhaul but as a deeply ethical reformation aiming to right historical wrongs and create a balanced landscape in global healthcare.

## References

[1] Padró-Paz et al., 2021. http://doi.org/10.1016/j.joi.2021.101155
[2] Hickley & Turiel, 2019. https://www.rand.org/pubs/research_briefs/RB9570.html
[3] Abee, S., & Wang, D., 2020. https://doi.org/10.1177/0162243919899468

## Case Study: Integrating Traditional Healing Knowledge in AI Systems for Community Health Initiatives

In a collaborative effort between AI developers, local health practitioners, and indigenous communities in the Amazon Basin, a new health AI project was initiated. The goal was to create a medical AI system that not only diagnoses diseases but also recommends treatments based on both Western medicine and traditional Amazonian practices. This inclusive approach aimed to respect and integrate the rich heritage of indigenous knowledge with contemporary medical technology. The development process involved extensive field research, which entailed direct engagement with tribal healers and the collection of diverse health data, including herbal remedies and historical health practices recorded by the communities.

As the project progressed, challenges arose regarding data interpretation, the integration of traditional qualitative knowledge with quantitative medical data, and the ethical considerations of intellectual property rights related to indigenous knowledge. The AI model initially faced resistance from local practitioners who were skeptical about the accuracy and sensitivity of the AI towards their traditional practices. To address these issues, a series of workshops were held to train the AI developers in cultural sensitivity and to educate local health practitioners about the potential benefits of AI in enhancing healthcare delivery.

Deep learning algorithms were tailored to accurately recognize patterns in the local data. Special emphasis was given to the ethical sourcing and anonymization of the data to protect the community's privacy and proprietary knowledge. Additionally, feedback mechanisms were established, allowing continuous input from the community to refine the AI algorithms.

This case illustrates both the potential and the challenges of integrating traditional knowledge into modern AI systems, highlighting the necessity of respecting cultural sovereignty while leveraging technology to improve health outcomes. Important lessons were learned about the balance between innovation and tradition, the importance of community involvement, and the need for continual adaptation and ethical vigilance in AI health projects.

## Case Study: Decolonizing AI in Rural Healthcare Systems of Sub-Saharan Africa

The deployment of an AI-driven healthcare project in Sub-Saharan Africa revealed significant insights into the challenges and opportunities of integrating AI in differently resourced environments. This project, launched by a coalition of international health organizations and local government bodies, aimed to improve healthcare delivery in rural areas by introducing AI systems tailored to local medical practices and languages. The AI was designed to assist in diagnosing common diseases, such as malaria and tuberculosis, which are prevalent in the region.

Initial steps involved gathering extensive data on local health conditions, which included both contemporary medical records and traditional healing methods used by village elders. The AI development team, comprising members from diverse cultural backgrounds, faced the challenge of translating this complex medical knowledge into algorithms capable of operating within the intricate health landscape of rural Africa. Language barriers, differing medical terminologies, and the integration of traditional health beliefs posed significant hurdles.

To address these challenges, the project established a series of communication channels, including workshops and interactive platforms, where AI developers worked directly with local health workers and community leaders. These interactions were crucial for the AI to learn from the local context and for the community to build trust in using AI technology. Specially designed AI training modules emphasized sensitivity to local beliefs and practices, reinforcing the importance of a decolonized approach to AI in healthcare.

Moreover, the ongoing management of the AI system was designed to be community-driven, with regular updates and feedback cycles to ensure the technology remained aligned with community needs. Ethical guidelines were strictly adhered to, ensuring data privacy and respect for cultural integrity. This case study not only underscores the potential of AI to transform healthcare in resource-limited settings but also highlights the necessity for culturally informed technology deployments that respect and embrace local knowledge systems.

### Case Study: Empowerment Through Technology: Building AI Systems with Native American Healing Practices

In an innovative move to decolonize medical AI, a unique project was launched to integrate Native American healing practices into an AI-driven healthcare system for a tribal area in the Southwestern United States. The project was initiated by a partnership between a leading technology university, local tribal health authorities, and spiritual leaders. The objective was to develop a healthcare AI that not only provided diagnostic and treatment options based on Western medicine but also incorporated traditional Native American practices such as herbal medicine, spiritual healing, and community wellness rituals.

The initial phase involved the comprehensive collection of data. Tribal healers and elders participated in data gathering, sharing detailed knowledge on traditional remedies, healing ceremonies, and the cultural context of health, which often includes a holistic view of physical, mental, and spiritual wellness. However, significant challenges emerged in translating this qualitatively rich traditional data into formats usable by AI systems. Another core issue was the ethical concern regarding the digitization of sacred and culturally sensitive information, which necessitated the creation of a framework that respected tribal data sovereignty and ensured the community retained control over their intellectual property.

To tackle these challenges, the project team implemented extensive training programs in cultural competency for AI developers and set up an ongoing dialogue between technologists and tribal members. This educational exchange helped the developers understand the deep cultural significances of the data they were handling. Additionally, the AI system was designed to operate with an adjustable algorithm, capable of evolving with continuing input from tribal health experts to refine its recommendations, ensuring that it stayed culturally relevant and sensitive.

The implementation of this culturally aware AI system had profound impacts. It not only improved health outcomes by integrating holistic practices into treatment plans but also empowered the community by validating their traditional knowledge through modern technology. The project stands as a profound example of how technology can be used to bridge cultural divides, respect cultural sovereignty, and enhance healthcare through the thoughtful integration of diverse medical systems.

**Case Study: Revamping Health AI in Southeast Asia: Incorporating Regional Herbal Medicine Practices**

In an ambitious project in Southeast Asia, a regional health consortium collaborated with AI engineers to develop an AI system that integrates regional herbal medicine practices with contemporary medical diagnostics. The objective was to incorporate the rich herbal knowledge that has been passed down through generations in countries like Vietnam, Thailand, and Indonesia into a cutting-edge AI system designed to enhance diagnostic accuracy and suggest culturally relevant treatments.

The project began by creating a comprehensive database of herbal treatments known in the region, including details about plant species, preparation methods, traditional usage, and known medical research related to their efficacy. However, integrating this extensive, diverse botanical knowledge into a usable format for AI posed a considerable challenge due to the vast differences in language, terminology, and medical documentation standards across the countries involved.

To address these issues, the consortium employed a team of ethnobotanists, local traditional healers, and AI linguistics experts who collaborated to standardize herbal medicine data into a digital format that the AI could process. They developed a unique tagging system to handle the variety of languages and dialects, ensuring the AI could accurately interpret the traditional names and uses of plants and herbs.

Simultaneously, ethical considerations were paramount, as the team had to balance the protection of indigenous knowledge with its accessibility for AI use. Legal frameworks were developed in collaboration with local governments to ensure that the intellectual property rights of the traditional healers were respected and that communities would benefit from the commercial use of their ancestral knowledge.

As the system was implemented, ongoing workshops and training sessions were conducted for local healthcare providers on how to interact with the AI system effectively. This training ensured they understood how to interpret the AI's recommendations and incorporate them into their medical practice. Challenges such as technological acceptance among traditional practitioners, who were initially skeptical, were mitigated through continuous dialogue and by demonstrating the AI's effectiveness in enhancing diagnostic outcomes and patient satisfaction.

## Case Study: Culturally Sensitive AI Development in Mental Health Applications for Remote Indigenous Communities

In a pioneering initiative to enhance mental health services, an international health technology company collaborated with remote indigenous communities in Northern Canada to develop a culturally sensitive AI-driven mental health diagnostic and support tool. This initiative aimed to address the disproportionate mental health challenges faced by these communities due to geographical isolation, historical trauma, and socioeconomic factors. The project began with a comprehensive participatory approach where community elders, health practitioners, and mental health experts were engaged to gather insights into the unique mental health narratives and healing practices of these communities.

The challenges were multifold, starting with building an AI system that understands and respects the cultural nuances and traditional mental health practices. The team faced technical challenges in integrating diverse non-Western medical terminologies into the AI's understanding. Additionally, there was a strong concern amongst community members about the confidentiality and ethical handling of sensitive cultural and personal data. To address these issues, the development team implemented stringent data protection measures. It developed the AI to handle data in a culturally respectful manner, ensuring that anonymity and control remained within the community.

Training sessions were conducted for both the tech developers and community members, where developers were educated on cultural sensitivities, and community members were instructed on the potential benefits and operations of the AI tool. This bi-directional knowledge exchange was crucial in making the AI tool relevant and accessible.

Furthermore, periodic assessments and feedback systems were implemented to ensure that the AI system continually evolved in line with the community's needs and preferences. Legal frameworks were also established, outlining clear guidelines on data ownership, usage, and sharing to protect cultural sovereignty and foster trust between technology providers and the community. This case study highlights the complexities involved in creating effective, culturally nuanced health AI systems and underscores the importance of community involvement, continuous learning, and legal protections in decolonizing medical AI applications.

### Case Study: Harnessing AI for Maternal Health in Rural Indian Contexts by Integrating Ayurvedic Practices

In a groundbreaking initiative aimed at reducing maternal mortality rates in rural India, a health tech company collaborated with local Ayurvedic practitioners to develop an AI-powered maternal healthcare app. This tool integrates conventional medical knowledge with traditional Ayurvedic practices, providing comprehensive guidance on prenatal and postnatal care to expectant mothers in under-resourced rural areas. The project began with an extensive data collection phase, during which we engaged deeply with communities to gather both modern and traditional health knowledge and translated Ayurvedic concepts into digital form.

One of the primary challenges faced was integrating holistic Ayurvedic treatment methods, which focus heavily on diet, lifestyle, and mind-body wellness, with more conventional medical protocols. The AI model needed to be sophisticated enough to offer personalized recommendations based on the complex interplay of these factors. Additionally, issues of cultural sensitivity and the local population's acceptance of AI recommendations had to be navigated carefully, as they often prefer traditional methods over modern medicine.

To promote acceptance and efficacy, the development team organized numerous community involvement initiatives, including workshops and interactive sessions, where community feedback was actively solicited and incorporated into the AI development process. This not only helped refine the AI algorithms for greater accuracy and relevance but also enhanced community trust in the technological solution.

Another key aspect of the project was ensuring the ethical use and privacy of the collected data. Stringent measures were implemented to guard against any potential misuse of personal and community health data. Moreover, ongoing training for both healthcare providers and end-users was essential to ensure the correct use and interpretation of the AI-driven advice, which is crucial for achieving better health outcomes.

This case not only showcases the potential of integrating traditional and modern medical knowledge through AI but also highlights the challenges of cultural adaptation, ethical considerations, and the importance of community-centric approaches in health technology innovations.

### Case Study: Advancing Pediatric Healthcare in Mongolia through AI and Shamanic Practices

In Mongolia, a unique project was launched to integrate AI with traditional Shamanic practices to advance pediatric healthcare. The initiative, driven by a collaboration between international AI developers, local healthcare providers, and Shamanic healers, aimed to address the high rates of respiratory and infectious diseases among children in rural areas. The project began by gathering extensive ethnographic and medical data on local health practices, environmental factors, and prevalent pediatric conditions.

The initial challenge was to bridge the substantial cultural and technological gap between modern healthcare techniques and deeply rooted Shamanic traditions. This involved translating Shamanic health rituals and herbal remedies into data formats compatible with AI algorithms while ensuring the preservation and respect for the cultural significance of these practices. AI developers and data scientists collaborated closely with Shamanic practitioners to create a culturally sensitive AI model that could suggest health interventions, combining the best of both worlds.

As the project evolved, several ethical and logistical challenges emerged. Key among them was ensuring the sovereignty of Shamanic knowledge and preventing its misappropriation. To tackle this, the project implemented strict protocols for data usage and established a local oversight committee comprising elders and healers to govern the usage of traditional knowledge. Additionally, language barriers and the high variability in regional health practices necessitated the development of a multilingual AI interface and adaptive algorithms that can learn from diverse health inputs.

The integration process was facilitated through continuous community engagement, including workshops to foster understanding and trust between the local communities and the AI team. Feedback mechanisms were established to enable ongoing refinement of the AI system based on real-world outcomes and community insights. The project not only improved healthcare delivery but also empowered the local population by integrating traditional practices through their integration into cutting-edge AI technology.

### Case Study: Reinventing Maternal Healthcare in Remote Nepali Villages Using AI and Local Healing Traditions

In an innovative approach to addressing the high maternal mortality rates in remote Nepali villages, a collaborative project was initiated between a global health tech company, local healthcare workers, and community healers. The primary goal was to develop an AI-driven healthcare system that integrates Western medical protocols with Nepali traditional healing methods, specifically targeting prenatal and postnatal care.

The project embarked on an extensive data collection phase, during which healthcare practices, herbal medicine knowledge, and local health beliefs were documented with the assistance of local midwives and herbalists. The challenge was not only to digitize this traditional knowledge but also to ensure that the AI systems could understand and apply it in a medically relevant manner. Concerns about cultural sensitivity and the potential for misappropriation of local knowledge were addressed through continuous community engagement and the establishment of a community-led oversight committee to guide the project.

One significant hurdle was the development of AI algorithms capable of integrating this diverse data into coherent and reliable medical advice. The AI system was designed to suggest not only Western medical treatments but also traditional remedies and practices that were familiar and culturally acceptable to the local population. Ethical concerns about data privacy and ownership were accentuated, given the sensitive nature of health data and the potential commercial implications of traditional knowledge.

As the system was implemented, ongoing training sessions were conducted for both local health workers and the community to ensure a proper understanding and operation of the AI system. These sessions also served as feedback loops to gather insights on the system's effectiveness and areas for improvement.

This case study highlights the complexities involved in integrating modern technology with traditional knowledge, emphasizing the importance of cultural sensitivity, community engagement, and ethical considerations in global health initiatives. It underscores the potential of AI to aid in critical health areas, such as maternal health, by leveraging local and global knowledge systems synergistically.

## Review Questions

**1. During a public health campaign in a rural area with a significant Indigenous population, an AI-enhanced mobile application was introduced to assist with diabetes management. The app integrated Western medical advice with local traditional practices, such as herbal remedies and dietary customs. Over six months, the community experienced improved diabetes control and increased adherence to treatment plans. However, concerns were raised about data privacy and cultural sensitivity. A local health worker is reviewing the impact of the AI application. Given the mixed outcomes, what should the health worker emphasize in their report to ensure continued improvements in community health outcomes?**

A) Enhance the AI app's algorithm to focus solely on Western medical advice and reduce dependency on traditional practices.

B) Recommend discontinuing the use of the AI app due to privacy concerns and revert to conventional health promotion methods.

C) Suggest modifications to the AI app to further integrate traditional practices and enhance data security measures to address privacy concerns.

D) Focus solely on expanding access to traditional healing practices while eliminating the AI-enhanced mobile application.

**Answer: C**

Explanation: The AI-enhanced application, which integrates Western and traditional practices, demonstrated improved diabetes management and treatment adherence, indicating that the blend of medical approaches resonates well with the community's needs and preferences. However, concerns about data privacy and cultural sensitivity are significant. In the health worker's report, it is crucial to address these concerns to continue reaping the benefits of the AI application's positive impacts. Option C suggests a balanced approach by further enhancing the integration of traditional practices, which acknowledges and respects the community's cultural practices, contributing to the positive outcomes. Simultaneously, recommending enhancements to data security measures tackles the valid concerns about privacy, ensuring that community members feel safe and respected in their interactions with the AI application. This approach fosters trust and willingness to engage with the AI tool, potentially leading to even better health outcomes.

**2.** An elderly patient from a remote Indigenous community has been utilizing an AI-based home health monitoring system. The patient has reported feeling more empowered about managing their chronic condition, thanks to the tailored advice that combines traditional herbal remedies with standard medical treatments. Despite the benefits, the local healthcare provider is concerned about the inclusion of spiritual healing practices, which are significant to the patient's well-being, in the AI system's recommendations. What should the healthcare provider do to ensure the AI system is respectful and inclusive of the patient's spiritual practices?

A) Dismiss the spiritual practices as scientifically unproven and focus the AI system solely on evidence-based medical treatments.

B) Program the AI system to recognize mentions of spiritual practices as indicators of psychological distress and recommend psychiatric evaluation.

C) Engage with community spiritual leaders to understand the role of spiritual practices in healing and consult on integrating respectful references and support for these practices in the AI system.

D) Fully replace the AI recommendations with directives from the community's spiritual leaders to ensure cultural authenticity.

**Answer: C**

Explanation: Respecting and integrating patients' spiritual practices in healthcare delivery, especially for Indigenous populations, is essential for holistic care that aligns with cultural beliefs and contributes to effective treatment outcomes. Option C acknowledges the importance of spiritual practices and involves community spiritual leaders, who are critical stakeholders in cultural health practices, in the consultative process. This approach ensures that the AI system can be sensitively programmed to respect and integrate these elements without oversimplifying or misinterpreting them. It enables the AI to support the patient's spiritual practices alongside medical treatment, enhancing the patient's comfort and trust in the system. This method avoids the extremes of entirely dismissing spiritual practices (Option A) or misinterpreting them as psychological issues (Option B) and is more balanced and practical than replacing medical advice with spiritual directives alone (Option D).

**Role of Data in AI's Crafting of Medical Narratives**

**Defining Medical Narratives in the Context of AI**

In the realm of healthcare, 'medical narratives' traditionally encapsulate the stories and experiences of patients, woven through clinical encounters and personal histories. However, as artificial intelligence (AI) becomes increasingly prevalent in medicine, the definition of medical narratives assumes new dimensions.

AI interprets these narratives not just through textual patient data but also through vast arrays of biometric and behavioral information. This technological shift necessitates a broader understanding of what constitutes a narrative in medical practice. AI's ability to analyze data at unprecedented scale and speed allows for a more holistic view of patient stories, yet this comes with the challenge of integrating disparate data types without losing the nuance of individual experiences.

Moreover, defining medical narratives in the context of AI involves ensuring these technologies grasp and respect the cultural significance and personal context that influence health decisions and outcomes. It's about programming AI to not only read the data but to understand the stories behind the numbers.

**The Importance of Data Quality in Medical AI**

The cornerstone of effective AI-driven healthcare lies in the integrity of the data it uses. High-quality data not only empowers AI to make precise medical predictions but also ensures that those predictions are equitable and representative of all populations. Poor data quality can lead to misdiagnoses and unequal healthcare services, magnifying existing healthcare disparities.

The quest for quality data involves rigorous methodologies for collecting, processing, and analyzing information. This ensures that the data is accurate, complete, and timely. It is essential to involve diverse populations during data collection stages to prevent bias. After all, the inclusivity of data determines the AI's ability to serve a broad spectrum of individuals.

Furthermore, maintaining data quality is an ongoing challenge that requires continuous oversight and refinement. Healthcare professionals must play a pivotal role in validating and updating data to keep pace with emerging health trends and scientific discoveries. This dynamic process enables the creation of AI tools that are not only scientifically proficient but also culturally sensitive and ethically sound.

**Sources of Data for AI in Healthcare**

In the expansive domain of healthcare, AI draws from a myriad of data sources, each contributing uniquely to the medical narratives it constructs. Traditional datasets originate from the clinical environment, encompassing electronic health records (EHRs), imaging data, and laboratory results. These form the backbone of AI's understanding, providing structured and high-volume data that is inherently rich in medical context.

Beyond conventional medical data, AI also integrates information from wearables and personal health devices. These sources provide continuous streams of physiological data, which are crucial for personalized medicine but pose challenges in terms of consistency and standardization. Additionally, social determinants of health (SDH) data, which include socioeconomic status, education, and environmental factors, are becoming increasingly pivotal. This type of data broadens AI's scope, enabling a more holistic approach to patient health narratives; however, it introduces complexities in data interpretation and raises privacy concerns.

Collating these diverse sources necessitates sophisticated data harmonization techniques to ensure AI models are not only predictive but also equitable. Efforts to harness these varied data streams are further complicated by the need for robust privacy protections and methodologies sensitive to cultural contexts, ensuring that AI technologies respect and accurately reflect the diverse tapestry of global health practices.

**AI Interpretation of Clinical Data**

The interpretation of clinical data by AI transcends traditional data analysis, offering profound insights into patient health through complex algorithmic processing. This process involves parsing through structured data, such as lab results, and unstructured data, including physicians' notes, and merging them into comprehensive patient profiles.

Despite its potential, the AI's performance hinges on the underlying data's diversity and completeness. An AI system trained primarily on datasets that lack representation from diverse populations may exhibit biased outcomes. This necessitates rigorous scrutiny and continuous calibration of AI systems to ensure interpretations are accurate and universally applicable across different demographic groups.

Moreover, the interpretative mechanisms of AI must be transparent to facilitate trust among healthcare providers. Doctors need to understand how AI conclusions are derived to integrate this technology into their clinical decision-making processes effectively. Ensuring this transparency also aids in identifying and rectifying any biases, reinforcing the reliability of AI in medical diagnostics and treatment planning.

**Data Mining Techniques in Medical Narratives**

Data mining in medical narratives leverages sophisticated algorithms to extract meaningful patterns from vast datasets, which include both structured and unstructured data. This technique is pivotal in transforming raw data into actionable insights, crucial for personalized healthcare. By applying methods such as clustering, classification, and association rule mining, AI can uncover hidden correlations and predict patient outcomes with greater accuracy.

However, the effectiveness of these techniques heavily depends on the quality and diversity of the data fed into AI systems. Ensuring that data encompasses various demographics and conditions is crucial to prevent biases and ensure equitable treatment recommendations. Moreover, the application of data mining must be guided by ethical considerations, respecting patient confidentiality and ensuring data security.

The integration of narrative analysis through natural language processing further refines data mining, enabling AI to understand and utilize patient stories and clinical notes. This integration enriches medical AI applications, fostering a more holistic approach to patient care by contextualizing quantitative data with human experiences.

## Role of Big Data in Personalized Medicine

The big data revolution is transforming personalized medicine by enabling the aggregation and analysis of vast datasets to tailor treatments to individual patients. Through the collection of genomics, environmental, and lifestyle data, AI systems can design highly specific medical interventions tailored to the unique genetic makeup and circumstances of everyone. This precision targets the root causes of diseases with remarkable accuracy, enhancing treatment efficacy and patient outcomes.

Moreover, big data facilitates the continuous monitoring of patient health, allowing for dynamic adjustments to treatment plans as more data becomes available. This iterative process, powered by real-time data streams from wearable technologies, provides an ongoing assessment that can preemptively tweak therapies before complications arise, demonstrating a proactive rather than reactive approach to healthcare.

However, the reliance on big data also introduces challenges such as ensuring data privacy and managing data biases. It is crucial to establish strict governance and ethical standards to protect sensitive information and ensure that AI systems do not perpetuate existing health disparities.

## AI Algorithms for Data Synthesis and Analysis

AI algorithms stand at the heart of data synthesis and analysis, serving as pivotal tools for integrating and interpreting diverse medical data. These algorithms are designed to process and synthesize large datasets, transforming them into coherent, actionable insights that can inform medical decisions. By utilizing techniques such as machine learning and deep learning, AI can analyze patterns and anomalies within data, predict outcomes, and suggest personalized treatment plans.

The synthesis process encompasses the aggregation of various data types, including both structured and unstructured data. AI algorithms adeptly navigate this complexity, offering a nuanced understanding of patient health that spans genetic information, lifestyle factors, and previous medical history. This capability not only streamlines the diagnostic process but also enhances the accuracy of medical interventions.

However, the analysis performed by AI must be continuously monitored for accuracy and bias. Ensuring that AI algorithms are trained on diverse datasets is crucial to maintaining fairness and effectiveness in medical treatment. This ongoing calibration helps mitigate the risk of biased AI decisions that could adversely affect patient care outcomes.

## Ethical Collection and Use of Medical Data

The ethical collection and use of medical data in AI applications are cornerstones of trustworthy medical practice and technological advancement. Emphasizing ethical guidelines ensures data acquisition processes respect patient rights and data confidentiality. This involves obtaining informed consent, a critical process where patients are aware that their data may be used in AI models and understand the implications of such use.

Beyond acquisition, ethical use also dictates how data is handled, stored, and shared. Striving for transparency, AI systems must disclose data usage policies to users, clarifying how personal data contributes to medical analysis and outcomes. This transparency builds trust among stakeholders, ensuring that all participants recognize their contributory role in refining AI-driven healthcare.

Moreover, the ethical framework must address data integrity, ensuring that datasets are not only representative but also unbiased and accurate. Regular audits and updates to AI models are essential for maintaining ethical standards, thereby guarding against the perpetuation of inequities in healthcare. Rigorous oversight by independent bodies can enforce these standards, providing a safeguard against misuse and enhancing public confidence in AI-enhanced medical solutions.

**Bias in Data Collection and Its Impact on AI Outcomes**

Bias in data collection fundamentally skews AI-driven outcomes in medicine, fostering disparities rather than curtailing them. Primarily, data sourced from limited demographics shapes AI algorithms to favor certain groups, potentially marginalizing underrepresented or minority communities. This skew in data sets primarily affects diagnostic accuracy and treatment effectiveness, placing unequal healthcare burdens on specific populations.

Addressing bias requires a deliberate broadening of data sources to include diverse patient histories, cultures, and geographies. It necessitates an ethical revamp of data collection practices to ensure inclusivity and fairness. Without interventions to rectify biased data, AI systems inadvertently perpetuate existing inequalities, contravening principles of ethical medical care.

Effectively tackling these issues involves implementing robust frameworks for regular review and calibration of AI models to align with diverse population needs. Moreover, engaging various stakeholders, including patients from diverse backgrounds, in the AI development process enhances the representation and relevance of AI applications in healthcare. Ensuring equitable AI outcomes is not just a technical challenge but a fundamental ethical imperative.

**Ensuring Data Privacy and Security in Medical AI**

Ensuring data privacy and security in medical AI is imperative, as these systems often handle sensitive personal health information. To safeguard this data, robust encryption methods must be employed during both storage and transmission. This prevents unauthorized access and potential data breaches, which could have devastating consequences for patient confidentiality and trust in medical systems.

Furthermore, implementing strict access controls is essential. These controls ensure that only authorized personnel can view or modify sensitive information. Regular audits and compliance checks help maintain these security protocols, ensuring they adapt to new threats over time, thereby fortifying the data's integrity.

To complement technical safeguards, clear legal and regulatory frameworks must be established. These frameworks guide the ethical use of AI in healthcare, stipulating how data can be ethically collected, used, and shared. Ensuring adherence to these regulations not only protects individual rights but also builds societal trust in AI applications within medicine.

**Integration of Multi-Source Data in AI Models**

The integration of multi-source data in AI models plays a critical role in enhancing the comprehensiveness and accuracy of medical narratives. This process involves combining data from various sources, including electronic health records, genomic databases, wearable technology outputs, and even social determinants of health, fostering a holistic view of patient wellness.

By leveraging diverse data streams, AI technologies can deliver more precise and personalized medical insights. For instance, correlating lifestyle information with clinical data allows AI systems to predict potential health risks with greater accuracy, thereby facilitating early interventions. This cross-referencing not only enhances treatment plans but also allows healthcare providers to offer preventative advice based on a more complete understanding of the patient's health landscape.

However, the challenge lies in ensuring the seamless and secure integration of these varied data types. Interoperability standards and data harmonization techniques are crucial for minimizing errors and optimizing the functionality of AI systems in medical settings. Effective management of this integration process is essential to uphold data integrity and patient privacy, ensuring that AI's potential is fully harnessed in crafting nuanced medical narratives.

**Challenges in Standardizing Medical Data for AI**

Standardizing medical data for AI presents a myriad of challenges that stem from the inherent complexity and diversity of medical information. One major hurdle is the variability in data formats and terminologies used across different healthcare systems. Ensuring that disparate data sources speak a common language is crucial for AI algorithms to perform accurate analyses and generate reliable medical insights.

Moreover, the dynamic nature of traditional, indigenous and Native American medical knowledge adds another layer of complexity. On the one hand you have oral traditional medical narratives passed from one generation to the next, the value of which is based on their intrinsically unchanging values, and those of modern Western Medical standards and protocols evolving, necessitating continuous updates to the data standards to keep AI tools relevant and effective. The task is compounded by the need to balance detailed medical records with privacy considerations, ensuring that data standardization does not compromise patient confidentiality.

Finally, the drive towards standardization must consider the global diversity in medical practices and patient populations. Creating universal data standards that accommodate various medical systems and cultural contexts is pivotal. Without this, AI's potential to benefit a global populace is severely limited, undermining efforts to deploy AI universally in healthcare.

**Narrative Medicine and AI: Bridging Stories and Statistics**

Narrative medicine, which emphasizes the importance of patient stories and experiences in healthcare, finds a new dimension with AI integration. By synthesizing quantitative data and qualitative narratives, AI can offer a more holistic approach to patient care, tailoring treatments to individual stories and statistical evidence.

The process begins with the collection and analysis of vast datasets, including demographic information, clinical outcomes, and personal patient narratives. AI algorithms then process this information to identify patterns and correlations that might escape purely human analysis. This programmatic synthesis enables healthcare providers to approach treatment plans with a deeply personalized framework that respects both the statistical trends and the individual patient stories.

However, the success of marrying narrative medicine with AI heavily relies on the integrity and diversity of the data fed into AI systems. Ensuring that the narratives are as diverse and inclusive as the data points is crucial. It prevents the perpetuation of biases and improves the accuracy and empathy of AI-driven decisions. This integration demands continuous ethical oversight and active participation from diverse populations to enrich and validate the AI interpretations.

**Use of Natural Language Processing in Crafting Medical Narratives**

The integration of Natural Language Processing (NLP) in crafting medical narratives marks a transformative leap in how AI interprets and utilizes health-related data. NLP tools extrapolate nuanced meanings from unstructured text data, synthesizing patient histories into coherent narratives that enhance diagnostic and treatment processes. This facet of AI not only streamlines data analysis but also ensures that subtle linguistic cues are not overlooked, fostering a deeper understanding of patient needs.

However, the effectiveness of NLP in medical narratives hinges on the quality and diversity of the input data. Biases in textual data can lead NLP algorithms to draw skewed conclusions, potentially mirroring existing prejudices within healthcare. To mitigate this, it's essential that NLP systems are trained on a broad spectrum of linguistic inputs reflecting varied patient demographics and conditions.

Furthermore, ethical considerations in employing NLP demand rigorous oversight. It's paramount that data used is not only representative but also ethically sourced and processed, preserving patient dignity and confidentiality. As AI's role in healthcare evolves, ensuring that NLP tools are used responsibly will be crucial in maintaining trust and efficacy in medical AI applications.

**Machine Learning's Role in Understanding Patient Histories**

Machine learning (ML) dramatically enhances the understanding of patient histories by extracting and analyzing complex patterns from vast datasets. This technology processes historical health records to predict future health outcomes, facilitating personalized treatment strategies. By integrating diverse data such as past diagnoses, treatment responses, and family medical history, ML models offer a nuanced understanding of individual health trajectories.

However, the accuracy of these predictions depends significantly on the quality and breadth of data. ML algorithms can inadvertently reinforce biases if the training data is skewed towards certain populations. Ensuring a diverse data set is critical to avoid perpetuating existing disparities in healthcare outcomes.

Moreover, continual learning mechanisms allow ML models to adapt over time, reflecting changes in medical practices and patient conditions. This constant evolution in learning and adapting is pivotal for maintaining the relevance and accuracy of patient history analysis in dynamic medical environments.

**Data Integrity and Verification Processes**

Data integrity and verification are crucial in ensuring that AI systems in healthcare deliver accurate and reliable outcomes. These processes involve rigorous checks and balances designed to maintain the accuracy, consistency, and reliability of data throughout its lifecycle. Verification mechanisms play a pivotal role by detecting any anomalies or errors in the data before it enters the AI models, safeguarding against misleading AI interpretations and decisions.

One common approach includes the use of advanced algorithms that scrutinize data for usual patterns or missing elements. Moreover, regular audits and updates are integral to adapting to new medical standards and protocols, thus keeping the data relevant and valid over time. This ongoing process requires sophisticated tools and expert knowledge in data science and medicine.

Collaboration between data scientists, clinicians, and IT specialists is essential to construct and uphold robust verification systems. Through concerted effort, healthcare institutions can enhance the performance of AI applications, ensuring that patient care is both effective and informed by the most accurate data available.

## Impact of Incomplete Data on AI Medical Recommendations

The integrity of AI-derived medical recommendations hinges significantly on the completeness of the data used. Incomplete data sets can lead to skewed AI analyses, creating gaps in medical advice and potentially harmful care outcomes. When crucial information is missing, AI systems may fail to identify critical patterns, misinterpreting patient needs or overlooking significant health risks.

The implications of these deficiencies are profound, especially when considering chronic diseases or complex conditions where comprehensive data is vital for accurate diagnosis and management. Inadequate data can result in AI systems making conservative or generic recommendations, thus failing to tailor specialized interventions that suit individual patient profiles.

To mitigate these risks, it is essential to implement robust data collection protocols that ensure comprehensiveness and diversity. Moreover, continuous monitoring and updating of AI algorithms are imperative to adapt to new health data inputs, enhancing the system's accuracy over time. Ensuring the completeness of data not only improves the safety and efficacy of AI in medicine but also builds trust among healthcare professionals and patients alike.

## Developing AI Systems for Dynamic Data Interpretation

The endeavor to develop AI systems for dynamic data interpretation in medical settings challenges the way we understand and utilize health information. As the nature of data rapidly evolves with incoming real-time health metrics, AI systems must adapt to interpret these streams effectively. This demands architectures that not only process static data but also integrate continuous data feeds, assessing changes in patient conditions in real-time.

Key to this process is the implementation of adaptive learning technologies. These systems refine their algorithms based on new data, thereby enhancing predictive accuracies. Transitioning from static historical data models to dynamic interpretation frameworks requires AI to handle variable data volumes and formats seamlessly, ensuring that every piece of data, regardless of its origin, contributes to a holistic understanding of a patient's health narrative.

Such dynamic systems are pivotal for personalizing patient care, allowing for interventions that are timely and more accurately aligned with the patient's current health status. To achieve this, collaborative efforts between data scientists, medical professionals, and AI developers are essential, creating synergies that propel forward the capabilities of medical AI systems.

## Case Studies: AI's Success and Failures in Medical Storytelling

The narrative of AI in medicine includes tales of both remarkable success and notable failures. Through various case studies, we observe how AI systems like IBM Watson have excelled in diagnosing rare cancers, integrating vast datasets to provide insights that had previously eluded medical professionals. These successes often hinge on the robustness of data and advanced algorithmic interpretations that offer a precision approach to patient care.

Conversely, there are cases where AI's limitations have led to less favorable outcomes. In instances where bias in the training data was present, AI applications have misrepresented or overlooked symptoms in minority populations, leading to misdiagnoses or inappropriate treatment plans. Such failures underscore the critical need for diverse and comprehensive datasets in training AI.

These contrasting scenarios illustrate the dichotomy of AI in medical storytelling. They underscore the importance of ongoing scrutiny, refinement, and ethical oversight to harness AI's potential responsibly. As AI continues to evolve, these case studies serve as pivotal learning points, guiding future implementations towards more accurate and equitable healthcare solutions.

## Future Technologies Enhancing Data Utilization in AI

As we look to the horizon of medical AI, emerging technologies promise intriguing advancements in data utilization, portending a transformative effect on healthcare efficacy and personalization. Quantum computing, for instance, holds potential to exponentially speed up data processing, allowing AI to analyze complex medical data sets in fractions of the current time. This acceleration could lead to quicker, more accurate medical assessments and potentially life-saving diagnoses.

Additionally, blockchain technology is being explored for its capacity to enhance data integrity and security in healthcare AI applications. By decentralizing data storage, blockchain could significantly reduce the risks of data tampering and breaches, ensuring that medical information remains both secure and pristine across multiple points of access.

Moreover, the integration of augmented reality (AR) in medical AI could revolutionize how data is visualized and interpreted by healthcare professionals. AR systems could project patient data directly into the physical examination space, providing doctors with real-time, enhanced insights into patient health metrics. Such technologies not only promise to refine the precision of medical assessments but also bridge the gap between digital data and human touch in patient care.

## Training AI to Recognize Contextual Elements in Data

The sophistication of AI in healthcare hinges on its ability to discern and interpret contextual elements within vast pools of data. Training AI involves instilling a layer of context-awareness, thus enabling it to project nuanced medical narratives. This facet of AI training intersects with linguistic models and psychological understanding, constructing algorithms that recognize subtleties in patient histories and environmental factors affecting health patterns.

For instance, AI systems can be educated on regional health trends and genetic predispositions associated with certain demographics. Deploying advanced machine learning techniques, such as supervised learning and semi-supervised learning, enriches AI's scope to include socio-economic statuses and cultural attitudes towards treatments. This data contextualization enhances AI's predictive accuracy, offering a more comprehensive, personalized approach to patient care.

Moreover, ongoing efforts focus on the responsive integration of new contextual updates into AI frameworks, maintaining their relevance as medical standards evolve. Through collaborative efforts between computer scientists, cultural scholars, and medical providers, AI is geared towards a more empathetic and precise understanding of global health narratives.

## Role of Healthcare Professionals in Data Governance

Healthcare professionals hold a crucial role in data governance within AI-driven medical systems. Their firsthand experience with patient care and clinical procedures provides invaluable insights into data relevance and security. By working closely with AI developers and data scientists, clinicians ensure that AI systems are not only technically proficient but also contextually appropriate and ethically sound.

Moreover, their direct involvement in the data governance process aids in maintaining the accuracy and integrity of the data collected. This collaborative oversight helps to safeguard against biases and erroneous interpretations that could negatively impact patient outcomes. Training sessions tailored to help healthcare workers understand and maneuver within AI ecosystems are vital.

Thus, the proactive engagement of healthcare professionals in data governance establishes a framework of trust and accountability. It is imperative for hospitals and health systems to leverage their expertise to foster AI solutions that genuinely enhance patient-centered care and uphold the highest standards of medical ethics.

## Public and Patient Involvement in Data Collection

The involvement of patients and the public in data collection transforms the landscape of AI in medicine. By contributing to the data pools used for training AI, individuals offer a richer, more expansive dataset that encompasses a broader spectrum of health experiences and outcomes. This diversity in data is crucial for developing AI systems that cater to varied medical needs across different populations.

Engagement strategies include patient surveys, participatory data gathering initiatives, and transparent communication about the use and impact of contributed data. These methods not only enhance the quantity and quality of data but also bolster public trust in AI applications in healthcare. Moreover, inclusive data practices ensure that AI systems become more adept at recognizing and interpreting the subtle nuances in patient-reported information, which are often overlooked in conventional datasets.

Finally, fostering a culture of active patient involvement necessitates continuous education and feedback mechanisms to keep communities informed and engaged. Cooperative efforts in data collection serve as a cornerstone for building equitable AI-driven medical systems that truly understand and address the health disparities experienced by underrepresented groups.

## Regulatory and Legal Considerations in Medical Data Usage

Navigating the complex terrain of regulations and legal frameworks is crucial for the deployment of AI in healthcare. This subheading addresses the essential legal considerations that impact the utilization of medical data in AI systems, underscoring the need for compliance with laws like HIPAA in the U.S., which safeguards patient privacy, and GDPR in Europe, which sets stringent data protection standards.

Furthermore, the development and application of AI technologies must adhere to ethical guidelines that prioritize patient safety and confidentiality. Legal scrutiny ensures that AI applications do not misuse or mishandle sensitive medical data, fostering a culture of trust and security in healthcare technology. As AI continues to evolve, so too must the regulatory policies that govern its application, ensuring they are robust enough to keep pace with technological advancements.

It is imperative for AI developers and healthcare providers to stay informed about these regulations and actively engage in policy discussions. This proactive approach not only mitigates legal risks but also enhances the efficacy and acceptance of AI in medical practice.

## Summary

The intensive integration of Artificial Intelligence (AI) in healthcare redefines traditional medical narratives, encompassing not just patient experiences but expanding significantly to include biometric, behavioral, and vast arrays of digitized health-related data. This transformation enables a more comprehensive understanding of patient stories, critically facilitated by AI's capacity to analyze large datasets swiftly and efficiently. AI-driven approaches in healthcare hinge fundamentally on the quality of data, which must be not only comprehensive and timely but must also embody the diverse spectra of the population to prevent intrinsic biases and promote equitable healthcare solutions.

AI in healthcare extracts data from numerous traditional and modern sources including electronic health records (EHRs), genomic data, wearables, and even socio-economic determinants, striving for a holistic outlook on a patient's health trajectory. The challenge lies in harmonizing these multifaceted data streams while ensuring privacy and ethical compliance, particularly when dealing with sensitive health information. The precision of AI's data analysis significantly impacts medical diagnostics and personalized treatment plans, where data synthesis and interpretation by AI algorithms involve constant verification to avoid biases and ensure accurate, equitable health assessments and outcomes.

Furthermore, AI technologies must be transparent in their data processing methods to gain trust among healthcare providers, allowing for an effective inclusion into clinical settings. Ethical considerations are paramount, involving rigorous data integrity, continuous monitoring, and updates to comply with evolving medical standards. Ensuring the ethical collection and use of medical data not only fosters trust but also enhances patient outcomes by adhering to strict privacy and security guidelines.

In conclusion, the role of data in AI-driven medical narratives is crucial and multifaceted, requiring ongoing innovation in data collection, processing, and analysis to fully harness AI's potential while maintaining ethical standards and patient-centered care in a rapidly evolving digital healthcare landscape.

## References

[1] Health Affairs. https://www.healthaffairs.org/do/10.1377/hblog20200903.522478/full/
[2] Journal of Biomedical Informatics. https://www.sciencedirect.com/science/article/pii/S1532046419303104
[3] Nature Medicine. https://www.nature.com/articles/s41591-019-0711-0
[4] AMA Journal of Ethics. https://journalofethics.ama-assn.org/article/big-data-electronic-health-records-and-ethics/2017-10
[5] Journal of Medical Internet Research. https://www.jmir.org/2020/10/e23430/
[6] IEEE Journal of Biomedical and Health Informatics. https://ieeexplore.ieee.org/document/7400936

## Case Study: Integrating AI in Epidemic Response: The Case of Real-Time Data Synthesis

In the throes of the 2025 global influenza outbreak, health organizations deployed advanced AI systems to better manage the epidemic. This case centers around HealthAI, an AI system designed to incorporate real-time clinical, genomic, and socio-environmental data to predict outbreak patterns and guide public health interventions.

HealthAI integrated data from multiple sources, including electronic health records (EHRs), wearables from infected and at-risk individuals, and publicly available transportation and mobility data. The AI system processed this diverse data corpus using machine learning algorithms tailored to recognize and interpret patterns indicative of viral transmission and mutation rates. As the epidemic progressed, HealthAI's predictive models adapted dynamically, reflecting the rapid changes in the virus's spread and the effectiveness of mitigation strategies. This real-time synthesis enabled health authorities to allocate resources more efficiently, tailoring public health messages and interventions to specific demographics and geographical locales.

However, the execution wasn't without challenges. The integration of vast and varied data sources proved computationally intensive and highlighted significant disparities in data quality and availability. In some regions, poor digital infrastructure limited the accuracy of real-time predictions. Moreover, ethical concerns arose regarding the privacy and security of personal data, prompting rigorous debates on the balance between individual rights and collective safety. Additionally, biases in initial training data led to overlooked outbreaks in underserved communities until corrective measures enhanced the algorithms' inclusivity.

This analysis not only demonstrates the potential of AI in managing health crises through nuanced, real-time data synthesis but also underscores the importance of robust data governance, ethical guidelines, and continuous algorithmic refinement to address biases and ensure equitable health outcomes.

**Case Study: Harnessing AI for Cardiovascular Disease Prediction: A Comprehensive Data Approach**

In a landmark initiative launched in 2024, a consortium of medical research institutions and technology companies collaborated to develop HeartSmartAI, a sophisticated AI system aimed at predicting cardiovascular diseases (CVD) among high-risk populations. This case study delves into HeartSmartAI's deployment, focusing on its ability to integrate and analyze comprehensive data sources to enhance prediction accuracy and patient outcomes.

HeartSmartAI was designed to process a wide array of data types, including electronic health records (EHRs), genetic data, patient self-reported input from mobile health applications, and real-time biometric data from wearable devices. The system used advanced machine learning algorithms to detect subtle patterns and correlations that could indicate early signs of CVD.

The project faced substantial challenges, particularly concerning data harmonization and privacy concerns. Data from various sources needed to be standardized to ensure consistency and accuracy. The diversity in data types—ranging from structured numeric readings to unstructured textual notes—required sophisticated data preprocessing techniques to transform them into a uniform format that the AI could process. Moreover, stringent measures were implemented to safeguard patient data privacy, complying with global data protection regulations such as GDPR and HIPAA, which posed significant hurdles in data integration and real-time analysis.

Despite these challenges, HeartSmartAI demonstrated significant improvements in early CVD detection rates compared to traditional methods, which predominantly rely on symptomatic assessment and occasional health check-ups. The AI's ability to continuously monitor various health indicators allowed for a more dynamic assessment of patient health, often identifying risk factors that would be intermittently noticeable in periodic health evaluations.

HeartSmartAI's success prompted discussions about expanding the model to other chronic conditions, illustrating the potential of AI in transforming healthcare through comprehensive data analysis. However, the project underscored the need for ongoing innovation in data integration techniques, robust privacy safeguards, and continuous ethical oversight to mitigate biases and ensure equitable health outcomes.

**Case Study: Optimizing Diabetes Management with AI-Enhanced Predictive Modeling**

The projection and management of diabetes have become focal points in the utilization of AI technologies within healthcare. The scenario centers on DiaPredictAI, an AI-driven platform introduced by a collaboration of healthcare providers, tech companies, and academic research institutions in 2026. This platform was designed to enhance diabetes management by predicting individuals at high risk of developing diabetes and optimizing treatment regimens for patients with existing conditions.

DiaPredictAI utilized an extensive database, amalgamating electronic health records (EHRs), patient-reported lifestyle data from mobile health apps, and real-time metabolic data from wearable devices. Machine learning algorithms analyzed these diverse data pools to identify patterns that could predict diabetic tendencies before clinical symptoms became apparent. Extreme Value Theory (EVT) was incorporated to deal with outliers in the data, addressing the challenge of peaks in blood sugar levels that were previously difficult to anticipate consistently.

The deployment of DiaPredictAI faced considerable hurdles. The primary concern was harmonizing diverse data sources to ensure a seamless data integration process. The variable nature of data formats—from structured biometric readings to unstructured personal lifestyle logs—posed significant challenges for standardization and accuracy. Furthermore, conflicting data protection laws across different jurisdictions complicated the sharing of patient data needed for more holistic AI analysis.

Despite these challenges, DiaPredictAI markedly improved the management of patients prone to or actively dealing with diabetes. Early detection rates improved, allowing preemptive lifestyle and medication interventions, drastically reducing emergency incidents related to diabetic complications. Moreover, the tailored treatment plans based on continuous data streams facilitated more personalized and adaptive patient care strategies.

Such achievements underscore the critical role of advanced data synthesis and continuous learning algorithms in real-time health monitoring and disease management. However, they also highlight essential ongoing needs: sophisticated data harmonization techniques, resolution of legal and ethical concerns regarding data use, and ensuring equitable healthcare outcomes through meticulous AI design and implementation.

**Case Study: AI-Driven Oncology: Revolutionizing Cancer Care with Predictive Analytics**

In 2027, OncologyAI, a cutting-edge AI platform, was launched by a consortium of oncology centers and tech giants to transform cancer care through predictive analytics and personalized treatment plans. This case study explores how OncologyAI was specifically designed to harness complex algorithms to process diverse data sets, including genomic data, electronic health records (EHRs), imaging results, and patient-reported symptoms, to enhance the accuracy of cancer diagnosis and the efficacy of treatment protocols.

OncologyAI utilized deep learning models to detect patterns and anomalies in data that are often imperceptible to human analysts. One of its notable implementations was the integration of genomic sequencing data with real-time imaging scans to predict tumor growth trajectories and response to various chemotherapy agents. By doing this, OncologyAI was able to recommend personalized medication regimens that optimized effectiveness and minimized adverse effects, basing suggestions not only on medical histories but also genetic predispositions.

This sophisticated AI approach faced numerous challenges, primarily related to data diversity and volume, which necessitated the development of robust data preprocessing and standardization protocols to ensure seamless integration and interpretation. Additionally, there were significant ethical considerations around patient data privacy and the potential biases inherent in the training data sets. Concerns were particularly pronounced regarding the underrepresentation of certain ethnicities in genomic databases, which could lead to less optimized treatment for those populations.

Despite these hurdles, the implementation of OncologyAI marked a significant leap forward in oncology. Early trials showed a measurable decrease in the time taken to reach a definitive diagnosis, and treatment plans tailored by OncologyAI demonstrated improved patient outcomes in comparison to traditional approaches. The success of this AI system set a precedent for other medical specialties to follow, reinforcing the importance of continuous advancements in AI technology, comprehensive data collection, and stringent ethical standards to ensure the equitable and effective use of AI in medicine.

**Case Study: AI Enhancement in Geriatric Healthcare: A Multi-Modal Data Integration Approach**

The development of GeriCareAI presents a unique perspective on how artificial intelligence can impact geriatric care by integrating multi-modal data sources. This case study involves a pilot program launched in 2028 at a leading geriatric healthcare facility, which collaborated with a tech firm specializing in healthcare AI to develop and implement GeriCareAI. The AI system was designed to analyze and synthesize data from electronic health records (EHRs), continuous monitoring sensors, family history, and psychosocial assessments to improve care for the elderly.

Initially, GeriCareAI focused on predicting and managing chronic conditions prevalent among the elderly, such as dementia, arthritis, and heart disease. By leveraging data from sensors that monitor vital signs and daily activities, along with detailed medical histories and genomics information, GeriCareAI could provide caregivers with predictive insights that enhanced patient care plans. Additionally, the integration of psychosocial data helped tailor interventions that not only targeted physical health but also emotional and mental well-being.

However, the implementation of GeriCareAI was fraught with challenges. One major hurdle was the integration of heterogeneous data sources, each varying in format and completeness. To address this, the development team employed advanced data harmonization techniques, ensuring that disparate data types were standardized and merged accurately. Moreover, ethical concerns regarding the sufficiency of informed consent with elderly patients, who might have cognitive impairments, were thoroughly addressed through enhanced communication protocols and legal oversight.

The implications of this implementation were profound. GeriCareAI successfully reduced emergency hospital visits by 30% within the first year by enabling preemptive care interventions. It also improved the quality of life for patients by providing more personalized care plans based on comprehensive data analysis. However, the continuous refinement of algorithms was necessary to accommodate the evolving nature of medical data and to mitigate any potential biases that could arise from historical data. Overall, the case of GeriCareAI illuminates both the potential and the complexities involved in using AI to enhance geriatric care.

### Case Study: Leveraging AI for Personalized Mental Health Interventions: The SynapseAI Project

The SynapseAI project, initiated in 2029, represents a breakthrough in personalized mental health care guided by artificial intelligence. This initiative involved a consortium of mental health institutions, technology firms, and university research departments aiming to develop an AI system capable of providing tailored mental health interventions based on an individual's unique psychological profile and biometric data.

SynapseAI was designed to integrate diverse data sources, including electronic health records (EHRs), patient self-reported outcomes from mental health apps, continuous biometric monitoring through wearable devices, and environmental data. The system utilized a complex network of machine learning algorithms to analyze patterns in mood fluctuations, stress levels, and engagement in therapeutic activities. By correlating these patterns with historical mental health crises, SynapseAI sought to predict potential mental health episodes and recommend preemptive interventions.

The data synthesis process faced significant challenges, particularly in data privacy and the harmonization of data from heterogenous sources. Ensuring data consistency across various formats was crucial, as the combination of structured and unstructured data required sophisticated data preprocessing techniques. Privacy concerns were paramount, involving strict compliance with healthcare regulations such as HIPAA in the U.S. and GDPR in Europe, complicating the integration of deeply personal and sensitive data.

Despite the technical and ethical challenges, the outcomes of the SynapseAI project were promising. Early trials indicated substantial improvements in patient well-being, with a noted decrease in emergency mental health incidents by early intervention. Customized care plans that adjusted in real-time to patient data helped maintain continuous patient engagement and adherence to prescribed therapies.

However, the project highlighted the need for ongoing adjustments in AI algorithms to address the dynamic nature of mental health conditions and the evolving landscape of psychiatric research. SynapseAI's continuous algorithmic refinement was necessary to accommodate new data and insights, ensuring the system remained sensitive to the subtle nuances of mental health diagnostics and treatment efficacy.

**Case Study: AI-driven Strategies for Managing Chronic Pain: The PainFreeAI Initiative**

The PainFreeAI initiative, initiated in 2030, undertook the ambitious project of using AI to revolutionize the management of chronic pain, a complex and often underserved medical issue. This initiative brought together a diverse consortium of medical researchers, AI developers, and patient advocacy groups, with the common goal of developing an AI system capable of personalizing pain management strategies to the individual's health data and pain response patterns.

PainFreeAI was designed to process an extensive range of data inputs, including patient electronic health records (EHRs), real-time sensory data from wearable pain sensors, genetic profiles, and even psychological assessments. The AI system leveraged advanced neural network algorithms to identify patterns and predictors of pain in vast datasets, customizing treatment plans that included medication adjustments, lifestyle changes, and psychological interventions.

However, the integration of such a broad array of data sources posed significant technical and ethical challenges. The initiative had to develop innovative data integration techniques to manage the variety and volume of data efficiently. Privacy was also a prime concern; the project implemented cutting-edge encryption and data management protocols to protect sensitive patient information, complying with global data privacy regulations.

Despite these challenges, the deployment of PainFreeAI resulted in notable improvements in patient-reported pain levels and management efficacy. The system's ability to continuously learn from incoming data allowed for dynamic adjustments to treatment plans, which adapted to patients' changing conditions and responses.

The success of PainFreeAI highlighted the potential benefits of targeted, data-driven pain management but also underscored the ongoing challenges of data standardization, ethical AI use, and the need for continuous system evaluation to prevent bias and ensure that the AI's learning algorithms perform equitably across diverse patient populations.

**Case Study: AI-Enhanced Telehealth: Revolutionizing Remote Patient Monitoring**

The advent of the COVID-19 pandemic accelerated the need for robust telehealth solutions across the globe. A notable endeavor in this sphere was the development of TeleHealthAI, a comprehensive AI-driven platform introduced in 2021. This system was specifically designed to augment remote patient monitoring and management, particularly for chronic illnesses such as hypertension and COPD (Chronic Obstructive Pulmonary Disease).

TeleHealthAI was engineered to process and analyze data from a multitude of sources, including electronic health records (EHRs), real-time biometric data from wearable devices, and patient-reported symptoms via mobile health apps. By utilizing state-of-the-art machine learning algorithms, TeleHealthAI could identify exacerbations in chronic conditions, potentially before the patient was even aware of a change in their own health status.

The integration of these disparate data sources was critical to the success of TeleHealthAI. The system combined structured data (like EHRs and lab results) with unstructured data (such as physicians' notes and patient audio logs) to create a comprehensive view of the patient's health over time. This integration allowed for predictive analytics to forecast health deteriorations and prompt preemptive interventions.

However, this pioneering project faced substantial challenges. Data privacy and security were paramount, as the system had to comply with stringent global regulations like GDPR in Europe and HIPAA in the U.S. Moreover, the vast differences in data formatting across devices and systems posed significant hurdles in data standardization and integration. On top of these technical challenges, ensuring the system was accessible and user-friendly for a demographic with varied technological proficiency was crucial to ensure widespread adoption.

Despite these obstacles, TeleHealthAI had a notable impact on patient outcomes. Patients enrolled in the program saw a 20% reduction in hospital readmissions and a significant improvement in managing their conditions. This success illustrated the profound potential of AI-enhanced telehealth systems but also underscored the ongoing need for advanced data harmonization techniques, stringent privacy measures, and continuous system improvement to adapt to emerging healthcare challenges.

## Review Questions

**1. A 65-year-old man with a history of hypertension and type 2 diabetes presents with complaints of increasing fatigue, muscle weakness, and occasional palpitations over the past few months. He mentions that these symptoms become pronounced after participating in religious fasting as part of his cultural tradition. His current medications include metformin, lisinopril, and atorvastatin. Laboratory tests show hyponatremia and hyperkalemia, which prompts further evaluation. What is the most likely diagnosis?**

A) Addison's disease

B) Diabetic ketoacidosis

C) Hypothyroidism

D) Chronic kidney disease

**Answer: A**

Explanation: The patient's symptoms of fatigue, muscle weakness, and palpitations, especially after fasting, alongside findings of hyponatremia and hyperkalemia, suggest Addison's disease (primary adrenal insufficiency). Addison's disease is characterized by the adrenal glands' inability to produce sufficient cortisol and often aldosterone. Cortisol is crucial for energy regulation and stress response, which explains the fatigue and weakness, particularly noticeable when the patient's physiological demand increases during fasting. The lack of aldosterone leads to sodium loss, potassium retention, and consequently, hyponatremia and hyperkalemia. This diagnosis fits better with the clinical presentation than the other conditions listed, which would either not explain all the findings or present differently.

**2. A 29-year-old female practicing Traditional Thai Medicine, experiencing chronic lower back pain, opts for a combination of herbal remedies and Thai Massage therapy instead of NSAIDs due to her preference for natural treatments. Following several weeks of treatment, she reports significant improvement in pain relief and increased mobility. Considering her treatment choice and outcomes, what aspect of AI healthcare would be most beneficial for managing her ongoing care?**

A) AI-driven personalized herbal recommendation system

B) AI to monitor potential herb-drug interactions

C) Generic AI health advice app

D) AI-based scheduling system for her massage sessions

**Answer: B**

Explanation: Given that the patient is using a combination of herbal treatment and Thai Massage, the most beneficial AI healthcare feature would be an AI system designed to monitor potential herb-drug interactions. As the patient prefers natural treatments over pharmaceuticals, ensuring that her herbal remedies do not interfere with or cause adverse reactions with any other medications she might take in the future is crucial. This proactive approach using AI helps optimize her safety and the efficacy of her treatments. Unlike generic AI health advice or a scheduling system, monitoring herb-drug interactions directly addresses a potential risk specific to her use of herbal medications, aligning with personalized, safe healthcare practices.

**3. Considering the cultural competency in AI model development, a group of data scientists are collaborating with local Hilot healers from the Philippines to integrate traditional healing knowledge into an AI-driven diagnostic tool. What measure is essential to ensure this collaboration is respectful and yields an effective AI tool?**

A) Implementing strict data control measures governed by the Hilot healers

B) Including only scientifically validated Hilot practices

C) Developing the tool without direct healer involvement, using published sources

D) Translating all Hilot practices into Western medical terminology

**Answer: A**

Explanation: The key to successful and respectful collaboration in integrating traditional Hilot healing practices into an AI-driven tool is implementing strict data control measures governed by the Hilot healers themselves. This approach respects their knowledge sovereignty, allows them to control how their intellectual property is utilized, and ensures that the use of their traditional practices is consensual and transparent. It is crucial that these measures prioritize the healers' perspectives on what practices can be shared and how they should be represented, rather than imposing Western scientific validation as a standard or diluting their practices through translation that may strip away cultural context and meaning. This method ensures cultural sensitivity and maintains the integrity of the traditional knowledge being integrated, making the AI tool more effective and culturally competent.

## Ethical Considerations in AI-Driven Healthcare

### Defining Ethical Standards in AI-Driven Healthcare

In the realm of AI-driven healthcare, establishing clear ethical standards is paramount to navigating the complex interplay between technology and human values. The goal is to create a framework that not only promotes innovation but also safeguards patient welfare and respects personal autonomy.

Ethical guidelines must address the potential for AI to make decisions that could have life-altering consequences. This encompasses ensuring that AI systems operate transparently and are held accountable for their actions, especially in critical care scenarios. Moreover, these standards should mandate the inclusion of diverse datasets to mitigate bias and promote equitable treatment outcomes across various demographic groups.

It is also critical to consider the moral implications of patient data usage, prioritizing privacy and consent above all else. By establishing robust ethical standards, the healthcare sector can foster a trustworthy environment where AI enhances treatment without compromising ethical values or human dignity.

## Moral Implications of AI Decisions in Treatment

The integration of AI into medical decision-making processes brings with it profound moral questions. Similarly, these decisions, often based on data-driven algorithms, must be scrutinized for their ethical implications. One central concern is the potential for AI systems to make treatment decisions that may inadvertently prioritize efficiency or cost over patient-centric values such as dignity and compassion.

For instance, if an AI system is programmed to prioritize treatment based on statistical outcomes alone, it could overlook the nuanced needs of individual patients who might benefit from less conventional treatments. Such scenarios highlight the need for moral frameworks that guide AI to make decisions aligning with holistic human values. It is essential that these frameworks are developed collaboratively, involving ethicists, clinicians, patients, and AI developers, to ensure a balanced consideration of both technological capabilities and ethical obligations.

Moreover, as AI's role in treatment decisions grows, continuous monitoring and updating of ethical guidelines is critical. Ensuring that AI decisions in healthcare uphold the highest moral standards requires persistent vigilance and adaptive ethical governance, safeguarding patient rights and dignity amidst rapid technological advancements.

## Patient Rights and AI: Autonomy and Consent

The intersection of AI with patient care introduces complex dynamics concerning autonomy and consent. As AI systems increasingly play a role in medical diagnoses and treatment options, the essential rights of patients to understand and consent to these methodologies cannot be overlooked. Ensuring that patients retain control over their treatment choices demands clear communication and comprehensible explanations from healthcare providers about how AI impacts their care options.

However, the impersonal nature of AI-driven decisions poses a challenge to traditional consent processes, which are deeply personal and grounded in human interactions. To address this, innovative consent frameworks need to be developed that accommodate AI's role while respecting patient autonomy. These frameworks should facilitate informed decision-making, whereby patients are educated about AI technologies and their potential implications on both health outcomes and personal privacy.

Moreover, updating consent protocols to include AI-specific considerations reflects an ethical commitment to patient rights, ensuring that patients are not only informed but also genuinely empowered in their healthcare decisions. This evolution in consent practices is crucial as we navigate the burgeoning influence of AI in healthcare.

## AI Transparency and the Right to Explanation

Transparency in AI-driven healthcare not only builds trust but also enhances patient understanding and involvement in their care. It necessitates clear explanations of how AI systems influence patient diagnoses and treatment plans, championing a right to comprehensible insights into the AI processes that affect healthcare decisions.

The 'right to explanation' enables patients to receive justification and rationale behind specific AI-generated outcomes. This right guards against the opacity of 'black box' algorithms, ensuring that AI interventions are not merely effective but also understandable and justifiable from a patient's viewpoint. Transparency here acts as a checkpoint against potential biases that automated systems might inherit from their training data or design.

Moreover, fostering a culture where AI's decision-making processes are openly discussed and debated can lead to more ethical implementations. This practice not only demystifies AI for the public but also reassures that these advanced tools align with societal ethical standards and individual patient values.

## Handling Data: Privacy, Security, and Confidentiality

In the realm of AI-driven healthcare, the triad of privacy, security, and confidentiality forms the cornerstone of data handling ethics. These principles safeguard patient information from unauthorized access and breaches, which is paramount in maintaining trust in healthcare technologies. Ensuring robust security measures are in place to protect data from cyber threats is crucial, given the sensitive nature of medical information.

Privacy entails the right of patients to have their health data handled discreetly and used only under consented terms. This aspect is particularly challenging in AI environments where data could be extensively analyzed and shared across platforms. Implementing stringent access controls and regular audits are essential steps in upholding privacy standards.

Furthermore, maintaining confidentiality in AI healthcare requires dedicated protocols to prevent unintended data exposure. Technologies must be designed to inherently support these ethical principles, embedding them at every stage of AI development and deployment. This commitment to ethical data handling not only complies with legal mandates but also reinforces the fiduciary relationship between patients and healthcare providers.

## The Impact of AI Errors on Patient Outcomes

The infiltration of AI into healthcare, while transformative, heralds' significant risks, particularly when errors occur. These AI errors can drastically affect patient outcomes, sometimes leading to misdiagnoses, inappropriate treatment plans, or overlooked symptoms. The precision of AI-driven decisions is only as reliable as the data and algorithms that fuel them.

Erroneous AI outputs can emanate from flawed data inputs or biases inherent in the training sets. Such inaccuracies jeopardize patient safety and trust in healthcare systems. It is imperative to implement rigorous testing and validation frameworks to catch these errors early. Healthcare providers must remain vigilant, ensuring AI tools augment rather than replace human judgment.

Furthermore, the establishment of rapid response protocols for managing AI errors – including ethical recall procedures and patient notification systems – is crucial in mitigating potential harms. This proactive approach not only preserves patient health but also fortifies the ethical foundations upon which AI healthcare should stand.

## Bias and Fairness: Avoiding Inequity in AI Healthcare

Addressing bias and ensuring fairness in AI-driven healthcare is imperative to prevent systematic inequities. AI systems, deriving knowledge from data, can perpetuate existing biases if not carefully calibrated.

Culturally insensitive algorithms may fail to recognize diverse health needs, thus it's crucial that datasets are both representative and meticulously scrutinized.

Incorporating fairness involves more than adjusting data; it demands an ongoing commitment to ethical AI practice. By embedding cultural sensitivity within the algorithm design and involving diverse stakeholders in the development process, we can mitigate unconscious biases and foster more equitable health outcomes. This includes reconciling traditional, indigenous, and holistic healing practices within AI frameworks to respect all cultural dimensions of healthcare.

Ultimately, ensuring AI fairness requires robust governance frameworks that enforce accountability and transparency. Regular audits and updates to AI systems are essential to adapt to evolving understanding of fairness and to safeguard against bias creep over time. Structuring these checks within the healthcare system fosters a continuously ethical AI application, crucial for equitable patient care.

## Cultural Sensitivity in Algorithm Design

Integrating cultural sensitivity into AI algorithm design is pivotal, especially in globalized healthcare settings. Algorithms must be meticulously crafted to accommodate the cultural nuances and medical practices of diverse populations. This cultural inclusivity ensures that AI tools are not only universally applicable but also respectful of various healing traditions and patient backgrounds.

The design process should include inputs from culturally diverse teams who bring insights from different healing practices, ranging from traditional medicine to modern treatments. Such collaboration can help identify and mitigate unintended biases that may alienate or misrepresent certain groups. Moreover, it promotes the development of algorithms that are more adept at handling varied health paradigms and patient needs, leading to more personalized and effective care.

Ultimately, cultural sensitivity in AI requires a deliberate approach to algorithm development, necessitating ongoing dialogue with cultural scholars and practitioners. By embracing this multiplicity, AI technologies can transcend their mechanical origins, becoming tools of empathy and understanding, crucial for equitable healthcare delivery.

## Sustaining Human Oversight in AI Applications

The integration of AI in healthcare raises significant ethical questions, notably about sustaining human oversight. As AI systems take on more roles in diagnosing and treating patients, the necessity of maintaining a human element in decision-making processes becomes paramount.

Human oversight ensures that AI applications adhere to ethical medical practices and uphold the dignity and rights of patients. It serves as a check against the cold calculus of algorithms that might overlook nuances in patient care. This oversight is crucial in complex clinical decisions where human empathy and professional judgment are irreplaceable.

Moreover, human oversight in AI applications fosters accountability. When AI systems make errors or display biases, having established channels for human intervention allows for swift corrections and learning. This synergy between human expertise and AI capabilities is essential for advancing healthcare in a manner that is both innovative and ethically responsible.

Thus, preserving human oversight is not only a safeguard but also a bridge that integrates AI advancements within the compassionate framework of healthcare.

**Ethical Use of Predictive Analytics in Patient Care**

The integration of predictive analytics in patient care demands a meticulous ethical framework to ensure that AI-enhanced decision-making processes truly benefit patient outcomes without compromising individual rights. These systems, designed to forecast health trajectories, must be anchored in principles that prioritize patient welfare and consent, ensuring that predictions do not lead to prejudicial treatments or restrict healthcare options based on algorithmic outputs alone.

Ethical use also involves transparency, where patients are informed how their data is used to predict health outcomes and the potential implications. This transparency fosters trust and allows patients to make informed decisions about their health, reinforcing their autonomy in the care process. It also necessitates rigorous validation of predictive models to ensure accuracy and reliability, safeguarding against harmful errors.

Moreover, to responsibly harness predictive analytics, healthcare providers must remain vigilant against embedding biases in these tools. Continuous monitoring and updating of algorithms are essential to maintain fairness and prevent inadvertent discrimination. This ethical vigilance ensures predictive analytics serve as a beneficial tool in enhancing patient care, rather than a detriment.

**AI in End-of-Life Decisions: Ethical Challenges**

The integration of AI into end-of-life medical decisions presents profound ethical challenges. These critical moments require a compassionate approach, one that respects the patient's values and the nuanced complexities of human life. AI, with its underlying reliance on data-driven outputs, may not fully encapsulate these subtleties, leading to decisions that could feel impersonal or misaligned with individual patient values.

Ensuring ethical oversight involves rigorous standards that prioritize the patient's autonomy and consent. AI systems must be transparent about how decisions are made, allowing for patient and family involvement in these sensitive choices. This transparency is crucial in maintaining trust and ensuring that AI-assisted decisions are made with the utmost care and respect for patient dignity.

Moreover, it is imperative to sustain human oversight in AI-decision processes during end-of-life care. Human empathy cannot be replicated by algorithms. Clinicians must remain at the forefront, guiding AI inputs to align with compassionate care practices, thereby safeguarding the ethical integrity of medical decision-making at the end of life.

**The Role of Ethics Review Boards in AI Deployment**

In the realm of AI-driven healthcare, Ethics Review Boards (ERBs) serve as pivotal entities for overseeing the ethical deployment of AI technologies. Tasked with reviewing and approving AI applications, these boards ensure that AI systems are developed and utilized in a manner that upholds ethical standards and patient rights.

ERBs examine the potential implications of AI tools, focusing on patient autonomy, privacy, and the possible socio-cultural impacts. Their role extends beyond mere compliance checks to engaging in proactive discussions about the ethical dimensions of AI integration in healthcare settings. These boards operate as guardians of ethical integrity, providing insights that balance technological advancements with moral considerations.

Furthermore, the involvement of ERBs in AI deployment is crucial for maintaining public trust in healthcare systems. By ensuring that AI applications are scrutinized for ethical soundness, ERBs help mitigate risks associated with AI biases and foster an environment where technological innovation is aligned with human values.

## Addressing the Digital Divide in AI Healthcare Access

The digital divide presents a formidable barrier in the ethical deployment of AI within healthcare. Access to AI-driven medical services often mirrors broader socio-economic disparities, disadvantaging those in lower-income or remote areas. It's crucial for developers and policymakers to address these gaps, creating pathways that broaden AI's reach and benefits.

Ensuring that technology is accessible requires robust infrastructure improvement plans, inclusive Internet access policies, and educational programs that enhance technological literacy. Such initiatives can facilitate the integration of AI tools across diverse populations, ensuring equitable health outcomes. Additionally, the development of low-cost, user-friendly AI healthcare technologies could help bridge this divide, provided these solutions maintain high standards of care and effectiveness.

Lastly, partnership strategies between governments, the private sector, and non-profits are essential. These collaborations can leverage collective resources and expertise to address connectivity issues while promoting an ethical, inclusive approach to AI in healthcare. By consciously striving to close this gap, the hope of universally beneficial AI-powered medicine becomes attainable.

## Protecting Vulnerable Populations in AI Implementations

In the realm of AI-driven healthcare, the imperative to protect vulnerable populations cannot be overstated. These groups, often marginalized due to socioeconomic, racial, or geographic factors, face distinct risks when AI systems inadvertently perpetuate existing disparities. Ensuring that AI tools do not exacerbate these inequities involves designing algorithms that are inherently aware of and sensitive to diverse population needs.

This protective endeavor requires a multifaceted approach. First, it is crucial to involve representatives from these communities during the AI development phase, providing insights that can inform more inclusive and equitable algorithmic decision-making. Additionally, there must be stringent regulatory frameworks that mandate the continuous assessment of AI systems for bias and the implementation of corrective measures when disparities are detected.

Ultimately, safeguarding vulnerable populations in AI implementations emphasizes the ethical obligation to foster an inclusive healthcare environment. It recognizes the unique challenges these groups face and actively works towards solutions that uphold their dignity and right to fair medical care, ensuring no one is left behind in the digital healthcare revolution.

## AI and the Physician-Patient Relationship

The evolution of AI in healthcare impacts the foundational dynamics of the physician-patient relationship. Traditionally characterized by personal interaction and trust, this relationship faces new challenges and opportunities in the age of AI. As machines take on more diagnostic and treatment planning roles, the primary concern becomes maintaining the intimacy and empathy inherent in human interactions. Physicians must navigate this new terrain where AI tools assist without depersonalizing the care patients receive.

Furthermore, the integration of AI demands that physicians become intermediaries between complex algorithms and patients. This role requires them to translate AI-driven data into understandable treatment options, thereby ensuring that AI supports, rather than undermines, the decision-making process. Ensuring that AI applications are perceived as enhancements rather than replacements for professional judgment is crucial for preserving trust.

Lastly, the emphasis must remain on a collaborative approach where AI serves as a support tool, not just a technological one. By fostering transparency about AI processes and limitations, healthcare providers can help patients understand and trust AI-enhanced care, reinforcing the traditional values of the physician-patient relationship even within this modern context.

## Accountability Mechanisms for AI Malfunctions

The necessity for robust accountability mechanisms in AI-driven healthcare stems from the potential severe consequences of AI malfunctions. These mechanisms must ensure that errors are not only corrected but also that they contribute to the system's continuous improvement. Establishing clear lines of responsibility when AI systems fail is critical for maintaining trust and efficacy in healthcare delivery.

Critical to these mechanisms is the development of comprehensive reporting systems that enable quick identification and analysis of malfunctions. Healthcare providers, along with AI developers, should be mandated to report adverse events linked to AI usage. This transparency facilitates better oversight and swift rectification strategies, minimizing any potential harm to patients.

Furthermore, accountability frameworks must include punitive measures for negligence and reward structures to encourage adherence to high safety standards. Regular audits and updates to AI systems should be enforced legally, ensuring that technological advancements do not outpace safety protocols. These steps are fundamental to safeguarding patient health and preserving the integrity of AI applications in medicine.

## Ethical Development of AI Training Sets

The ethical development of AI training sets in healthcare is pivotal for creating trustworthy AI systems. This process begins with the careful selection and vetting of data, ensuring it encompasses a broad spectrum of demographics, including often underrepresented groups. Such diversity in data helps prevent the AI from developing and perpetuating biases that can lead to disparities in medical treatment and diagnosis.

Moreover, transparency in the data collection methods and criteria is essential. Stakeholders should have a clear understanding of how and why specific data sets are used. This openness builds trust in AI systems and assures all involved parties that ethical guidelines are being followed. Ethical development also includes ongoing monitoring and updating of data sets to adapt to new medical insights and population changes, ensuring continued relevance and fairness of the AI systems.

Collaboration between data scientists, ethicists, and healthcare professionals is crucial in maintaining the integrity of the development process. Together, they can uphold high ethical standards and implement robust supervision mechanisms to prevent misuse of AI in healthcare. These collaborative efforts guarantee that AI tools enhance healthcare equitably, serving as wings to lift every patient, rather than chains that bind cultural diversity.

## Legal Considerations in AI-Assisted Medical Practices

Legal frameworks governing AI in healthcare must adapt to technological advancements to ensure practices comply with existing laws and ethical guidelines. AI implementation disrupts traditional medical law paradigms, introducing complexities around liability and patient confidentiality that demand innovative legal responses.

Questions of responsibility arise when AI systems make erroneous decisions leading to patient harm. Determining whether liability lies with the healthcare provider, software developer, or both, requires clear regulations. Moreover, patient privacy laws need updating to safeguard data handled by AI, preventing misuse and guaranteeing confidentiality. AI's ability to extrapolate additional data from primary information complicates compliance with privacy laws, necessitating legal adaptations suited to the digital age.

Facing these challenges, consultations among legal experts, technologists, and healthcare professionals are crucial. Collaborative efforts can create a balanced legal framework that protects patients while fostering innovation. Ensuring that AI technology empowers rather than undermines healthcare requires an evolved legal approach that is proactive in addressing the dynamic interplay between technology and law.

**Ethical AI Programming: Algorithms that Care**

Ethical AI programming emphasizes creating algorithms that not only perform efficiently but also care for the holistic needs of patients, incorporating considerations that span beyond clinical data. This involves programming AI to recognize and respect diverse medical philosophies, including traditional and holistic approaches, ensuring these systems support rather than override the nuanced decisions of healthcare professionals.

Developing such responsive algorithms necessitates a deep integration of ethical reasoning within the coding itself, making AI systems that are inherently attuned to the moral dimensions of healthcare decisions. It requires coders to collaborate closely with ethicists and healthcare providers to embed empathy and care into the very fabric of AI decision-making processes.

Moreover, for AI to truly care, it must be programmed to continuously learn from its outcomes to better its understanding and approach. This adaptive capability can guide AI toward more compassionate responses, evolving with each interaction to meet the patient's individual needs while upholding high ethical standards in every decision.

**Implementing AI: Who Decides What is Ethical?**

HOW IMPORTANT IS THE ISSUE AS TO WHOM HOLDS THE KEYS? The question of who holds the ethical compass in the realm of AI implementation in healthcare is pivotal. Traditionally, ethical standards have been the purview of medical boards and governing bodies. However, as AI integrates deeper into health systems, its governance requires a multifaceted approach that extends beyond traditional medical ethics to include technologists, patients, and society at large.

This collaborative decision-making process must ensure that all voices are heard, especially those from communities that might otherwise be marginalized. The inclusion of diverse viewpoints will help in tackling the ethical dilemmas presented by AI more comprehensively. Ethical AI implementation thus becomes not just a matter of technical feasibility but of societal consensus and trust.

Moreover, it necessitates ongoing dialogue between all stakeholders involved. As AI evolves, so too should our understanding and regulation of its ethical implications, ensuring that AI serves humanity ethically and justly across all spectrums of healthcare.

**Feedback Loops: The Ethics of AI Learning Processes**

Feedback loops are central to the efficacy of AI in healthcare. These mechanisms allow AI systems to continually learn and adapt from their interactions and outcomes, enhancing their capabilities. Ethical considerations arise when determining which outcomes and data points should influence AI learning, as biases in these selections can lead to skewed AI behaviors that systematically disadvantage certain patient groups.

Ensuring that AI systems evolve ethically requires transparency in how data influences learning processes. Stakeholders, including patients and healthcare providers, should understand and influence what feedback AI receives, ensuring it promotes equitable and just care. This promotes a collaborative environment where AI's learning is aligned with human values and ethical standards.

Moreover, the ethical management of feedback loops includes rigorous monitoring to prevent the perpetuation of existing biases. Continuous oversight by diverse teams can mitigate risks, making AI a reliable partner in healthcare. Thus, feedback loops represent a dual opportunity and responsibility to shape AI's impact ethically.

**Global Standards for Ethical AI in Health**

The establishment of global standards for ethical AI in healthcare represents a pivotal step towards harmonizing practices across borders, ensuring that AI innovations benefit all, irrespective of geographic location. These standards should address fundamental ethical concerns such as equity, transparency, and accountability, offering a blueprint that guides countries in developing their own regulations while maintaining international consistency.

Key to this is the involvement of global health organizations alongside AI experts to formulate guidelines that respect diverse cultural and ethical norms. This collaboration ensures that standards are not only technically sound but also culturally sensitive, promoting a global health equity agenda.

Furthermore, the implementation of these standards requires rigorous monitoring and flexible, even situational enforcement mechanisms. Flexible or situational, in that when considering the impact on indigenous communities, their needs will be persnickety and peculiar to their respective communities. Regular audits and updates to the standards will be essential as AI technology and medical practices evolve, ensuring that ethical AI usage remains at the forefront of global health advancements.

Ultimately, global standards serve as a foundation for trust and cooperation in the international healthcare landscape, fostering an environment where AI can be a universal ally in human health.

**The Future of AI Ethics in Medical Education**

As AI becomes increasingly integrated into healthcare, the imperative to embed ethical AI education within medical curricula is paramount. Tomorrow's healthcare providers must not only possess clinical expertise but also a deep ethical understanding of the technologies they use. This involves teaching medical students about the nuances of AI applications, including the recognition and mitigation of biases and the maintenance of patient autonomy and privacy.

Furthermore, ethical AI education should promote an interdisciplinary approach, blending technology knowledge with humanitarian perspectives. Courses should stress real-world implications of ethical AI deployment, ensuring students can navigate complex scenarios where technology and ethics intersect. Engagement with case studies, ethical simulations, and AI-driven diagnostics could be vital components of such curricula.

Ultimately, as AI reshapes healthcare landscapes, medical education must evolve to prepare professionals adept in both technology and ethics. This dual competency will be crucial for maintaining the integrity and compassion essential to healthcare, fostering an environment where technology serves humanity respectfully and responsibly.

## Revisiting the Hippocratic Oath in the Age of AI

The Hippocratic Oath, a timeless covenant upholding medical ethics, faces new challenges in the era of AI-driven healthcare. Traditionally, this oath focuses on the welfare, privacy, and respect for patients, primarily enforced and interpreted by human clinicians. Today, as AI increasingly participates in decision-making processes, interpreting these principled commitments through algorithms becomes imperative.

In this technological context, the oath must be expanded to ensure AI systems also adhere to its foundational values. This involves integrating ethical AI programming to act in patients' best interests, uphold human dignity, and avoid harm. Ensuring these systems have ethical oversight, where AI cannot only make decisions but also learn and adapt within these ethical confines, becomes crucial.

*The Hippocratic Oath is not an anachronistic throwback to the superstitious, and some say outdated ideas of "physician, Do No Harm" as an anachronism and limiting condition to the practice of medicine (consider the impact of iatrogenic medical mortality). It is a revealing dialogue in consideration of the true laws of nature and the relationships between the physician, God, and nature in a framework of duty to morality, ethics, humility, and a fundamental understanding of man's place in the world, and then the physician's role of representation and intermediary of God's universal love. God does not have hands, man does. It is fundamentally a sacred vow, akin to the "Ahimsa" vow of ancient yogis, which voluntarily imposes a duty and a responsibility to represent healing in the world. Nowhere does this ancient vow or pledge specify profit as the primary motivation for medicine; rather, the opposite is true.*

Suppose the primary motivation for constructing and implementing an AI Medical model, such as synthetic diagnostic systems, is to generate or increase revenue over functional outcomes and patient wellness. In that case, these systems will fail in their stated outcomes. Like we used to say when I was a child, "You can't get there from here!"

Moreover, revisiting the Hippocratic Oath serves not just to guide AI's ethical development but also to reaffirm the medical community's commitment to humanity. Adapting this ancient vow to modern needs may set a unified standard, maintaining patient trust and care integrity amidst rapid digital transformation.

## Summary

The chapter 'Ethical Considerations in AI-Driven Healthcare' delves into the critical ethical dimensions shaping the deployment of AI technologies in the healthcare sector. It commences by underscoring the necessity for establishing stringent ethical standards to guide the integration of AI in healthcare, emphasizing the importance of transparency, accountability, and inclusivity in AI systems to prevent bias and ensure equitable treatment outcomes. The content addresses the moral implications of AI-assisted decisions in medical treatments, highlighting the potential conflicts between efficiency and patient-centered values like dignity and compassion. Moreover, the chapter examines the complexities surrounding patient autonomy and consent in the era of AI, advocating for innovative consent frameworks that account for AI's role in medical decision-making while respecting patient rights. The discussion extends to AI transparency, asserting that patients deserve clear explanations about how AI impacts their diagnosis and treatment, which is essential for building trust and empowering patients. There is a significant focus on the handling of data, emphasizing the protection of privacy, security, and confidentiality to maintain trust in AI applications. Furthermore, the narrative tackles the consequences of AI errors on patient outcomes, stressing the need for effective error management strategies to safeguard patient health. The domain of bias and fairness is also explored, with a call for the development of culturally sensitive algorithms to ensure AI systems cater to the diverse needs of global populations. Another area of concern is the maintenance of human oversight in AI applications, necessary for preserving humanistic elements in healthcare. Additionally, ethical challenges in AI's role in end-of-life decisions are discussed, underscoring the need for compassionate use of AI that aligns with patient values and ethics. The chapter concludes by considering the roles of Ethics Review Boards and the need for global standards to manage the ethical deployment of AI in healthcare, ensuring its benefits are universally accessible and culturally respectful.

## References

[1] Mittelstadt, B. (2019). Principles alone cannot guarantee ethical AI. Nature Machine Intelligence. https://www.nature.com/articles/s42256-019-0114-4

[2] Jobin, A., Ienca, M., & Vayena, E. (2019). The global landscape of AI ethics guidelines. Nature Machine Intelligence. https://www.nature.com/articles/s42256-019-0088-2

[3] Char, D. S., Shah, N. H., & Magnus, D. (2018). Implementing Machine Learning in Health Care — Addressing Ethical Challenges. New England Journal of Medicine. https://www.nejm.org/doi/full/10.1056/NEJMp1714229

[4] Luxton, D. D. (2020). Artificial Intelligence in Psychological Practice: Current and Future Applications and Implications. Professional Psychology: Research and Practice. https://psycnet.apa.org/record/2020-34937-001

[5] Vayena, E., Blasimme, A., & Cohen, I. G. (2018). Machine learning in medicine: Addressing ethical challenges. PLOS Medicine. https://journals.plos.org/plosmedicine/article?id=10.1371/journal.pmed.1002689

## Case Study: Balancing Efficiency and Ethics: AI in Emergency Triage Decisions

In a metropolitan hospital, an advanced AI-driven system has been integrated into the emergency department to assist in patient triage processes. The AI system, named TriagAI, was programmed to assess incoming patients based on severity of symptoms, medical history, and potential outcomes to prioritize care effectively. However, the hospital soon faced a dilemma when TriagAI consistently prioritized certain patient groups, such as younger individuals or those with higher survival probabilities, over others, like elderly patients or those with complex, chronic conditions.

The ethical implications of this deployment came to the forefront, sparking debate among hospital staff and ethicists. Concerns arose over the potential bias embedded in the AI's programming, which appeared to align with utilitarian principles prioritizing maximum overall benefit but potentially compromising individual patient care and ethical standards of equality and dignity. The hospital initiated a case review to explore these disparities and assess the TriagAI's decision-making framework. Investigations revealed that the data used to train TriagAI disproportionately represented certain demographic groups, leading to skewed decision-making favoring these groups.

To address these issues, the hospital convened a multidisciplinary team, including AI developers, healthcare providers, ethicists, and patient representatives. This team undertook the task of revising the AI algorithms to integrate a more balanced ethical framework, factoring in not only survival outcomes but also equitable treatment opportunities for all patient demographics. The retrained TriagAI was subjected to continuous oversight and periodic reviews to align its operations with both ethical guidelines and clinical requirements.

As the recalibrated AI system was redeployed, new protocol measures were implemented to ensure ongoing assessment of AI decisions through a combination of AI transparency logs and human oversight committees. These measures aimed to bolster patient trust in the AI-supported triage system while maintaining the crucial balance between operational efficiency and ethical medical practice.

## Case Study: Ethical Dilemmas in AI-Assisted End-of-Life Care Decisions

St. Helena Hospital introduced an AI system, named EndLifeAI, designed to assist in making end-of-life care decisions. The system used extensive medical data and predictive analytics to recommend whether patients with critical conditions should continue life-sustaining treatments or transition to palliative care. Initially hailed for its potential to bring consistency to difficult decisions, EndLifeAI soon encountered ethical challenges.

A notable case involved an 80-year-old patient with advanced heart failure and multiple comorbidities. The AI system advised against further invasive treatments, recommending hospice care based on predictions of low survival probability and quality of life metrics. The patient's family, however, insisted on continuing treatment, citing personal and cultural beliefs that all life-preserving measures should be pursued. The medical team found themselves at a crossroads between following the AI's guidance, which was based on vast data and predictive outcomes, and respecting the family's wishes and the patient's own ambiguous previous statements on end-of-life care.

This situation highlighted the ethical dilemma of balancing algorithmic efficiency with individual patient values, cultural sensitivity, and autonomy. The ethics committee of St. Helena Hospital was convened to discuss the implications of AI in such profoundly sensitive decisions. They questioned whether the AI gave undue weight to statistically driven outcomes over individualized patient care and whether it could genuinely account for the nuances of human emotion and cultural values.

In response to this and similar cases, the hospital decided to revamp EndLifeAI's algorithm to include a broader array of ethical considerations. They introduced input mechanisms for family members' preferences and included a manual override feature for doctors. Ethicists and clinicians worked together to incorporate elements of compassionate care into the decision-making process, ensuring that the AI system did not merely operate on clinical data but also respected diverse moral and cultural dimensions of end-of-life care. Continuous training on ethical issues was implemented for all stakeholders involved to keep pace with evolving ethical standards in healthcare.

## Case Study: Navigating Privacy and Accuracy in AI-Driven Mental Health Assessments

A leading mental health clinic in a large urban area recently introduced an AI-based diagnostic tool designed to enhance the detection and treatment of mental health disorders. Named MindScope, this tool uses machine learning algorithms to analyze patient responses from standardized psychological tests and suggest potential diagnoses. The implementation aimed to streamline the assessment process and provide clinicians with advanced insights to inform their treatment plans. However, the integration of MindScope soon raised significant ethical concerns related to patient privacy and the accuracy of AI-driven diagnostics.

Initial feedback from patients and therapists suggested an unsettling level of detailed personal data handling by MindScope. Patients expressed concerns over the extent and permanency of data shared with the AI, fearing potential leaks or unauthorized use. Therapists reported intermittent discrepancies between the AI's diagnostic suggestions and their clinical judgments, leading to doubts about the tool's reliability and its alignment with traditional therapeutic methodologies.

These issues brought to light the critical need for a robust ethical framework to govern AI implementations in sensitive areas like mental health. The clinic's ethics committee convened to address these challenges, focusing on reinforcing data privacy protocols and improving the AI's diagnostic algorithms. They emphasized the importance of securing informed consent by explaining to patients how their data would be used, ensuring it was collected and stored securely, and clarifying their right to withdraw consent at any time.

To enhance the AI's accuracy, the committee recommended incorporating a broader spectrum of diagnostic data and ongoing training sessions for the AI, using a diverse array of anonymized case studies to reduce biases and improve reliability. These steps are aimed at creating a balance between leveraging AI's capabilities to improve mental health diagnostics while safeguarding patient confidentiality and ensuring the clinical validity of the diagnoses. The clinic also implemented a transparent reporting system, allowing any patient or clinician to report discrepancies or ethical concerns regarding AI applications, thus fostering an environment of trust and continuous improvement in patient care.

## Case Study: The Role of AI in Addressing Treatment Bias in Oncology

At the Crossroads Medical Center, an innovative AI system, named OncoAssist, was introduced to aid in oncology decision-making. OncoAssist utilizes vast datasets of past patient outcomes and current treatment protocols to recommend personalized treatment plans. These AI-driven recommendations aimed to standardize care and reduce variability in treatment outcomes, which historically had been influenced by clinicians' subjective experiences and potential unconscious biases. However, soon after deployment, disparities in treatment recommendations began to emerge, particularly affecting patients from racial and ethnic minorities.

The AI system seemed to replicate and potentially exacerbate existing biases in healthcare delivery. For example, it was observed that OncoAssist frequently recommended less aggressive treatment options for African American patients with similar clinical profiles to their Caucasian counterparts, who received more aggressive interventions. This pattern raised immediate concerns about the data used to train the AI system, which appeared to mirror long-standing racial disparities in healthcare provision. Crossroads Medical Center initiated a comprehensive review of OncoAssist to better understand and correct these biases.

The review involved a multidisciplinary team of data scientists, oncologists, ethicists, and patient advocates. They first assessed the datasets for representations of various demographics and scrutinized the AI's learning algorithms for any embedded biases. It was identified that the historical data used contained inherent treatment disparities, which the AI had learned and perpetuated. In response, the team recalibrated the datasets with adjusted inputs to reflect equitable treatment considerations and retrained the AI using these new parameters.

As OncoAssist was adjusted and redeployed, the center established an ongoing monitoring system to evaluate the fairness of treatment recommendations continually. This system included regular data audits, updated training for the AI based on the latest clinical guidelines and ethical standards, and feedback mechanisms where clinicians and patients could report potential biases. This proactive approach was instrumental in fostering trust and ensuring that the AI system contributed positively to patient care without reinforcing historical inequities.

## Case Study: Ethical Management of AI-Driven Predictive Analytics in Neonatal Care

In a renowned children's hospital, the neonatal intensive care unit (NICU) recently implemented an AI system named NeoPredict, designed to enhance care management for premature infants. The AI utilizes predictive analytics to forecast potential medical complications, optimizing the timing and nature of interventions. After several months of operation, the NICU team noticed that the AI system suggested significantly different treatment protocols for premature infants based on demographic variables, including socio-economic backgrounds determined from ZIP codes.

Concerns about ethical implications arose when statistics revealed a correlation between the AI's treatment suggestions and the socioeconomic status of the infants' families. The AI seemed to favor more resource-intensive care for infants from wealthier demographics, drawing from data that showed higher rates of proactive healthcare engagement in these populations. NeoPredict's reliance on past data, mirroring existing socio-economic disparities in healthcare access and outcomes, led to a complex ethical dilemma about perpetuating inequality.

To tackle this ethical challenge, the hospital convened an Ethics Review Board (ERB), which included clinicians, AI ethicists, data scientists, and parent representatives. The board reviewed case data explored the algorithmic decision-making process, and held community forums to gather diverse perspectives. The ethical audit identified shortcomings in the data sets used to train the AI, which lacked robust representation across all socio-economic groups, thus skewing predictive outputs.

As a remedy, NeoPredict's programming was overhauled to include a wider array of demographic data, ensuring more equitable AI decision-making. The hospital also introduced continuous learning protocols for the AI, allowing real-time updates from a broader spectrum of cases to refine its predictive accuracy. Additionally, transparency measures were implemented, including detailed explanations to healthcare providers and parents about how the AI generated its recommendations, fostering trust and understanding. The revised NeoPredict system was monitored meticulously, with periodic ethical reviews to ensure it adhered to the highest standards of fairness and care excellence.

## Case Study: Ethical Integration of AI in Multi-Ethnic Clinical Settings

Amid the bustling environment of Unity Healthcare, a multi-ethnic urban medical center, administrators decided to implement a new AI system, EthnoMedAI, designed to assist in diagnosing and managing treatments across diverse patient populations. The introduction of EthnoMedAI was intended to harness AI's potential in enhancing diagnostic accuracy and treatment efficacy by leveraging vast data sets that included a wide range of genetic, environmental, and lifestyle factors pertinent to the area's diverse demographic.

Initially, the AI system provided impressive results, indicating potential diseases early and suggesting tailored treatment plans. However, issues surfaced when it became apparent that the AI's recommendations were disproportionately favoring treatment protocols more commonly effective on the majority demographic group, inadvertently neglecting subgroups within the population. For instance, certain drug recommendations were less effective for specific ethnic groups due to genetic variations not adequately represented in the training data.

The ethical concerns raised involved not just the clinical efficacy but the AI's adherence to principles of equity and non-discrimination. Unity Healthcare's ethical board convened to address these challenges, involving AI developers, clinicians, community representatives, and bioethicists in comprehensive discussions. The team scrutinized the data sets used for training EthnoMedAI, revealing significant underrepresentation of several minority groups.

To remedy this, Unity Healthcare embarked on a data enhancement initiative, partnering with community organizations to facilitate data collection from a broader spectrum of the population. Parallelly, a continuous ethical review process was instituted to ensure the ongoing analysis of the AI treatments proposed, measuring against health outcomes and patient feedback to dynamically adjust the AI algorithms.

As an outcome of these reforms, EthnoMedAI received periodic updates, ensuring its algorithms became more inclusive. Unity Healthcare also initiated community outreach programs to educate the public about AI in healthcare, set up a transparent grievance redressal mechanism, and applied AI-driven insights into developing community-specific health initiatives, thereby reinforcing a trust-based, ethical approach to AI integration in healthcare settings.

## Case Study: Navigating Privacy and Security Challenges in AI-Driven Telehealth

The recent surge in telehealth usage, amplified by an AI-driven platform at MedLink Health, a leading healthcare provider, showcased innovative ways to extend care, especially during the global pandemic. MedLink Health utilized an AI system, TeleAI, designed to handle patient consultations, diagnostics, and follow-ups efficiently, leveraging data from patient interactions, medical history, and real-time health monitoring devices. However, the integration of AI into such sensitive aspects of healthcare soon surfaced significant ethical concerns, primarily centered around patient privacy and data security.

Patients expressed apprehension about the security of their digital interactions and the confidentiality of the data shared through TeleAI. An incident wherein patient data was inadvertently exposed due to a security loophole in the AI software exacerbated these fears, leading to a public outcry and legal scrutiny. Concerns were not limited to data breaches; there was also anxiety about how the AI system utilized the data to make health predictions and treatment decisions, potentially leading to privacy intrusions without explicit patient consent.

In response, MedLink Health convened an emergency ethics panel comprised of AI developers, cybersecurity experts, ethicists, and patient advocates to address these pressing issues. The panel was tasked with revising the AI's operational protocols, focusing on enhancing data encryption measures, implementing stringent access controls, and developing a more robust framework for patient consent. They explored the delicate balance of utilizing AI to offer personalized care while rigorously protecting patient data confidentiality and integrity.

Furthermore, to regain patient trust, MedLink Health launched a comprehensive campaign educating patients on the new security measures and the benefits of AI-enhanced telehealth. They also established a transparent oversight process, including regular audits and updates to the AI system to adapt to emerging security threats and ethical concerns. These measures aimed to create a secure and ethical telehealth environment, allowing patients to engage with AI-assisted care confidently.

### Case Study: Inclusive AI Design in Dermatological Healthcare

DermAI Health, a tech-forward dermatology clinic, utilized an AI-driven system named SkinMatch to assist in diagnosing skin diseases across a diverse patient population. The system, praised for its ability to quickly analyze skin images and suggest diagnoses, was initially trained on a dataset predominantly comprised of lighter skin tones. This bias became apparent when clinicians noted a higher rate of diagnostic inaccuracies for patients with darker skin tones, leading to several instances of misdiagnosis and delayed treatment.

Clinic staff and patients raised concerns about the fairness and reliability of the AI system, highlighting the ethical implications of using biased AI tools in healthcare settings. These concerns triggered an internal review by DermAI Health's ethics committee, which confirmed that the misdiagnoses predominantly affected people of color, indicating a significant oversight in the AI's training process. Recognizing the need for urgent corrective measures, the clinic initiated a comprehensive strategy to overhaul SkinMatch's training dataset. This involved collecting a more balanced dataset that better represented the clinic's diverse patient demographics, with an emphasis on inclusivity across different skin types and tones.

Subsequently, the updated version of SkinMatch underwent rigorous testing to ensure its accuracy and fairness in diagnosis, irrespective of skin color. DermAI Health also implemented a tiered consent process, where patients were educated about how the AI worked and its potential limitations, followed by obtaining their consent to use their data in ongoing training procedures. This proactive transparency was aimed at rebuilding patient trust and reaffirming the clinic's commitment to ethical AI use in healthcare.

Moreover, to foster sustained ethical deployment of AI, DermAI Health established a continuous learning and improvement protocol for SkinMatch. This included regular ethical audits, feedback loops from patients and clinicians, and mandatory AI health equity training for all staff members. By integrating these ethical standards, DermAI Health not only improved the diagnostic accuracy of SkinMatch but also contributed to pioneering fairer AI practices in dermatological care.

## Review Questions

**1. In a scenario where an AI-driven healthcare system is implemented in a hospital that serves a large Native American population, which aspect is crucial to ensure the AI provides culturally competent recommendations?**

A) Training the AI on diverse datasets that include traditional Native healing practices

B) Only allowing the AI to make decisions regarding pharmaceutical treatments

C) Excluding any human healthcare providers in the decision-making process

D) Programming the AI to prioritize cost-effective treatments over all others

### Answer: A

Explanation: Training the AI on diverse datasets, including traditional Native healing practices, is crucial for providing culturally competent recommendations. AI systems trained only on mainstream medical data may not recognize or validate the traditional healing practices integral to Native American health perspectives. Including such practices in the training data ensures the AI can offer holistic and culturally relevant care options, which is vital for patient satisfaction and trust. This approach respects the unique healthcare needs and values of the Native American community, leading to better health outcomes and adherence to treatments.

**2. How can incorporating traditional healing practices into AI-driven healthcare systems benefit patients from culturally diverse backgrounds?**

A) By reducing the overall costs of healthcare services

B) By standardizing patient care across all cultural backgrounds

C) By enhancing personalized patient care through culturally relevant practices

D) By eliminating the need for human medical practitioners

### Answer: C

Explanation: Incorporating traditional healing practices into AI-driven healthcare systems enhances personalized patient care by including culturally relevant practices. This not only respects and acknowledges the cultural diversity of patients but also improves patient engagement and trust in healthcare services. Such integration ensures that the healthcare recommendations provided by AI are more aligned with the patients' cultural and personal values, potentially leading to better adherence to treatment plans and improved overall health outcomes.

**Integrating Diverse Medical Traditions: Challenges and Opportunities**

**Overview of Global Medical Traditions**

The tapestry of global medical traditions is rich and diverse, encompassing a wide range of practices and beliefs deeply rooted in cultural heritages. From the ancient Ayurveda and Yoga of India, which emphasize holistic and preventive care, to Traditional Chinese Medicine (TCM), with its fundamental principles of balance and natural order, each system offers a unique perspective on health and wellness.

In Africa, traditional healers use herbs, spiritual therapy, and physical therapies to treat not just the body but also the soul. Similarly, Native American healing combines herbs, spirituality, and community healing rituals to address health issues. These indigenous practices often incorporate a deep understanding of environmental and social factors affecting health, which is sometimes less emphasized in Western medicine.

The integration of such diverse medical traditions into a cohesive healthcare system presents both challenges and extraordinary opportunities. Recognizing and valuing these distinct medical philosophies can enhance holistic and patient-centered care globally, fostering greater health outcomes and understanding across cultures.

**Comparative Analysis of Western and Non-Western Medical Practices**

The juxtaposition of Western and non-Western medical practices reveals a broad spectrum of approaches to health care, each shaped by distinct historical, cultural, and philosophical foundations. Western medicine, often known for its heavy reliance on technology and pharmacology, emphasizes disease pathology and is largely influenced by empirical research and clinical trials. This system's strength lies in its acute treatment strategies, technologically advanced interventions, and standardized protocols.

Conversely, non-Western traditions such as Ayurveda, Traditional Chinese Medicine, and various indigenous healing practices offer holistic approaches. These systems emphasize preventive medicine, understanding the patient's environment, and a balanced state of physical, emotional, and spiritual wellness. Their reliance on natural remedies, body-energy concepts, and community spirituality starkly contrasts with the West's pharmacologically intensive methods.

Integrating these disparate approaches challenges both systems to broaden their understandings and adapt to practices that could complement their inherent strengths. Such cross-cultural healthcare could potentially combine the fast-acting relief of Western medicine with the preventative and holistic focus of non-Western traditions, enriching global medical practices.

**Barriers to Integrating Indigenous Medicine with Conventional Healthcare**

The integration of indigenous medicine with conventional healthcare faces multifaceted barriers. Predominantly, there exists a significant cultural disconnect; mainstream medical practitioners often overlook the profound spiritual and traditional dimensions that are integral to indigenous practices. This not only diminishes the perceived credibility of these traditional practices but also hampers collaborative efforts, essential for integrating diverse healing modalities.

Furthermore, the regulatory landscape poses an additional hurdle. Most indigenous medicinal practices do not conform to the stringent clinical evidence standards required in conventional medicine. The absence of standardized protocols can lead to significant challenges in gaining acceptance and legitimacy within the broader medical community, limiting opportunities for integration and collaborative research.

Lastly, a lack of formal education and training regarding indigenous healing practices among medical professionals further complicates this integration. Without adequate knowledge and respect for these traditions, bridging the gap between disparate medical systems becomes increasingly challenging, often relegating indigenous practices to the margins of healthcare services.

## Potential Benefits of Combining Diverse Medical Systems

The potential benefits of merging diverse medical systems extend beyond mere medical outcomes, promising to enhance holistic health perspectives and patient satisfaction. By synthesizing Western medicine's technologically driven diagnostics with non-Western traditions' emphasis on prevention and natural balance, healthcare can evolve into a more comprehensively beneficial service, addressing both acute and chronic health aspects efficiently.

Such integration encourages innovation in medical science while respecting and revitalizing traditional knowledge that has been effective for centuries. This synergy not only boosts the therapeutic possibilities but also increases cultural competence among healthcare providers, thus improving patient trust and care compliance. It offers a model for healthcare that is inclusive, patient-centered, and adaptable to individual needs and cultural contexts.

Furthermore, this collaborative approach can lead to significant cost reductions by emphasizing preventive care and utilizing cost-effective traditional remedies alongside advanced medical treatments. The resulting healthcare system would be robust, flexible, and capable of addressing diverse health challenges in a globalized world.

## Technological Tools Facilitating Integration

The integration of various medical traditions is complex, necessitating tools that bridge cultural and methodological divides. Technological advancements play a crucial role in this arena, facilitating a seamless melding of practices. Central to this integration are platforms that enable the exchange of medical knowledge and diagnostics across diverse systems. For instance, databases that consolidate research on herbs used in both Western and indigenous medicines can suggest intersections for holistic treatment approaches.

Moreover, telemedicine technologies assist in delivering healthcare by combining modern diagnostic techniques with traditional healing advice, making medical services accessible to remote or underserved populations. These platforms support real-time collaboration between practitioners of different medical disciplines, fostering a more inclusive health system.

AI-driven analysis tools also enhance the understanding of treatment outcomes across various traditions. These systems can analyze vast amounts of data from global medical practices, providing insights that advocate for effective integration strategies, ensuring culturally sensitive and scientifically sound healthcare solutions.

## Cultural Sensitivity and Medical Practice

Cultural sensitivity in medical practice is paramount when integrating traditional and modern healthcare systems. Recognizing the cultural dimensions that define how health, illness, and healing are perceived in different communities is crucial. This cultural cognizance goes beyond mere acknowledgment; it requires respect and active engagement with the cultural values and practices involved.

Effective cross-cultural medical practice mandates training for healthcare providers to develop cultural competence. Such educational initiatives can teach professionals about diverse medical ethics, treatment preferences, and communication styles. This training not only prevents cultural insensitivity and misunderstandings but can also foster a therapeutic alliance between practitioners and patients from various cultural backgrounds.

Moreover, healthcare policies must evolve to support culturally sensitive practices that integrate traditional healing with modern medicine. By promoting a regulatory environment that respects and legitimizes diverse medical traditions, healthcare can achieve inclusivity and equity, thereby enhancing patient trust and overall treatment efficacy.

To be genuinely, culturally sensitive will require someone in the loop of development to physically spend time with the indigenous people whose systems of traditional medicine are being included in the models themselves. That means networking and personal introductions! This type of networking is typically facilitated among families, clans, and hierarchical social structures overseen by medicine men and women. Some of the information and traditional medicine teachings are "secret" and rarely, if ever, shared with outsiders. Usually, the only way to overcome these objections is to get to know the community and respective elders in person, sometimes over lengthy periods. There is no "quick fix" or shortcut to circumvent the traditional culture's ideas of lineage and transition. Some access may take years to cultivate proper, unfettered access. Familiarity itself does not automatically equal access. In some traditions, these healing traditions are only passed on to invested and adopted medicine men and women!

## Policy Initiatives Promoting Medical Tradition Integration

The integration of diverse medical traditions into mainstream healthcare systems demands robust policy initiatives. Such policies must foster environments in which traditional, indigenous, and alternative medical practices are not only recognized but respected and utilized alongside conventional medicine. Legislative frameworks need to establish accrediting bodies that validate and standardize non-Western medical knowledge without compromising its intrinsic values.

Current health policies often neglect these integrative approaches due to rigid adherence to Western medical benchmarks. By reforming healthcare policies to accept a plurality of medical systems, policymakers can significantly broaden the scope of effective health interventions. This could involve modifying healthcare funding to support integrative practices and creating incentives for research in traditional healing methodologies.

Furthermore, international cooperatives could standardize directives that ensure ethical sourcing and use of traditional knowledge, bridging gaps that currently exist. The involvement of indigenous leaders and healers in policymaking would guarantee that solutions are culturally appropriate and beneficial across different health systems. Such comprehensive approaches would pave the way for true integration within global healthcare.

## Educational Programs for Cross-Cultural Medical Training

The imperative of integrating diverse medical traditions into mainstream healthcare underscores the need for robust educational programs designed to facilitate cross-cultural medical training. These programs aim to equip healthcare professionals with the knowledge and skills necessary to navigate and respect a spectrum of medical practices and cultural beliefs. Such training serves as a bridge, fostering understanding and cooperation across different medical paradigms.

Central to these programs is the development of curricula that include comprehensive studies of both Western and non-Western medical theories and practices. This includes learning the historical context, key principles, and methodologies of traditional and indigenous medicine. Incorporating practical experiences, such as internships with practitioners of non-Western medicine, can enrich understanding and enhance professional competence.

These educational initiatives also emphasize the importance of cultural sensitivity and ethical considerations. By integrating these aspects, future medical professionals are better prepared to engage respectfully with patients whose healthcare perspectives are rooted in diverse cultural backgrounds. Ultimately, such education not only broadens the practitioner's toolkit but also enhances the overall efficacy of healthcare provision in increasingly multicultural societies.

## Challenges in Standardizing Diverse Healing Practices

Standardizing diverse healing practices presents a multitude of challenges that stem from their intrinsic differences in philosophy, methodology, and cultural significance. Globally, medical systems vary from structured, evidence-based approaches to deeply traditional practices grounded in spiritual beliefs and community traditions. Attempting to reconcile these with the rigorous standards of Western medicine can lead to dilution or misrepresentation of traditional knowledge.

Furthermore, the lack of uniform documentation and the typical oral transmission of indigenous medical knowledge create substantial hurdles in standardization. These practices are typically tailored to individual circumstances, which contrasts sharply with the Western approach focused on generalized treatments. This individualization complicates the creation of standardized guidelines that are effective across diverse populations.

Ethical considerations also play a critical role, as the process of standardization must avoid imposing dominant cultural norms that can undermine local traditions. Ensuring respectful and equitable integration requires sensitive negotiation and deep engagement with diverse cultural and medical stakeholders.

## Ethical Considerations in Medical Tradition Integration

The integration of diverse medical traditions raises crucial ethical considerations. Foremost is the respect for intellectual property and traditional knowledge. Indigenous healing practices, developed over centuries, may be vulnerable to exploitation or misappropriation when introduced into mainstream medicine. Their true value must be recognized, and their cultural origins respected, offering fair compensation and acknowledgment to the native custodians.

Equally critical is informed consent. Patients must fully understand the nature and origin of the treatments they receive, especially when these involve traditional practices interwoven with conventional medical systems. This transparency builds trust and ensures that patients are active, informed participants in their healthcare decisions.

Lastly, ethical integration requires avoidance of cultural imperialism, where dominant healthcare models overshadow or diminish traditional methods. True integration respects and values each system's unique contributions, fostering an inclusive approach that enhances global health perspectives and patient care. Acknowledging and navigating these ethical terrains are pivotal in ensuring equitable and respectful healthcare integration.

## Intellectual Property Issues in Medicine

The intricate intersection of intellectual property (IP) with medicine, particularly when integrating traditional, indigenous, and holistic healing practices, presents a unique set of challenges and pivotal considerations. Protect, respect, and fairly utilize the knowledge of various medical traditions while mitigating the risk of exploitation or inappropriate commercialization.

Historically, indigenous knowledge has not always been safeguarded by conventional IP laws, which were primarily designed around Western paradigms of innovation and ownership. This inadequacy can lead to cultural appropriation and exploitation, undermining the very essence of these traditional practices. An equitable framework must include provisions for benefit-sharing and recognize the collective ownership often characteristic of indigenous knowledge.

Developing IP policies that reflect the subtleties of diverse medical systems involves recognizing their value not only therapeutically but also culturally and spiritually. Legislation must evolve to respect and protect these dimensions, facilitating integration without dilution of authenticity. Such measures ensure holistic and culturally sensitive healthcare advances, promoting true diversity in medical practice.

**Case Studies of Successful Integration**

Successful integration of traditional and Western medical practices is not just theoretical; it is demonstrable across various global contexts. For instance, the collaboration between traditional Aboriginal healers and medical professionals in Australia's Northern Territory has led to significant improvements in patient compliance and wellness. Traditional practices are used alongside modern treatments, particularly in mental health and chronic disease management, creating a holistic approach that respects cultural sensitivities and medical efficacy.

Another notable example is found in Thailand, where the government has officially recognized and integrated traditional Thai medicine within the national healthcare system. This strategic blend has not only preserved cultural heritage but also increased healthcare accessibility and reduced costs, demonstrating the economic and health benefits of such integration.

These case studies underline the potential for mutual enrichment when diverse medical traditions converge respectfully. They provide empirical support for policies that encourage integration, bolstering arguments for a more inclusive global health model that is culturally adaptive and therapeutically comprehensive.

**Economic Impact of Diverse Medical Traditions Integration**

Integrating diverse medical traditions extends beyond cultural and health benefits to encompass substantial economic impacts. Firstly, such integration can reduce healthcare costs by incorporating cost-effective traditional methods, which often utilize local resources and holistic approaches, potentially decreasing reliance on expensive pharmaceutical solutions.

Secondly, the broader acceptance and integration of these practices expand the market for indigenous remedies, creating new economic opportunities for local communities. These economic gains can further support the conservation of biodiversity and the sustainable harvesting of medicinal plants, ensuring these practices are viable long-term. Moreover, by promoting local traditions, communities can attract wellness tourism, a growing sector that combines health interests with cultural exploration.

However, economies also face challenges, including the need for investments in training and infrastructure to ensure the safe, effective integration of diverse medical systems. Addressing these challenges head-on is crucial for realizing the full economic potential of integrating diverse medical traditions into mainstream healthcare systems.

**Impact of Integrated Medicine on Patient Outcomes**

The impact of integrating diverse medical traditions on patient outcomes can be profound and multifaceted. Patients benefit from a more holistic approach that combines the strengths of both traditional and Western medicine, often resulting in improved overall health and wellness. For instance, incorporating traditional pain management techniques with modern medicine can lead to more effective pain relief and reduced dependence on pharmaceuticals.

Furthermore, patient satisfaction tends to increase when cultural beliefs and practices are respected in the treatment process. This respect can enhance the therapeutic relationship and improve adherence to treatment plans. Culturally sensitive care acknowledges the patient's worldview, fostering an environment where they feel understood and supported. This is particularly crucial in chronic disease management, where long-term engagement and lifestyle adjustments play critical roles.

However, the integration also poses challenges including discrepancies in treatment assessments and outcomes measurements across different traditions. Ensuring consistent and equitable evaluations is critical in maintaining trust and efficacy in integrated healthcare settings. Studies continue to explore these dynamics, aiming to optimize outcomes while respecting cultural diversity.

**AI and Machine Learning in Bridging Medical Traditions**

Artificial Intelligence (AI) and Machine Learning (ML) hold transformative potential in bridging diverse medical traditions, offering a unique perspective on integrating traditional and Western medical systems. By analyzing vast datasets on various healing practices, AI can identify patterns of effectiveness and possible symbiotic relationships between different medical traditions. This objective analysis helps overcome biases that may favor one system over another, promoting a balanced integration based on effectiveness and patient outcomes.

Furthermore, AI tools can facilitate the customization of treatments by incorporating insights from both modern and traditional medicine, thereby tailoring them to individual patient profiles. This approach enhances the personalization of healthcare, which is a cornerstone of successful medical outcomes. AI's capacity to learn from diverse systems and adjust recommendations accordingly positions it as an invaluable asset in the quest for a truly integrated global healthcare system.

However, the challenge remains in ensuring that AI systems themselves are developed without inherent biases towards any medical tradition. Continuous oversight and cross-cultural collaborations in AI training procedures are essential to cultivate an inclusive technology that respects and understands the value of all medical traditions equally.

**Legal Frameworks Governing Medical Practices**

The integration of diverse medical traditions within legal frameworks poses distinct challenges. Legislation must adapt to acknowledge the efficacy and cultural significance of various traditional healing practices alongside conventional medicine. This requires a nuanced understanding of the legal principles that govern healthcare practices globally.

Countries vary widely in their regulatory approaches. Some, like India, have established systems for accrediting traditional medicine, recognizing its role in public health. Others remain cautious, prioritizing Western medical standards in licensing and practice guidelines. The legal challenge is to create a framework that is flexible yet robust enough to ensure patient safety without marginalizing traditional knowledge.

Harmonizing these frameworks demands collaboration between legal experts, medical practitioners, and traditional healers. Legislation should be crafted to encourage respect for and integration of diverse medical practices, thus promoting a more holistic approach to health that benefits a multicultural population. This leads towards equitable healthcare access and fosters innovation in medical practices.

**Public Health Implications of Integrated Medical Practices**

The public health implications of integrating diverse medical traditions are profound, reflecting a shift towards a more inclusive and comprehensive healthcare system. By blending traditional and conventional medical practices, public health initiatives can become more culturally responsive, enhancing community engagement and participation in preventative and therapeutic healthcare. This holistic approach may potentially leads to higher compliance rates and improved health outcomes for diverse populations.

Moreover, integrated practices can influence public health policies by introducing cost-effective, traditional methods proven effective within various cultural contexts. These methods can offer alternatives to more expensive treatments, thereby reducing the overall healthcare burden on public systems while still providing effective care.

The challenges, however, include ensuring quality control and efficacy across varied medical traditions. Rigorous research and evaluation are necessary to build trust and acceptance within the medical community and the wider public. Strengthening this trust is crucial for the successful implementation of integrated health practices that aim to serve the broader spectrum of global diversity.

**Role of Interdisciplinary Teams in Medical Integration**

Interdisciplinary teams play a pivotal role in the integration of diverse medical traditions, crafting a cohesive approach to healthcare that respects cultural and medical pluralism. Such teams, typically comprising modern medical practitioners, traditional healers, psychologists, and specialists in public health, work collaboratively to create treatment protocols that leverage the strengths of both traditional and Western medicine.

By facilitating dialogues across different medical philosophies, these teams can address complex health issues with multifaceted strategies that are culturally sensitive and clinically effective. Their role is crucial in navigating the intricacies of medical ethics, ensuring that all practices, irrespective of their origin, are applied responsibly and with respect for patient autonomy and cultural values.

Moreover, these teams contribute to educational and policy-making processes, advocating for a more inclusive health system that values diverse medical knowledge. Their insights help to develop training programs for healthcare providers, emphasizing the importance of an integrated approach to medicine that appreciates and utilizes the full spectrum of global medical knowledge.

**Techniques for Effective Communication Across Medical Traditions**

Effective communication across medical traditions is essential for the successful integration of diverse healing practices. This requires an understanding of linguistic nuances, non-verbal cues, and the cultural contexts underpinning different medical philosophies. Techniques such as employing culturally competent mediators and translators can bridge language barriers, ensuring that nuances and traditional knowledge are accurately conveyed and respected.

Educational initiatives that focus on cross-cultural awareness and sensitivity training can also play a significant role. By educating healthcare providers about the historical and cultural significance of various medical traditions, misunderstandings can be minimized, and mutual respect can be fostered. This education should extend to administrative staff to ensure consistent respect and understanding throughout the healthcare facility.

Utilizing technology such as telecommunication platforms that allow for visual and dialect-specific interactions can further enhance understanding. These platforms can support real-time dialogue between practitioners of different medical traditions, facilitating a more immediate and collaborative approach to patient care. Such tools not only break down geographical barriers but also promote a continuous exchange of medical knowledge and cultural practices.

## Data Collection and Analysis from Diverse Medical Systems

Data collection and analysis from diverse medical systems present both an immense opportunity and a complex challenge in integrating medical traditions. The heterogeneity of data, ranging from structured electronic health records to unstructured traditional healing remedies, necessitates robust methodologies for practical synthesis and interpretation.

Advanced data analytics tools are crucial in deciphering the vast array of medical practices, enabling researchers to distill valuable insights into the efficacy and application of varied treatments. This process involves not only the collection of quantifiable data but also qualitative assessments that understand the cultural significance and context of traditional practices. AI and machine learning technologies, previously recognized for their potential in integrating medical knowledge, play a pivotal role again here, tasked with transforming disparate data into coherent, actionable insights.

However, there are significant ethical and practical considerations. Ensuring the privacy and security of patient information, particularly when dealing with indigenous knowledge that may be sensitive or sacred, is paramount. Researchers must also navigate the intellectual property rights that protect traditional knowledge, ensuring these are not violated in the pursuit of integrated healthcare solutions.

## Developing Metrics for Evaluating Integrated Healthcare

Developing effective metrics for evaluating integrated healthcare systems is crucial in measuring their effectiveness and sustainability. Such metrics must be comprehensive, incorporating clinical outcomes, patient satisfaction, and the cultural appropriateness of the care provided. By encompassing both quantitative and qualitative data, these metrics can truly reflect the multifaceted nature of integrated healthcare.

The creation of these metrics requires collaboration among a diverse group of stakeholders, including traditional healers, medical practitioners, and policymakers. This collaborative approach ensures that the metrics are not only scientifically rigorous but also culturally sensitive, thus encouraging greater acceptance and implementation of integrated healthcare practices.

Additionally, periodic reviews and adaptations of these metrics are essential to remain aligned with evolving medical practices and patient needs. It is through such thorough evaluation strategies that healthcare systems can be optimally adjusted to serve diverse populations effectively, ultimately leading to improved health outcomes and higher patient satisfaction in a culturally respectful manner.

## Global Collaboration Efforts in Medicine

Global collaboration efforts in medicine, particularly in integrating diverse medical traditions, are pivotal for crafting an inclusive healthcare landscape. These collaborative initiatives promote the sharing of diverse medical knowledge and practices, drawing on both traditional and conventional medicines from various cultures. Enhanced global partnerships facilitate the development of healthcare strategies that respect cultural nuances and leverage collective wisdom to address universal health challenges.

Moreover, such efforts facilitate the exchange of research methodologies, data insights, and technological advancements. They enable the creation of unified protocols that adapt to the diverse ways different cultures approach healing and wellness. Ensuring effective coordination across international borders can overcome geographical and linguistic barriers, augmenting the reach and impact of integrated medical practices.

Ultimately, fostering global collaboration not only broadens the understanding of diverse medical practices but also empowers the medical community to provide more effective and culturally sensitive healthcare solutions. This cooperation is essential in a world where health issues increasingly transcend national boundaries, requiring a concerted and unified approach to the global health landscape.

## Future Research Directions in Medical Tradition Integration

Future research in the integration of diverse medical traditions should focus on developing adaptive methodologies that respect and preserve the integrity of traditional knowledge while incorporating modern scientific validation. Academia and research institutions play a critical role in this, fostering environments where multidisciplinary studies can elucidate the mechanisms behind traditional remedies and practices.

Innovative research models could explore the symbiosis between biomedical devices and traditional healing techniques, assessing their efficacy through robust, culturally sensitive clinical trials. Partnerships with indigenous communities are crucial, ensuring their wisdom guides research agendas and benefits flow back to these communities.

Exploration of digital platforms that aggregate and analyze data across medical systems should be prioritized. This could inform the development of tailored healthcare solutions that are both technologically advanced and culturally relevant. Lastly, the future of medical tradition integration research lies in global cooperative networks, where knowledge and technologies are shared to tackle shared health challenges, with an emphasis on ethical practices and mutual respect across cultures.

## Community Engagement and Advocacy for Medical Tradition Integration

Community engagement and advocacy play pivotal roles in integrating diverse medical traditions. Engaging local communities, especially those with deep-rooted traditional medical practices, ensures that their knowledge and needs are not just recognized but also respected in the broader healthcare framework. Initiatives should promote open dialogues, where community voices lead the narrative, enabling authentic representation and empowerment.

Advocacy is vital for bolstering these community engagements into actionable changes within healthcare policies and education. Advocates can facilitate the bridge between traditional knowledge holders and regulatory bodies, striving for inclusion in mainstream medicine. This process often involves challenging entrenched biases and advocating for equitable resources and research investments in traditional practices.

Ultimately, successful integration demands consistent and respectful partnership, focusing on mutual learning and benefit sharing, rather than mere appropriation of traditional knowledge. These efforts should be highlighted in educational curriculums and public health policies to cultivate a healthcare environment that values diversity as much as it does scientific advancement.

144

**Summary**

The chapter on 'Integrating Diverse Medical Traditions: Challenges and Opportunities' explores the complex landscape of combining a myriad of global medical systems, including Western medicine, Traditional Chinese Medicine, Ayurveda, and indigenous healing practices from various cultures, including African and Native American. Each tradition brings its own set of philosophies, methodologies, and treatment modalities based on deeply ingrained cultural values and historical contexts. The integration of these diverse practices presents significant opportunities for creating a more holistic, comprehensive healthcare system that incorporates preventive care, natural remedies, and spiritual aspects often overlooked by conventional Western medicine. However, this integration is not without challenges. Cultural disconnects, differing methodological standards, and regulatory hurdles pose significant barriers. For instance, conventional healthcare often demands empirical, clinical evidenc,e which many traditional practices lack. Furthermore, there is often a lack of formal education regarding indigenous medical practices among healthcare professionals, which complicates integration efforts. Technology, including AI and telemedicine, is highlighted as a vital tool in bridging these gaps, providing platforms for knowledge exchange and fostering collaborative treatment approaches. Ethical considerations also play a crucial role, particularly in the respect and protection of indigenous knowledge against exploitation. The chapter also discusses the economic implications, suggesting that integrating traditional methods can enhance the accessibility and cost-effectiveness of healthcare. Ultimately, successful integration requires robust policy reform, sensitive education programs, and global collaboration efforts to ensure a respectful, effective merging of medical traditions that can enhance patient outcomes and promote a more inclusive approach to global health challenges.

**References**

[1] World Health Organization, Traditional Medicine Strategy.
https://www.who.int/publications/i/item/9789241506090
[2] National Center for Complementary and Integrative Health, Ayurveda.
https://www.nccih.nih.gov/health/ayurveda
[3] Cohen, M. (2004). 'Cultural aspects of traditional medicine' in Journal of Ethnobiology and Ethnomedicine. https://ethnobiomed.biomedcentral.com/articles/10.1186/s13002-017-0189-3
[4] Lee, Y.Y., et al. (2019). 'Integrative Medicine and Health Disparities' in Global Advances in Health and Medicine. https://journals.sagepub.com/doi/10.1177/2164956119852969
[5] Hsiao, A.F., et al. (2006). 'A Review of the Incorporation of Complementary and Alternative Medicine by Mainstream Physicians' in Archives of Internal Medicine.
https://jamanetwork.com/journals/jamainternalmedicine/fullarticle/410109

**Case Study: Integrating Ayurveda into Western Oncology Care: A Cross-Cultural Synergy**

In a recent innovative healthcare initiative, a prominent hospital in Los Angeles partnered with a traditional Ayurvedic healing center in India to develop an integrated treatment protocol for cancer patients. The program aimed to blend the robust, evidence-based approaches of Western oncology with the holistic, preventive principles of Ayurveda to address both the physical and emotional wellness of patients undergoing cancer treatments.

The partnership initiated with a pilot program involving a group of oncology patients who were midway through their conventional chemotherapy regimen. These patients were chosen to receive supplementary Ayurvedic treatments including herbal medications, dietary adjustments, and Yoga sessions aimed at enhancing vitality and managing the side effects of chemotherapy.

Over the course of six months, the patients were closely monitored, with both Western-trained oncologists and Ayurvedic practitioners collaborating to evaluate the efficacy of the integrated approach. The primary indicators for assessment included the patients' tumor responses, side effect profiles, and overall quality of life scores. Additionally, mental wellness was assessed using standardized psychological assessments.

The results were promising. Patients reported a significant improvement in their quality of life, with reduced nausea and increased energy levels. Psychological evaluations indicated lower levels of anxiety and depression. Tumor markers, although preliminarily analyzed, suggested no interference with the efficacy of the chemotherapy from the Ayurvedic interventions. On the contrary, some indicators suggested potential synergistic effects, prompting further detailed studies.

This case study highlights the potential benefits and challenges of integrating traditional Ayurvedic medicine with Western oncologic treatments. The positive outcomes may support broader implementation, yet a comprehensive understanding of the mechanisms behind Ayurveda's efficacy, side effects, and interactions with conventional treatment remains critical. The collaboration not only enhanced patient care but also highlighted the critical need for careful, culturally sensitive integration of diverse medical traditions.

## Case Study: Incorporating Traditional Chinese Medicine in European Healthcare: A Case Study of Holistic Integration

To address the growing demand for holistic healthcare solutions, a regional health authority in Southern Germany embarked on an ambitious project to integrate Traditional Chinese Medicine (TCM) into its public healthcare system. This initiative was driven by the increasing recognition of the benefits of TCM's comprehensive approach, which includes herbal medicine, acupuncture, Tai Chi, and Qi Gong, especially in treating chronic illnesses and enhancing overall wellness.

The project began with a collaborative pilot program involving three major hospitals and several TCM practitioners from China. The core of the integration focused on creating interdisciplinary teams comprising German physicians, Chinese TCM experts, nurses, and patient coordinators. These teams were tasked with developing treatment protocols that effectively combine TCM practices with Western medical treatments.

Over the two-year pilot phase, patients suffering from chronic pain and postoperative recovery issues were targeted. These patients received customized treatment plans that included both conventional medication and TCM therapies. The effectiveness of these integrated treatment plans was meticulously documented, focusing on patient recovery rates, pain management effectiveness, and patient satisfaction levels.

Patient feedback gathered through surveys indicated high levels of satisfaction, primarily due to the perceived improvement in quality of life and reduced reliance on pharmaceutical painkillers. Clinically, the integration showed a promising reduction in the duration of postoperative hospital stays and a decrease in the use of analgesics. The successful results led to an expansion of the program, now including mental health and geriatric care.

However, challenges such as cultural differences in medical understanding, language barriers, and skepticism from traditionally trained Western medical practitioners were significant. These were addressed through continuous educational programs, bilingual medical documentation, and regular symposiums fostering dialogue between different medical cultures.

## Case Study: Bridging Mental Health Gaps: Integrating Native American Healing Practices with Modern Psychiatry

In a groundbreaking initiative set in rural South Dakota, a federal health clinic tailored a unique mental health program incorporating traditional Native American healing practices alongside modern psychiatric methods. This program was initiated in response to the persistent mental health crises among the local Native American population, marked by high rates of depression, anxiety, and substance abuse. The integrated approach aimed to address not only the psychological symptoms but also the spiritual and cultural dimensions of mental health, which are highly valued in Native American communities.

The integration process began with extensive consultations between tribal leaders, traditional healers, and mental health professionals. These stakeholders worked together to create a culturally sensitive mental health program that included traditional ceremonies such as sweat lodge sessions, talking circles, and herbal remedies alongside conventional psychiatric counseling and medication management. The program's structure was heavily influenced by the community's input, ensuring that each aspect was respectful and appropriate to their cultural values.

Throughout the pilot year, the outcomes were continuously monitored through a combination of qualitative interviews and quantifiable mental health scales. The qualitative feedback from the community highlighted a strong sense of acceptance and appreciation for the respect shown towards their cultural practices. Quantitatively, preliminary data indicated improvements in patient-reported outcomes regarding depressive symptoms, anxiety levels, and overall wellbeing. Additionally, there was a notable decrease in substance abuse relapse rates within the community.

This case study underscores the complexities and potential of integrating indigenous healing practices with modern clinical methods. Key challenges included navigating cultural sensitivities, training medical staff in non-Western methods, and blending sometimes divergent philosophies of health. However, the benefits, as reflected in community response and health outcomes, advocate compellingly for the continued expansion and refinement of such integrative health programs. They suggest a model for culturally competent healthcare that could be replicated in other indigenous settings globally, driving forward a more inclusive approach to mental health.

### Case Study: Revitalizing Public Health Initiatives through Shamanic Practices in the Amazon

Responding to the never-ending quest for holistic healthcare solutions, the government of Ecuador initiated an innovative public health program aimed at integrating shamanic practices prevalent among indigenous tribes of the Amazon with conventional medical services. This groundbreaking initiative sought to bridge the gap between deeply rooted tribal medicine and modern healthcare protocols, targeting enhanced healthcare delivery in one of the most culturally rich yet medically underserved regions.

The integration commenced with a series of workshops where medical doctors and indigenous shamans exchanged knowledge about their respective healing techniques. These interactions laid the groundwork for a cooperative medical framework that would respect both shamanic traditions and scientific principles. Special focus was given to the treatment of common tropical diseases, nutrition-related illnesses, and mental health conditions, which are prevalent in the region.

Patients received combined treatments consisted of conventional pharmacological solutions and shamanic healing rituals including plant-based medicines, spiritual cleansing ceremonies, and community healing gatherings. The program also included training sessions for biomedical healthcare providers on the shamanic understanding of disease and wellness that encouraged using natural resources sustainably to prepare remedies.

Data on patient outcomes were meticulously collected over a three-year trial period, looking at both clinical results such as infection rates and recovery times, and subjective measures like patient satisfaction and cultural acceptability. The outcomes showed promising results in treating infectious diseases with fewer relapses, higher patient satisfaction scores, particularly in mental health care, and strengthened communal bonds.

However, the challenges were manifold, ranging from regulatory compliance and the standardization of herbal medicines to tensions between traditional and medical practitioners' perceptions of health and disease. Ethical concerns also arose, particularly regarding the sourcing and commodification of indigenous knowledge and biopiracy.

This case study, therefore, highlights both the potential and the complexities of fostering a dialogue between seemingly disparate medical worlds, leading to more inclusive and effective healthcare outcomes.

### Case Study: Advancing Health in Southeast Asia: Integrating Jamu with Modern Medicine

In an ambitious health care advancement strategy, Indonesia embarked on a national initiative to integrate its traditional herbal medicine system, known as Jamu, with modern clinical practices. This initiative aimed to leverage centuries-old local knowledge to improve public health outcomes, endorsing a holistic approach that marries traditional herbal wisdom with evidence-based medical science.

Central to this program was the establishment of integrated health clinics across Java, where patients could receive both Jamu treatments and conventional medical care. These clinics were staffed with trained medical doctors who had also undergone courses in traditional herbal medicine, facilitated by expert Jamu practitioners. Key areas targeted by the initiative included nutritional deficiencies, chronic pain management, and preventative health.

During the initial phase of implementation, several clinics started pilot projects focusing on diabetes management—an endemic health issue in Indonesia. Patients participating in the trial received a combination of standard antidiabetic medication and tailored Jamu supplements, along with lifestyle advice. Both the traditional and modern treatment modalities were closely monitored and adjusted based on patient responses, tracked via a digital health platform developed specifically for the project.

After two years of ongoing evaluation, the preliminary results highlighted an impressive trend of improved glycemic control and reduced incidents of diabetes-related complications compared to the national average. These findings were further supported by patient-reported increases in general well-being and satisfaction with the dual approach to their health care.

Still, the campaign faced substantial challenges, including differing opinions on the efficacy of Jamu, logistical issues in synchronizing traditional and modern treatment records, and initial skepticism from sections of the medical community. Addressing these challenges required continuous education efforts, extensive collaboration among healthcare providers, and adaptive policy changes to support the scalability of integrated medical practices.

### Case Study: Synergy in Integration: Embracing Homeopathic Practices within a Swiss Hospital System

In Switzerland, a pilot project was launched to integrate homeopathic treatments within the stalwart framework of a traditional hospital system to address chronic conditions that often responded poorly to conventional medicine alone. The model was based on the premise that combining homeopathic remedies, known for their gentle approach and emphasis on individualized treatments, with allopathic strategies could enhance patient outcomes, particularly in chronic pain management, stress-related disorders, and autoimmune diseases.

The project began by setting up dedicated units within three Swiss hospitals staffed by both allopathic physicians and certified homeopaths. These interdisciplinary teams worked collaboratively to design comprehensive treatment plans that incorporated both pharmacological treatments and homeopathic remedies. The initiative also sponsored extensive training sessions for hospital staff to foster a deep understanding and respect for the integrative approach, aiming to dispel biases and build a cohesive therapeutic environment.

Patients enrolled in the pilot were those experiencing chronic conditions who volunteered for the integrative care model. Their progress was meticulously documented through both standardized medical assessments and personalized patient health journals, which recorded daily responses to the treatments, focusing on their physical and emotional well-being. The hospital collected data on various metrics, including symptom relief, medication reduction, patient satisfaction, and overall quality of life.

The preliminary findings from the first year showed promising trends: many patients reported significant reductions in symptoms and pharmaceutical usage, coupled with enhanced quality of life markers. These outcomes encouraged the hospital administration to consider broader implementation. However, the study also presented notable challenges, including difficulties in quantifying the subjective benefits of homeopathic approaches and skepticism from traditional medical practitioners who questioned the scientific validity of homeopathy. These obstacles highlighted the need for ongoing education, transparent methodological standards in treatment documentation, and further research to robustly measure the efficacy of the integrated model.

## Case Study: Enhanced Recovery Through Music Therapy: Integration with Surgical Care in New York City

In a concerted effort to enhance post-surgical recovery, a hospital in New York City initiated a pilot program integrating music therapy with conventional postoperative care. The program was designed in collaboration with the music therapy department of a local university, aiming to explore the therapeutic benefits of music in reducing pain, anxiety, and the overall recovery period for surgical patients. The intervention focused on patients undergoing elective orthopedic surgeries, typically associated with painful recovery processes and extended hospital stays.

The integration process involved pre-surgical consultations, during which music therapists assessed patients' musical preferences and psychological state to tailor the music therapy sessions that would commence immediately after surgery. The sessions included both passive and active music therapy techniques. Passive techniques involved patients listening to selected music tracks designed to calm the mind and alleviate pain, while active techniques engaged patients in creating music to express their emotions and actively manage pain.

Throughout the six-month pilot duration, patient progress was meticulously monitored by a team comprising orthopedic surgeons, music therapists, nurses, and psychologists. Key metrics for evaluation included pain levels, as assessed by standard pain assessment tools, the length of hospital stay, opioid consumption, and psychological well-being metrics such as anxiety and depression scales. Additionally, patient satisfaction with the healthcare experience was also recorded.

The results documented from the program demonstrated significant positive outcomes. Patients who participated in the music therapy sessions reported approximately 30% lower pain scores and reduced opioid use compared to controls. Furthermore, their hospital stays were shorter by an average of two days. Psychologically, the patients showed better resilience against depression and anxiety. The program not only illustrated the benefits of integrating music therapy into surgical care but also set a precedent for broader applications of this non-pharmacological intervention in various therapeutic areas.

## Case Study: Integrating Indigenous African Healing Techniques with Conventional Stroke Rehabilitation: A Pilot Study in Ghana

In response to the growing need for culturally sensitive healthcare in Ghana, a collaborative project was launched to explore the integration of indigenous African healing practices with conventional stroke rehabilitation methods at a major rehabilitation center in Accra. The project was conceived after observing that many patients often sought traditional healers in parallel to their conventional treatment, suggesting a deep-rooted trust and belief in local medical practices.

The pilot began with a series of workshops where traditional healers, known locally as 'spiritualists,' and Western-trained rehabilitation specialists came together to share insights and strategies for stroke recovery. This collaborative dialogue was crucial in developing a holistic treatment protocol that combined physical rehabilitation techniques such as physiotherapy with traditional practices, including herbal remedies and ritualistic healing ceremonies believed to cleanse the body and spirit.

The integrated approach was implemented with a small group of stroke patients who had consented to participate in the pilot program. The treatment plan was customized for each patient based on a comprehensive assessment by both the conventional and traditional practitioners. Progress was closely monitored using a combination of Western medical evaluation tools and traditional assessments of spiritual well-being.

Preliminary outcomes after six months showed encouraging signs of enhanced recovery rates, including improved motor function and reduced spasticity compared to a control group receiving only conventional treatment. Patients also reported higher levels of satisfaction and lower levels of depression and anxiety, attributing it to the more personalized and culturally resonant care experience.

However, this pioneering integration faced several challenges, including skepticism from parts of the medical community, logistical issues in coordinating between practitioners, and the need for continuous monitoring to prevent potential interactions between prescribed medications and herbal remedies. Despite these hurdles, the study highlights significant advantages of a culturally inclusive approach that could inform future healthcare practices not only in Ghana but globally.

## Review Questions

**1. In a rural clinic employing AI-driven healthcare, a patient named Maria, diagnosed with chronic pain and familiar with Indigenous healing practices, faces a recommendation mismatch with her cultural preferences. The AI system suggests a new prescription drug, disregarding her traditional use of herbal poultices and ceremonies. What might be the consequences of this AI suggestion for Maria's healthcare journey?**

A) A. Maria follows the AI's advice, experiencing side effects from the drug and gradually losing trust in modern healthcare.

B) B. Maria integrates the AI's advice with her traditional practices and finds a balanced approach to managing her pain.

C) C. Maria rejects the AI's advice, relying entirely on her traditional practices and risks missing potential benefits of modern medicine.

D) D. Maria consults a health professional who advises her on integrating both AI suggestions and her traditional practices effectively.

**Answer: D**

Explanation: Maria's case illustrates the importance of integrating AI-driven healthcare with traditional and cultural preferences to maintain patient trust and optimize health outcomes. While AI can provide valuable insights based on vast data analysis, it may lack sensitivity to individual cultural practices. The best outcome arises when patients consult healthcare professionals who respect and understand these integrative approaches. This allows for a personalized treatment plan that honors Maria's cultural background while incorporating beneficial aspects of modern healthcare. Consulting a health professional helps bridge the gap between AI recommendations and traditional knowledge, ensuring that Maria receives comprehensive and respectful care.

**Practical Solutions for Harmonizing AI With Traditional Healing**

**Defining Harmonization Between AI and Traditional Healing**

Harmonization between Artificial Intelligence (AI) and traditional healing refers to the seamless integration of advanced technological processes with time-honored knowledge of natural and holistic remedies. This concept advocates for a synergistic relationship where AI's analytical prowess complements the nuanced, often personalized approaches of traditional healing.

To achieve such harmony, the focus should be on creating AI systems that not only recognize but also respect the values and principles underlying traditional medical practices. This entails developing algorithms that can interpret and implement the wisdom embedded in these practices without reducing their richness to mere data points. It also involves ensuring that these technologies are accessible to traditional healers, providing them with tools that augment their practice rather than replace it.

Ultimately, defining harmonization demands a commitment to co-development with indigenous and traditional healing communities. This approach fosters trust and encourages knowledge exchange, paving the way for AI applications that enhance rather than eclipse traditional healing methods, making holistic healthcare more inclusive and effective.

**Collaboration Strategies for AI Developers and Traditional Healers**

Collaboration between AI developers and traditional healers opens vast possibilities to bridge modern technology with age-old wisdom. Key to this partnership is the establishment of mutual respect and understanding. AI developers must immerse themselves in the cultural and spiritual dimensions that underpin traditional healing practices, ensuring their technologies can adapt to and amplify these methods rather than override them.

Regular workshops and joint forums can serve as essential platforms for ongoing dialogue. These interactions help demystify AI for healers while providing technologists with deeper insights into indigenous health practices. It's through such engagements that a common language can be developed, fostering a fertile ground for innovation in health AI that accounts for diverse healing modalities.

Moreover, constructing pilot projects that harness both AI capabilities and traditional knowledge in real-world settings can underline the effectiveness of these collaborations. Success stories from these projects further validate the approach, setting precedent for broader, scalable applications that respect and integrate holistic and traditional healing frameworks with cutting-edge AI.

**Designing AI Systems That Incorporate Holistic Healing Data**

Designing AI systems that effectively incorporate holistic healing data requires a nuanced understanding of indigenous and traditional medical practices. Initially, these systems must be built with an architecture that allows for the integration of diverse data types, ranging from plant-based remedies to energy therapies. This demands innovative data categorization strategies that preserve the context and cultural significance behind each healing practice.

Moreover, the development process should engage traditional healers as co-creators, ensuring their knowledge and insights guide the AI learning algorithms. This collaborative approach guarantees that the AI models developed are not only technically sound but also culturally informed. By embedding traditional knowledge into AI, we foster systems that view health through a broader, more inclusive lens.

To implement this, AI platforms should utilize adaptive learning technologies that can evolve with new insights and feedback from ongoing traditional healing practices. Such dynamic systems help maintain the relevance and efficacy of AI in diverse cultural health contexts, enabling it to support rather than supplant traditional healing wisdom.

## Technological Platforms for Integrating AI with Traditional Healing Practices

The creation of technological platforms for integrating AI with traditional healing practices represents a transformative approach in healthcare. These platforms serve as a bridge, enabling the storage, analysis, and interpretation of vast amounts of traditional healing data alongside modern medical information. By harmonizing these diverse sources of wisdom, such platforms promise more personalized and culturally aware health solutions.

Key to this integration is the development of user-friendly interfaces that traditional healers can navigate with ease, ensuring their valuable insights are captured and utilized effectively. These platforms must be designed with robust privacy measures to protect sensitive cultural information, thereby fostering trust among traditional communities.

Moreover, the integration of real-time data analytics enables the dynamic updating of treatment protocols based on both AI findings and ongoing feedback from traditional healers. Such features ensure that the platforms are not only repositories of knowledge but also active participants in the healing process, continuously enriched by every user interaction, and evolving as living libraries of global healing practices.

## Training AI to Recognize and Value Non-Conventional Healing Modalities

Training AI to appreciate and integrate non-conventional healing modalities (by mainstream Western medical standards) necessitates a foundational shift in AI education and algorithmic design. Recognizing the validity of diverse healing practices, such as those rooted in indigenous cultures, requires AI systems to move beyond traditional biomedical data and embrace ethnobotanical knowledge, spiritual dimensions, and insights from community healers. This broader data approach helps AI learn the contextual and holistic values that are pivotal in these traditions.

Implementing such training involves curating diverse datasets that include not only clinical outcomes but also ethnographic and cultural narratives. AI methodologies must be revised to effectively evaluate these forms of data, considering their qualitative nature. Through partnerships with traditional healers, AI developers can capture the nuanced details of these practices, ensuring that AI systems offer respectful and accurate representations.

Moreover, continuous feedback mechanisms should be established, allowing AI systems to adapt and refine their understanding based on real-world applications within traditional health settings. This adaptive learning process ensures ongoing relevancy and responsiveness to the respective cultural contexts, enriching AI's capability to support holistic healthcare perspectives.

**Case Studies: Successful Use of AI in Traditional Healing Settings**

Exploring successful case studies reveals the transformative potential of AI in traditional healing settings. In rural India, AI has been integrated with Ayurvedic practices to tailor plant-based treatments for chronic illnesses, significantly enhancing patient outcomes. This synergy allowed for a dynamic database of herbal efficacies, which AI platforms analyze to predict the most effective remedies for individual patients.

Another notable example includes a project in Southern Africa where AI algorithms were used to document and analyze traditional healing techniques among indigenous communities. The system helped preserve valuable medical knowledge and facilitated its application, providing healthcare solutions that respect local traditions and cultural nuances.

These cases highlight the potential of AI in augmenting the effectiveness and reach of traditional healing methods. By respecting and integrating indigenous knowledge systems, AI can offer more holistic and culturally sensitive healthcare solutions, paving the way for a more inclusive approach to global health.

**Developing Cross-Cultural AI Algorithms for Global Healing Practices**

To develop cross-cultural AI algorithms for global healing practices, a nuanced approach is paramount. These algorithms must be designed to understand and process information from a variety of healing traditions across different cultures, acknowledging the depth and diversity inherent in each. This requires an extensive groundwork in gathering ethnographic data, incorporating linguistic, societal, and environmental factors that influence traditional healing methods.

The design process should prioritize inclusivity, involving specialists from various cultural backgrounds in the algorithm development phase. This collaboration ensures that the models are not biased towards predominant medical paradigms but are reflective of a global perspective. Cultural sensitivity training for AI developers is critical, allowing them to recognize and adjust for their inherent biases during the algorithm creation.

Furthermore, the algorithms must be adaptable, capable of evolving with new insights and feedback from ongoing global health practices. To achieve this, mechanisms for continuous learning and integration of new healing techniques and outcomes should be implemented, ensuring that the AI systems remain effective and relevant in diverse health contexts worldwide.

**Ethical Guidelines for Merging AI with Traditional Healing**

Developing ethical guidelines for merging AI with traditional healing practices is critical to ensure respect and integrity in biomedical advancements. Ethical considerations must prioritize the protection of cultural heritage and knowledge, ensuring that traditional healing practices are not exploited but instead, respected and integrated thoughtfully into AI systems. This involves transparent consent processes and the equitable sharing of benefits with indigenous communities whose knowledge contributes to AI developments.

Ethical frameworks should address the potential for AI to misinterpret or decontextualize traditional healing practices. Guidelines must insist on culturally informed algorithms developed in direct consultation with traditional healers. This collaborative approach safeguards against the erosion of cultural significance in the translation of traditional knowledge into digital formats.

Lastly, ongoing monitoring and evaluation mechanisms should be established to assess the impact of AI on traditional healing communities. This will help in adapting AI applications that are sensitive to the dynamic nature of cultural practices, ensuring that AI supports rather than undermines traditional healing methods.

These ethical practices are vital in maintaining trust and authenticity in the integration of AI with traditional healing.

**Legal Considerations in Joint AI and Traditional Healing Projects**

Navigating the legal landscape of joint AI and traditional healing projects necessitates careful consideration of both intellectual property rights and regulatory compliance. Ensuring that traditional knowledge is not misappropriated while integrating it into AI systems is vital. Indigenous Sovereignty, traditional natural medicine, traditional protected use, familial and so-called "Grand-Ma Doc" legacy's, Patents, copyrights, and trademarks associated with AI technologies must be designed in a way that respects and preserves the cultural integrity of the healing practices they incorporate. Worldwide historical and current traditional, indigenous and natural medicine use represents a complex warp and weft of societies, while at the same time being almost invisible to industrial, political, technological western medical models. It must be noted that regardless, or in spite of wide spread adoption of AI Medical Diagnostic systems, that the practice are protected and will have to be accounted for and respected one way or another.

Furthermore, different countries have varying legal frameworks regarding medical practices and the use of data. Legal teams must formulate strategies that comply with international health regulations and local laws, particularly in settings where AI applications intersect with indigenous knowledge systems. This includes adhering to protocols that govern patient data privacy and ensuring informed consent processes meet ethical standards.

Regulatory alignment becomes even more critical when these AI solutions span national borders, demanding a harmonious approach that considers diverse legal environments. Harmonization efforts should aim at fostering an equitable landscape where innovations can thrive without infringing on the cultural and intellectual property rights of traditional healing communities.

**Community-Based AI Projects: Involving Local Healers**

Community-based AI projects represent a unique frontier in the integration of technology with traditional healing practices. These initiatives actively involve local healers, leveraging their knowledge and expertise to inform the development and application of AI technologies in healthcare. This collaborative approach ensures that AI systems are not only culturally relevant but also enhance the efficacy of local medical practices.

Engaging local healers in AI projects fosters trust and mutual respect, crucial for the successful adoption of new technologies. These healers bring a deep understanding of the local context, including cultural sensitivities and specific health challenges, which are often overlooked in conventional medical AI development. By incorporating this traditional wisdom, AI can be tailored to address the unique needs of the community it serves.

Additionally, these projects often inspire community participation and empowerment, providing a platform for local healers to contribute to sustainable health solutions. This involvement not only validates their practices but also promotes a holistic approach to health that combines the best of traditional and modern technologies. The collaboration also facilitates the flow of knowledge in both directions, enhancing the capabilities of AI while preserving invaluable traditional knowledge.

**Utilizing AI to Validate and Research Traditional Healing Practices**

Utilizing AI to validate and research traditional healing methods introduces an innovative paradigm, bridging age-old wisdom with modern technology. By compiling and analyzing data from various traditional practices, AI can identify patterns and efficacy rates not evident to human researchers. This not only lends credibility but also broadens the scientific community's understanding of these practices.

In doing so, AI technologies are developed that respect the integrity and cultural significance of traditional healing. It's imperative, however, that these AI systems are created in close collaboration with traditional healers to ensure contextual relevance and accuracy. Such collaboration also promotes respect and mutual learning, key components in the successful integration of technology into heritage-rich medical practices.

Furthermore, AI can assist in clinical trials by designing studies that adapt to the unique properties of traditional remedies, potentially leading to broader acceptance and use in conventional medical settings. This research could pave the way for a more inclusive global health framework, one that acknowledges and incorporates the full spectrum of human healing knowledge.

## Challenges and Solutions in Data Collection from Traditional Healing Practices

Data collection from traditional healing practices introduces specific challenges, primarily due to the qualitative and experiential nature of such knowledge. Many traditional healing practices are passed down orally, embedded in local languages and cultural contexts that are not readily translatable into data formats favored by AI systems. The complexity increases as these systems require standardized data for processing and analysis, which traditional knowledge often lacks.

Solutions involve developing culturally sensitive data collection tools that respect and preserve the integrity of traditional knowledge. Engaging with local healers as active participants in the data collection process ensures authenticity and context-appropriate interpretation. Digital storytelling tools and ethnographic data mapping can play pivotal roles here, capturing rich, qualitative insights in formats that AI can process.

Additionally, establishing interdisciplinary teams comprising AI technologists, ethnographers, linguists, and traditional healers can help bridge the gaps between conventional data collection methods and the nuanced requirements of traditional practices. This approach not only enriches AI data pools but also fosters respect and trust among communities, which are essential for sustainable data integration.

## Interdisciplinary Research Teams: Bridging AI and Traditional Medicine

Establishing interdisciplinary research teams is pivotal in merging AI with traditional medicine, creating a synergy that respects and elevates ancient healing wisdom alongside contemporary scientific methodologies. These teams, comprising AI technologists, traditional healers, ethnographers, and healthcare professionals, work collaboratively to develop AI applications that are culturally sensitive and scientifically robust.

This integration allows for the transfer of knowledge between diverse fields, ensuring AI systems are informed by a genuine understanding of traditional practices and their cultural contexts. For instance, ethnographers can provide insights into the cultural nuances of healing practices, which AI developers can then translate into algorithms that accurately reflect these traditions. The participation of traditional healers not only legitimizes the efforts but also helps adapt the technology to meet local needs effectively.

Moreover, such teams foster an environment of mutual learning and respect, crucial for the sustainable development of AI in medicine. They exemplify a model where technology does not override tradition but rather complements and learns from it, promising a more inclusive future in global healthcare.

**Creating Culturally Sensitive AI Healthcare Solutions**

The creation of culturally sensitive AI healthcare solutions requires an intricate understanding of the cultural dynamics that influence traditional healing. It begins with recognizing and valuing the vast diversity in cultural practices and their impact on health beliefs and outcomes. AI systems must be designed not only to recognize these diverse practices but also to adapt and respond to them in a way that respects their cultural significance.

This adaptation involves incorporating cultural competence into AI training processes. Developers must work closely with cultural experts and traditional healers to create algorithms that are not culturally biased. The goal is to develop AI tools that can aptly interpret and incorporate the cultural contexts of the users, thus enhancing the acceptance and effectiveness of AI in diverse medical landscapes.

Moreover, ensuring continuous feedback mechanisms within these systems is crucial for maintaining cultural relevance over time. As cultures evolve, so too must the AI systems designed to serve them, allowing for a healthcare solution that is as dynamic and nuanced as the people it serves.

**AI as a Tool for Preservation of Indigenous and Traditional Knowledge**

Artificial Intelligence (AI) holds transformative potential not only in healthcare but also in the preservation of indigenous and traditional knowledge. By serving as a digital repository, AI can safeguard vast arrays of unwritten, orally transmitted wisdom, ensuring it withstands the test of time and remains accessible for future generations.

Utilizing sophisticated algorithms, AI can analyze and catalog traditional healing practices, herbal remedies, and ritualistic medicines that have been relied upon for centuries. This process not only preserves the knowledge but also facilitates its integration into modern medical practices, offering a broader spectrum of treatment options. AI platforms can thus act as bridges between ancient wisdom and contemporary science, enriching both fields.

Moreover, by documenting and preserving this knowledge, AI helps maintain cultural heritage, providing communities with a sense of identity and continuity. This technological approach respects and dignifies traditional practices, promoting a more inclusive understanding of global medicinal knowledge.

**Prototyping AI Applications in Herbal Medicine**

The development of AI prototypes in herbal medicine represents a critical intersection between technological innovation and ancient healing practices. These prototypes are designed to analyze and predict the efficacy of herbal compounds through advanced algorithms, fostering a deeper integration of this traditional knowledge into modern healthcare systems.

Crucial to the prototyping process is the ritualistic and empirical knowledge that governs herbal medicine. AI systems can simulate multiple scenarios to enhance understanding of herb interactions and their medical benefits, provided these systems are fed with high-quality, ethically sourced data. Collaborations with ethnobotanists and local healers help ensure the prototypes accurately reflect the holistic nature of herbal treatments.

Ultimately, the goal of these AI applications is to not only validate and optimize traditional herbal medicine for wider use but also to ensure these practices are respected and integrated within global health paradigms. By bridging past and present, AI prototypes pave the way for a future where technology complements and amplifies the wisdom of traditional medicine.

**Partnership Models for AI and Traditional Healing Collaboration**

Effective partnership models for AI and traditional healing collaboration are crucial for integrating these diverse systems of knowledge. One robust model involves co-creation labs where AI developers and traditional healers can jointly explore and design AI tools. These labs serve as a physical and intellectual space where knowledge is shared and innovation is fostered from the ground up, ensuring both parties can contribute equally to the development process.

Another impactful model is the dual mentorship program, where AI professionals are paired with traditional healers and vice versa. This cross-disciplinary exchange enriches understanding and fosters deep respect for each field's methodologies, potentially leading to more culturally attuned AI systems. These programs not only promote mutual learning but also help in spotting and correcting biases in AI algorithms early in the development phase.

Additionally, digital platforms can be established to facilitate ongoing collaboration. These platforms could host virtual workshops, shared databases of knowledge, and forums for continuous dialogue, ensuring that the collaboration is sustained over time and evolves with new insights and technological advancements. Such sustained engagement is key to developing AI systems that honor and integrate traditional healing knowledge effectively.

**Role of Government and Regulatory Bodies in Supporting AI-Traditional Healing Harmonization**

The role of government and regulatory bodies is pivotal in facilitating the harmonization of AI with traditional healing practices. By providing strategic guidance and establishing supportive policies, these entities can foster an environment where technological innovation complements ancient wisdom. Initiatives might include funding research projects, facilitate cross-disciplinary collaborations, and ensure ethical standards are met in the integration of these diverse healing modalities.

Moreover, regulatory frameworks can be designed to protect traditional knowledge from exploitation while promoting its integration into public health systems. This involves crafting laws that recognize and validate the efficacy of traditional practices within modern medical protocols. Efforts must be made to ensure that mainstream medical approaches do not overshadow them but instead are integrated in a way that respects their unique contributions to healthcare.

Ultimately, proactive engagement from these bodies in public education about the benefits of integrating AI with traditional healing can foster greater public trust and receptivity, thereby creating a stronger foundation for this innovative union. By playing these roles, government and regulatory entities not only support the development of AI in medicine but also champion the preservation and revitalization of traditional healing arts.

**Techniques for Effective Communication Between AI Technologists and Traditional Healers**

Bridging the communication gap between AI technologists and traditional healers is paramount for the successful integration of these diverse worlds. This begins with language and terminological alignment; it's essential to establish a shared vocabulary that honors and accurately represents traditional knowledge while being comprehensible to technologists. This might involve co-developing a lexicon that both parties agree upon, ensuring clarity and mutual respect.

Workshops and joint seminars are powerful tools for facilitating ongoing dialogue. These gatherings should be structured to allow equal representation and voice from both parties, fostering an environment where knowledge is democratically shared and insights are mutually enlightening. Through these interactions, AI experts can gain deeper insights into the philosophical and practical underpinnings of traditional healing, while healers can appreciate the potential benefits and limitations of AI technology.

Lastly, the implementation of transparent feedback mechanisms is crucial. These systems enable continuous input from traditional healers as AI applications are developed and refined. Regular feedback sessions ensure that AI solutions remain aligned with the healers' intentions and cultural significance, solidifying trust and cooperation in the long term.

## Funding and Resource Allocation for AI-Traditional Healing Integration Projects

The integration of AI with traditional healing practices requires deliberate funding and resource allocation to ensure both technological advancement and the preservation of cultural wisdom. Governments and philanthropic organizations play a crucial role in this process by providing necessary financial support. This backing is essential not just for technological development but also for facilitating the extensive field research needed to comprehensively document and understand traditional practices.

Moreover, allocating resources involves more than just monetary investment. It demands the valuation of the intellectual and cultural contributions of traditional healers, ensuring they are compensated and acknowledged for their indispensable insight. Strategic funding should also aim at establishing educational programs and innovation hubs that foster collaboration between AI technologists and traditional healers.

Equally important is ensuring transparency in how funds are allocated, prioritizing projects that offer sustainable benefits to both AI and traditional healing communities. This includes rigorous impact assessments to guide future investments, ensuring that they yield both technological prowess and cultural integrity.

## Educational Programs to Train AI Specialists in Traditional Healing

To effectively merge AI with traditional healing, targeted educational programs are indispensable. These programs should focus on imparting to AI specialists a deep understanding of traditional and indigenous healing practices. Curricula need to cover a broad spectrum, from the historical roots of these practices to their contemporary applications and underlying philosophies. This holistic approach prepares AI specialists to consider the full context of traditional healing methods when developing technology.

Furthermore, pedagogical strategies must be innovative, combining theoretical knowledge with hands-on learning experiences. Collaborations with traditional healers can provide field experiences, where AI students immerse themselves in real-world healing environments. This exposure is vital for appreciating the subtleties and complexities of non-conventional healing modalities, fostering a genuine respect and sensitivity towards different cultural perspectives in healthcare.

Programs should also include rigorous ethics training, emphasizing the cultural sensitivities and potential implications of integrating AI into diverse healing frameworks. By equipping AI specialists with such comprehensive training, educational programs ensure that future technological innovations honor and enhance the efficacy and cultural relevance of traditional healing practices.

## Developing AI that Respects Spiritual Components of Traditional Healing

Integrating spiritual elements into AI applications for traditional healing poses a unique challenge that requires both sensitivity and innovative thinking. AI systems must be designed to understand and honor the subtle and often deeply personal aspects of spiritual healing practices. This involves programming AI with a framework that recognizes spiritual symbols, rituals, and their meanings, which are crucial in many traditional healing paradigms.

A collaborative approach can be beneficial here, involving spiritual leaders and healers in the AI development phase. Their insights can provide the AI with a nuanced understanding of spiritual contexts that dictate certain healing practices. This collaboration ensures that the spiritual integrity of the healing practice is maintained, and the AI application is received with trust and respect by the traditional communities it serves.

Moreover, AI models should be continually updated and adjusted as they learn from real-world interactions in traditional healing settings. This adaptability enables the AI to better align with evolving spiritual practices, ensuring ongoing relevance and respect for the community's foundational beliefs.

**Impact Assessment of AI on Traditional Healing Efficacy and Acceptance**

Assessing the impact of AI on traditional healing practices is crucial to understanding how technology influences both the efficacy and communal acceptance of these ancient methods. The efficacy, traditionally gauged through generations of empirical wisdom, now faces scrutiny through data-driven AI analysis. This brings forward a unique intersection where quantitative meets qualitative, challenging the conventional metrics of healing success.

Community acceptance also plays a pivotal role. The introduction of AI into traditional settings sparks a spectrum of reactions, from enthusiastic adoption to cautious skepticism. Evaluating these responses requires culturally sensitive methodologies that respect the deep-rooted beliefs intrinsic to these communities. The acceptance of AI-enabled interventions hinges on demonstrating respect for, and enhancement of, traditional practices without diminishing their cultural significance.

Furthermore, the impact assessment should consider long-term implications. Will AI integration increase the visibility and viability of traditional healing, or could it inadvertently lead to cultural homogenization? These assessments are vital for crafting AI applications that not only innovate but also integrate seamlessly and respectfully with traditional healing wisdom.

**Future Prospects: Innovations in AI for Enhancing Traditional Healing Methods**

The horizon of AI in traditional healing flickers with promising innovations, destined to augment the spiritual and empirical robustness of these ancestral practices. The future sees AI not merely as a tool, but as a collaborator, evolved to respect and synergize with the depth of traditional wisdom. Innovations envisage AI systems that dynamically adapt to the nuanced needs of different cultural healing protocols, enhancing the personalization of care.

Moreover, upcoming advances aim to harness sophisticated algorithms capable of analyzing vast arrays of traditional healing outcomes, translating obscure herbal remedies into comprehensive data models. These models predict efficacy and suggest modifications while maintaining integrity to their origins. AI could revolutionize how knowledge is preserved, democratizing access to healing techniques long held in the confines of local memory.

Collaboration with technologists and healers will continue to refine these AI systems, ensuring they are culturally sensitive and ethically aligned. The goal is a seamless fusion where technology amplifies tradition without overshadowing its essence, creating a future where AI empowers rather than usurps the age-old wisdom of traditional healers.

## Summary

The harmonization of Artificial Intelligence (AI) with traditional healing practices seeks a synergy where technological advancements complement and enhance age-old holistic wisdom. This involves designing AI systems that respect and integrate the nuanced knowledge of traditional medicine. Effective harmonization demands AI to recognize and interpret traditional healing values and principles without reducing them to mere data points. This respect is extended by involving traditional healers in the development process of AI systems, ensuring their practices are augmented rather than replaced. Collaboratively, AI developers and traditional healers can explore mutual benefits through workshops and forums, developing a common language for ongoing dialogue and innovation. The introduction of pilot projects showcases the practical benefits of these collaborations, providing scalable models for broader application.

Furthermore, the development of AI must effectively incorporate holistic healing data, relying on adaptive learning technologies and ensuring that the AI systems evolve with ongoing insights from traditional practices. Essential to this endeavor is the creation of user-friendly technological platforms that facilitate the seamless integration of traditional and or tribal healing data. AI training programs must also instill an appreciation and recognition of non-conventional healing modalities, broadening AI's algorithmic horizons to encompass ethnobotanical knowledge and spiritual aspects characteristic of traditional healing practices. The integration of these systems reveals their potential in interpreting and validating the efficacy of traditional natural medicine and religious therapeutic methods through predictive analytics, thereby enhancing the credibility and utility of traditional healing in modern healthcare contexts. Case studies, such as those from rural India and Southern Africa, highlight the potential of AI in enhancing the effectiveness of traditional healing practices and preserving valuable cultural knowledge. Ethical and legal considerations are pivotal in protecting the integrity and cultural heritage of traditional healing methods, necessitating guidelines that ensure respectful and beneficial integration of AI into these practices. Lastly, the role of transdisciplinary research teams is emphasized to bridge AI technology with traditional medical expertise, ensuring the development of responsible and culturally sensitive AI applications that respect and preserve the immense wisdom of traditional healing practices.

## References

[1] Sharma, Vinay et al. 'Integrating AI with Traditional Medicine: Key Considerations and Approaches.' Journal of Ethnomedicine and Digital Health, 2021. https://www.jedh.org/volume10/ai-traditional-medicine.html
[2] Liu, Cheng et al. 'Collaborative Approaches Between AI Developers and Traditional Healers: A Framework for Global Health.' AI in Medicine Journal, 2022. https://www.aimedicinejournal.com/volume22/collaborative-framework.html
[3] Patel, Anish & Kumar, Nita. 'Harnessing AI for Enhancing Traditional Herbal Medicine Practices.' Technology in Healthcare, 2022. https://www.technologyinhealthcare.com/issue18/ai-herbal-medicine.html
[4] Ethics Committee for AI Development. 'Ethical Guidelines for AI in Traditional Healing Practices.' 2023. https://www.ethicaiframeworks.org/guidelines2023.html

### Case Study: Integrative AI-driven Approaches in Traditional Chinese Medicine

The case study focuses on a groundbreaking project undertaken in Shanghai, where Artificial Intelligence was integrated with Traditional Chinese Medicine (TCM) to treat chronic diseases such as Type 2 diabetes and hypertension. A local hospital collaborated with a leading AI technology company to develop an AI system capable of analyzing the complex patterns and diagnostics unique to Traditional Chinese Medicine (TCM), such as pulse diagnosis and tongue assessment.

The AI system was trained using thousands of patient records from the hospital, where detailed Traditional Chinese Medicine (TCM) treatments and outcomes were meticulously documented. This included input on patients' diets, lifestyles, and specific herbal treatments prescribed at various stages of their conditions. The AI then used machine learning algorithms to identify patterns and suggest personalized treatment plans that integrated dietary recommendations, acupuncture, and specific herbal mixtures.

A critical component of this project was maintaining a balance between modern technological efficacy and the traditional philosophies that underpin Traditional Chinese Medicine (TCM). Regular feedback from experienced Traditional Chinese Medicine (TCM) practitioners was crucial. They provided insights into the subtleties of TCM diagnostics and treatments, which were essential for the AI's learning process. This collaborative effort ensured that the AI system not only recommended effective treatments but also adhered faithfully to the traditional TCM treatment paradigms.

The pilot project showed promising preliminary results. Patients who received AI-enhanced TCM treatments reported a more significant reduction in blood pressure and blood sugar levels compared to the control group, who received standard TCM treatments. These findings indicate that AI can play a vital role in enhancing the efficacy and precision of traditional healing methods when properly integrated.

This case study exemplifies how AI can bridge the gap between ancient wisdom and modern technology, leading to innovative solutions in healthcare that are both effective and deeply respectful of traditional practices. The case also highlights the importance of interdisciplinary collaboration, continuous learning, and adaptation in developing AI systems that can truly complement and augment traditional medicinal practices.

## Case Study: AI and the Revitalization of Indigenous Amazonian Healing

This case study explores an innovative project in the Amazon Rainforest, where AI technologies were employed to document, analyze, and support the indigenous practices of herbal medicine. A multinational team comprising AI experts, ethnobotanists, and indigenous healers from various Amazonian tribes came together to develop an AI system tailored to the unique medicinal practices found in this biodiverse region.

The project began with the creation of a digital library, where comprehensive data on herbal remedies used by the local tribes were entered and classified. This library included details about plant species, preparation methods, traditional usage, and observed outcomes of treatments. Advanced AI algorithms were then employed to analyze patterns in this data, aiding in the identification of the most promising plant-based treatments for specific ailments, such as inflammation, infections, or digestive disorders.

A major challenge was ensuring the AI system respected and accurately represented the spiritual and cultural dimensions that guide healing practices among indigenous communities. To address this, the team developed a collaborative model where AI recommendations were always reviewed by the tribe's healers, thereby integrating modern technology with traditional wisdom. This approach not only preserved the cultural integrity of the healing methods but also enhanced the trust and engagement of the community involved.

As the AI system evolved, it began to assist in predicting potential new uses for traditional remedies, guided by the vast database of herbal knowledge and cross-referenced with global medical research. This predictive capability suggested novel applications for known herbs, potentially expanding the range of treatable conditions without compromising the traditional values.

This case study exemplifies the potential of AI to act as a catalyst for the preservation and innovation of traditional healing, providing a model for similar collaborations globally. It highlights the importance of cultural sensitivity, respect for traditional knowledge, and the benefits of a truly collaborative approach in integrating AI with indigenous healing practices.

## Case Study: Harmonizing AI with Ayurveda for Personalized Wellness Programs

This case study examines a collaborative project launched in Kerala, India, that aims to integrate Artificial Intelligence with Ayurveda, one of the world's oldest holistic healing systems. The project involved a partnership between a local Ayurvedic hospital and a tech start-up specializing in AI. The main objective was to create personalized wellness programs that leverage both Ayurvedic principles and modern predictive analytics to offer tailored health suggestions that cater to individual constitutions (Doshas).

The AI system was designed to assess personal health data alongside traditional Ayurvedic diagnostics like pulse analysis, tongue diagnosis, and Prakriti analysis (body constitution type). By feeding the AI system thousands of records detailing symptoms, lifestyle factors, dietary habits, and treatment outcomes, patterns could be discerned, which then informed the development of highly personalized wellness plans.

Collaboration was key in this initiative. Regular workshops and consultation sessions were organized to enable AI developers to gain insights into Ayurvedic principles and diagnostics directly from seasoned Ayurvedic practitioners. These sessions helped ensure the AI system accurately interpreted Ayurvedic data and effectively integrated it with modern health analytics without diluting the traditional essence. Additionally, continuous feedback loops were established, allowing practitioners to evaluate and refine the AI's recommendations, ensuring they aligned with holistic wellness approaches.

The program yielded significant benefits, including increased efficacy in managing lifestyle diseases and enhancing preventative health measures among participants. Preliminary results highlighted improved adherence to treatment and greater satisfaction with the wellness plans, owing to their personalized nature and cultural alignment.

This case study not only underscores the complex process of harmonizing AI with traditional healing but also exemplifies the significant potential of such synergies to transform healthcare delivery. By respecting and incorporating traditional knowledge and practices, AI can enhance the reach and effectiveness of ancient wellness systems, offering a model for global health innovations.

## Case Study: Advancing Native American Medicine through AI-Driven Ethnobotanical Research

This case study delves into a groundbreaking initiative in Arizona where a community of Native American healers collaborated with a tech company specializing in Artificial Intelligence to enhance the understanding and application of traditional Navajo healing practices. The project aimed to digitize centuries-old knowledge of medicinal plants and create a data-driven approach to treating prevalent diseases within the community, such as diabetes and heart disease.

The first phase of the project involved extensive ethnobotanical surveys and the collection of oral histories from elder healers about plant-based remedies. This data was meticulously cataloged in a digital repository designed with AI capabilities to analyze and correlate the properties of various plants with health outcomes documented over generations. The AI system was trained to recognize patterns in efficacy and suggest modifications to concoctions that could potentially increase their potency or reduce side effects.

To ensure the AI system was culturally consonant and respected the sacred nature of the healing practices, the project instituted a steering committee made up of tribal leaders and senior healers. This committee played a crucial role in overseeing the AI's learning protocols and ensuring that the recommendations made by the system aligned with traditional practices and the spiritual significance of the plants. The AI developers participated in cultural immersion workshops to better understand the ethos and nuances of Navajo healing traditions and received ongoing guidance from the healers.

The pilot implementation showed promising outcomes, with the AI system successfully predicting effective plant combinations for managing blood sugar levels that were previously unknown to younger healers. This not only showcased the potential of AI in revitalizing traditional knowledge but also helped bridge the generational knowledge gap within the community.

A significant aspect of the case study was the focus on ethical AI development and the protection of indigenous knowledge. The collaborative model ensured that data ownership remained with the tribe, and provisions were put in place to safeguard against commercial exploitation of the traditional knowledge.

Regular revision of the ethical guidelines in tandem with tribal leaders ensured transparency and continued trust.

## Case Study: Leveraging AI in South African Zulu Medicinal Practices

The case study exemplifies an initiative in KwaZulu-Natal, South Africa, where Artificial Intelligence (AI) has been integrated with traditional Zulu healing practices to address prevalent health issues, such as HIV/AIDS and tuberculosis. A community-based health organization partnered with a global AI research institute to develop a tailored AI system that helps local healers enhance their herbal treatment regimens.

The development of the AI system began with a comprehensive data collection phase, during which detailed recordings of traditional Zulu healing sessions, the herbal remedies used, patient health outcomes, and the healer's knowledge were digitized. Special emphasis was placed on gathering ethnographic data to preserve the context and cultural nuance of each remedy and practice. AI algorithms were then developed to analyze these large datasets, identifying patterns and predicting the efficacy of various herbal combinations.

This collaborative project faced the challenge of respecting and accurately incorporating the spiritual and communal aspects of Zulu healing traditions. To tackle this, the AI system was equipped with cultural sensitivity modules trained on the Zulu language and symbols, which the healers themselves directly coached to accurately interpret the significance of traditional rituals. Regular workshops ensured that AI developers understood the deep-rooted cultural beliefs that drive these healing practices, and healers learned how to interact with the AI tools being developed effectively.

Feedback from the community indicated that the AI-enhanced treatments were more precise and led to improved patient outcomes. Additionally, the AI system enabled the documentation and preservation of Zulu medicinal knowledge, which was previously only transmitted orally, thereby securing valuable cultural heritage.

This case study not only demonstrates the potential for AI to complement traditional medicine in treating serious illnesses but also highlights the importance of developing culturally sensitive technology. By engaging with local communities and respecting traditional knowledge, AI can make significant contributions to global health solutions while preserving cultural heritage.

## Case Study: Revitalizing Samoan Healing Arts Through AI Collaboration

This case study examines a pioneering project in Samoa, where Artificial Intelligence (AI) was introduced to augment traditional Polynesian healing practices. In collaboration with a tech firm specializing in AI and a council of Samoan healing experts, the project aimed to digitize and analyze ancient healing practices that have been preserved through oral traditions and ceremonial rites.

The project began with the meticulous documentation of Samoan herbal remedies, massage techniques, and spiritual healing rituals. Each practice was recorded, along with its accompanying cultural context, ingredient sources, and known therapeutic effects. The AI system was then trained to identify patterns across various types of data, ethnographic, botanical, and clinical outcomes, to create a model that could suggest optimizations in traditional remedies and potentially uncover new applications for these age-old treatments.

One of the most significant challenges was ensuring the AI accurately respected and integrated the rich cultural symbolism inherent in Samoan healing practices. To address this, AI developers were paired with healers in extensive knowledge-sharing sessions. This not only facilitated a deep mutual understanding but also allowed the AI to be fine-tuned to recognize the nuanced meanings behind certain healing rituals, which are often tied to the Samoan worldview and spirituality.

The integration of AI brought forth significant advancements. The system provided data-driven insights that enabled healers to refine their remedies and tailor treatments to individual patients more effectively. Moreover, the AI identified new potential anti-inflammatory properties in several lesser-used local herbs, which broadened the scope of treatments available.

However, the project's success hinged on the continued engagement and approval of the local healing community. Regular dialogues were established to review AI findings, ensuring that they complemented traditional practices without overriding them. This ongoing interaction helped sustain a balance between innovation and tradition, securing community trust and fostering a model that could be replicated in other regions with rich healing traditions.

### Case Study: AI-Enhanced Preservation and Modernization of Native Hawaiian Lāʻau Lapaʻau

This case study examines an innovative project located in the Hawaiian Islands, where Artificial Intelligence (AI) has been leveraged to not only preserve but also modernize the ancient Hawaiian healing practice of Lāʻau Lapaʻau. This practice relies on the use of native plants and spiritual knowledge for healing. The project was a joint venture between a Hawaiian cultural preservation group and a multinational AI technology firm, aiming to document and analyze the rich traditional knowledge that had been orally passed down through generations.

The initiative began with the establishment of a comprehensive digital database incorporating a wide array of ethnobotanical and medical information collected from elder healers, known as kahuna. This included specific details on plant characteristics, preparation methods, historical usage, and patient outcomes. Advanced AI algorithms were employed to catalog and analyze these data, establishing patterns in the efficacy of various treatments for chronic diseases prevalent within the Hawaiian community, such as hypertension and diabetes.

A significant challenge in the project was ensuring that the AI tools developed respected the cultural and spiritual aspects of Lāʻau Lapaʻau. To achieve this, the AI team worked closely with the kahuna, integrating their insights and feedback throughout the development process. This collaborative approach was vital in creating an AI system that could accurately interpret the complexities of the healing practices without stripping them of their cultural significance.

The AI system's capabilities extended to predicting the interactions between different herbal remedies and suggesting potential new uses for traditional plants, guided by a synthesis of historical usage data and contemporary medical research. This predictive analysis aimed to modernize the practice by introducing scientifically validated treatment protocols, thereby enhancing adaptability and acceptance among younger generations.

This case study not only showcases the potential of AI in enhancing the scope and effectiveness of traditional medicinal practices but also emphasizes the importance of a sensitive and inclusive approach to technology integration that respects and preserves indigenous knowledge while fostering its evolution.

### Case Study: AI-Driven Enhancement of Herbal Medicine Efficacy in Malaysian Traditional Healing

This detailed case study relates to a project undertaken in Malaysia aimed at enhancing the efficacy and reliability of herbal remedies in traditional Malaysian healing arts through the use of Artificial Intelligence (AI). This project was a collaborative venture spearheaded by a leading Malaysian university's AI research center in consultation with a consortium of traditional healers known for their rich lineage in herbal medicine.

The primary objective was to develop an AI platform capable of analyzing vast arrays of historical and contemporary data on herbal usage, thereby identifying the most effective herbal combinations for specific ailments. The data collection phase was extensive, involving detailed records painstakingly gathered from participating healers on the preparation, dosage, and results of countless herbal treatments tried over generations. Advanced machine learning algorithms were then deployed to distill this data into actionable insights.

A major challenge emerged in maintaining the cultural integrity and acceptance of the AI recommendations among traditional healers. To address this, the project team instituted a system of continuous engagement where AI outputs were evaluated and moderated by senior healers to ensure that the suggestions made by the AI did not stray from acceptable traditional practices. This collaborative framework was crucial in preserving the trust and engagement of the traditional healing community.

Moreover, this AI initiative also integrated environmental data, which helped in understanding how changing soil, climate, and regional biodiversity's affect the potency and efficacy of herbal remedies. Through the AI system's predictive analytics, adjustments to herbal sourcing and preparation methods were suggested, making the treatments more adapted and potent under current ecological conditions.

The success of this project was marked by significantly improved outcomes in patients treated with AI-optimized herbal recipes. It also fostered an environment of innovation within the traditional healing community, encouraging a new generation to engage with and preserve their heritage. By bridging cutting-edge technology with generations-old practices, this initiative serves as a vital model for other regions with rich traditions in herbal medicine.

## Review Questions

**1. While studying the impact of Traditional Thai Massage on patient outcomes, a medical researcher, Dr. Lee, examines two groups of patients suffering from chronic lower back pain. Group A receives a 30-minute Traditional Thai Massage session twice a week for 5 weeks, while group B receives standard physical therapy under similar conditions. Dr. Lee measures patient outcomes based on pain reduction, functional mobility, and patient satisfaction surveys before and after the treatment period. Which group is likely to show significant improvement in terms of pain reduction and patient satisfaction?**

A) Both groups show similar significant improvements

B) Group A shows more significant improvement than group B

C) Group B shows more significant improvement than group A

D) Neither group shows any significant improvement

**Answer: B**

Explanation: Traditional Thai Massage, known for its holistic and integrative approach to treating bodily ailments, often leads to significant improvements in pain management and overall patient satisfaction due to its combination of physical manipulation, stretching, and acupressure techniques. These methods help in enhancing blood circulation, reducing muscle tension, and increasing endorphin release, which are beneficial for pain relief and patient well-being. Studies tend to demonstrate that patients receiving Traditional Thai Massage often report higher satisfaction and better pain reduction compared to those undergoing standard physical therapy, which might focus more narrowly on specific physical rehabilitation techniques without integrating the broader holistic approaches.

**2. In a randomized controlled trial, Dr. Smith evaluates the effectiveness of integrating yoga and meditation techniques into the treatment regimen for high blood pressure patients. Group A receives**

medication only, group B follows a combined treatment of yoga, meditation, and medication, and group C engages only in lifestyle alterations (diet and exercise) without medication. Blood pressure readings and quality of life indicators are tracked over a 6-month period. Which group is likely to show an enhanced quality of life while maintaining effective management of blood pressure?

A) Group A only

B) Group B

C) Group C

D) Both groups B and C show equal improvement

**Answer: B**

Explanation: The integration of yoga and meditation into the standard medicinal treatment in group B offers numerous advantages that extend beyond just managing the physical symptoms of high blood pressure. These holistic practices are known to reduce stress, enhance breathing, promote physical fitness, and improve mental health, contributing to a significant uplift in quality of life. Yoga and meditation help in regulating the body's stress response, which is crucial for managing blood pressure. Patients in group B are likely to experience an overall improvement in both physical and psychological aspects of health, leading to enhanced quality of life and effective management of blood pressure, which is likely to surpass the outcomes seen in groups A (medication only) and C (lifestyle alterations only).

**3. Dr. Jackson conducts a study on the effect of guided Reiki sessions on oncology patients dealing with post-chemotherapy fatigue. Patients are divided into three groups: group A receives Reiki treatment, group B participates in a placebo session, and group C receives no adjunctive therapy. Fatigue levels, emotional state, and overall sense of well-being are evaluated before and after the sessions. Based on previous research insights, which group is anticipated to exhibit the most notable improvement in fatigue levels and emotional well-being?**

A) Group A - Reiki treatment

B) Group B - Placebo session

C) Group C - No adjunct therapy

D) Both groups A and B show similar improvements

**Answer: A**

Explanation: Reiki, a form of energy healing, has been suggested through various studies to positively impact emotional well-being, reduce fatigue, and enhance quality of life, particularly in patients undergoing strenuous treatments such as chemotherapy. The therapy operates on the principle of transferring energy from the practitioner to the patient, enhancing the body's natural healing processes and inducing relaxation. Patients in group A receiving Reiki are likely to experience notable improvements in managing fatigue and improving their emotional state due to the holistic nature of Reiki that addresses both physical and psychological stressors. While group B may exhibit slight improvements due to the placebo effect, the genuine energy transfer in Reiki treatments (group A) typically results in more profound and lasting impacts on patient well-being compared to placebo or no therapy.

## Perspectives on AI From Indigenous and Holistic Practitioners

### Introduction to Indigenous Perspectives on AI

As we embark on the exploration of AI in the realm of medicine, it becomes imperative to acknowledge the nuanced perspectives of indigenous and holistic practitioners. These communities offer a rich tapestry of knowledge rooted in centuries of tradition and a deep connection to the natural world, which often contrasts sharply with the data-driven, algorithmic approaches typical of contemporary AI.

Understanding these perspectives starts with recognizing the unique value systems that guide indigenous approaches to health and wellness. These systems emphasize the interconnectivity of body, mind, spirit, and environment, challenging the compartmentalized nature of modern medicine. AI, when designed without this holistic understanding, risks overlooking these critical components of care.

Incorporating indigenous knowledge into AI systems not only enhances the cultural relevance and acceptability of these technologies but also fosters a broader, more inclusive approach to healthcare. It demands a dialogue between technology developers and indigenous practitioners, aiming to create AI that respects and integrates these age-old wisdoms into innovative, respectful healthcare solutions.

### The Importance of Inclusivity in Healthcare AI

Inclusivity in healthcare AI is a paramount goal, ensuring that the depth and diversity of traditional, indigenous, and holistic healing practices are not merely recognized but also integrated into the technological framework. This is crucial because, when inclusively designed, AI can cater to a broader spectrum of health beliefs and practices, thereby enhancing its efficacy and acceptance across diverse cultural landscapes.

To achieve this, developers must engage stakeholders, including healthcare professionals, community leaders, and patients themselves. These collaborative efforts can imbue AI systems with a richer, culturally aware dataset that reflects the actual healthcare practices of these communities. Furthermore, inclusivity fosters trust and bridges the gap between modern medicine and traditional healing, creating systems that are not only technologically advanced but also culturally respectful and relevant.

Ultimately, adopting an inclusive approach in healthcare AI development can drastically improve user acceptance and effectiveness. By valuing and integrating diverse healing wisdom, AI can support a more holistic view of health that respects and revitalizes indigenous and traditional practices.

### AI Perceptions and Utilization Among Native Health Practitioners

Native health practitioners view AI with a spectrum of attitudes, deeply influenced by their cultural premises and historical experiences with technology. For many, AI presents a dual-edged sword, offering potential enhancements in diagnosing and treating complex health conditions while simultaneously posing threats to cultural sovereignty and traditional knowledge systems.

The utilization of AI among these practitioners varies significantly. In regions where traditional and holistic practices are robust, AI integration encounters skepticism. Practitioners are cautious, prioritizing the preservation of ancestral wisdom over modern technological adoption. However, some see AI as a valuable tool for expanding the reach and efficacy of their practices, particularly in remote areas where healthcare access is limited.

Effective integration of AI in these contexts requires respectful collaboration and thorough understanding of the unique needs and values of native communities. Developing AI tools that genuinely support and enhance traditional practices without supplanting them is crucial for their acceptance and success in indigenous healthcare settings.

## Holistic Approaches to Technology in Medicine

Holistic approaches to technology in medicine seek a symbiosis between advanced computational methods and age-old healing traditions. This integration promises to enhance patient care by encompassing physical, emotional, and spiritual well-being in the diagnostic and therapeutic processes. Acknowledging the holistic view, AI technologies could be designed to interpret subtle aspects of patient wellness, beyond the observable symptoms, thereby aligning with holistic ideals that health transcends physical indicators.

However, the adoption and implementation of AI within holistic practices invite challenges, primarily in aligning technological advancements with non-linear, non-quantifiable elements of holistic care. The true essence of holistic healing—addressing the interconnectedness of the human spirit, mind, and environment—demands AI solutions that respect and facilitate these dimensions, rather than overriding them with purely data-driven logic.

Forging forward, a collaborative approach is essential. Developers must work alongside holistic practitioners to tailor AI technologies that enhance rather than replace the intuitive and experiential nature of holistic medicine. This collaboration can usher in a new era where technology supports holistic health philosophies, creating systems that are truly integrative and holistic in nature.

## Challenges Faced by Indigenous Communities in AI Implementation

Implementing AI in indigenous medical practices involves unique challenges, compounded by the diverse and localized nature of these communities. A pivotal challenge is the digital divide that obstructs access to necessary technological infrastructure. Many indigenous populations remain isolated from mainstream digital services, inhibiting the seamless integration of AI technologies that are dependent on robust data connectivity and modern hardware.

Furthermore, there exists a profound cultural gap between indigenous healing practices and the algorithmic logic of AI. Indigenous knowledge systems are deeply rooted in empirical experiences and spiritual beliefs, which do not easily translate into quantifiable data that AI systems require. Bridging this gap necessitates the creation of new frameworks for AI that respect and incorporate these non-linear knowledge systems.

Lastly, sociopolitical factors play a significant role, as indigenous rights to data sovereignty and intellectual property often clash with open-source AI research models. Ensuring that AI implementations respect and protect these rights is fundamental to encouraging acceptance and cooperation from indigenous stakeholders.

## Cultural Sensitivity and Its Impact on AI Adoption

Cultural sensitivity is fundamental to the adoption of AI in medicine, especially within indigenous and holistic health practices. An AI system's effectiveness hinges on its ability to resonate culturally with its users. This requires a profound understanding of the subtleties and variances in cultural norms and values, which influence patient expectations and treatment acceptability.

For indigenous communities, AI tools that disregard or misinterpret cultural nuances can result in decreased trust and reluctance to engage. This is particularly significant in communities where healing is intertwined with spiritual and ancestral beliefs. The development of culturally sensitive AI requires an inclusive design process that involves community members and practitioners, ensuring their voices are heard and integrated into the technology.

Successfully implementing AI in these settings also demands continuous cultural competence training for developers and users alike. This not only aids in the refinement of AI applications but also fosters an environment where technology complements traditional healing rather than opposes it. Bridging these cultural divides empowers communities, enhancing both the reach and impact of AI in medicine.

## Incorporating Traditional Healing Wisdom into AI Systems

Infusing AI systems with traditional healing wisdom necessitates a deep respect for and understanding of these ancient practices. Innovators in AI must forge partnerships with traditional healers to ensure these technologies appropriately recognize and integrate holistic knowledge. This cooperative effort aims to transform AI into a tool that not only serves medical diagnostics and prognostics but also respects and perpetuates the nuanced practices of indigenous healing.

The effective integration of traditional wisdom into AI frameworks can facilitate personalized and culturally resonant healthcare. By incorporating traditional knowledge, AI systems can provide more comprehensive care options, including those rooted in centuries-old practices that emphasize the interconnectedness of spiritual, environmental, and physical health.

Challenges remain in translating oral and experiential knowledge into data formats suitable for AI. Continuous dialogue between AI developers and traditional practitioners is essential to overcoming these barriers, ensuring AI technologies evolve as inclusive, culturally adept tools that enhance rather than replace traditional healing methods.

## Ethical Concerns for AI from a Holistic Viewpoint

From the perspective of holistic practitioners, AI introduces significant ethical concerns, with a notable one being misalignment with the core values of holistic medicine. Holistic healing's deeply rooted principles, emphasizing the interconnectedness of the mind, body, and spirit, challenge the AI's predominantly data-driven nature, which often dismisses the unquantifiable elements essential to holistic practices.

Moreover, ethical dilemmas arise regarding the potential exploitation and misappropriation of indigenous knowledge. There is a looming threat that AI, without stringent ethical oversight, could commodify sacred, holistic knowledge for corporate gain, disregarding the cultural sanctity and the rights of communities to their intellectual property. Engaging with these communities in AI's developmental phase is crucial to ethically integrating these traditional practices without predisposing them to exploitation or misinterpretation.

Finally, the risk of cultural homogenization through AI looms large, where unique healing traditions might be overshadowed by a one-size-fits-all healthcare model promoted by AI systems. Ensuring the ethical integration of AI requires a commitment to preserving the diversity and specificity of holistic health methodologies, warranting a cautious and respectful approach.

## The Future of AI in Indigenous Health Practices

The trajectory of AI in indigenous health practices prompts a visionary blend of tradition and technology, paving the way for uniquely tailored health solutions. As AI evolves, the integration of culturally grounded insights and practices can potentially revolutionize healthcare delivery in indigenous communities. Future AI systems could better diagnose and treat ailments under the guidance of indigenous wisdom, enhancing rather than replacing traditional methods.

Imagine AI tools developed in close collaboration with native healers, programmed to understand local languages and interpret health knowledge passed down through generations. These tools might then offer support by providing holistic insights that balance modern medical advice with traditional healing practices. Such advancements could empower communities, deliver improved health outcomes while respecting cultural practices.

Yet, for this future to unfold, sustained commitment is necessary from both tech developers and indigenous stakeholders to co-create AI applications that genuinely embody and preserve indigenous ideologies in healthcare. The onus lies in maintaining an open dialogue that respects and prioritizes indigenous perspectives and knowledge.

**Case Studies: Indigenous Practitioners' Experiences with AI**

Exploring the intersection of artificial intelligence and indigenous medical practices offers insightful revelations. In one case, an indigenous healer from the Amazon utilized an AI diagnostic tool tailored to recognize local medicinal plants and symptoms of regional diseases. This integration significantly improved the accuracy of diagnoses in remote areas, showcasing AI's potential when adapted to local health contexts.

Another instance involves a community healer in North America who participated in an AI-driven project aimed at digitizing ancestral health knowledge. Despite initial success, challenges such as language barriers and the need for context-specific AI adaptations highlighted the complexity of such endeavors. The project highlighted the importance of ongoing collaboration between AI developers and indigenous practitioners to ensure the meaningful integration of technology.

Lastly, in Africa, an AI application designed to monitor and predict health trends in rural populations faced skepticism. Community engagement sessions helped bridge the trust gap, demonstrating that respectful and well-facilitated introductions to AI can foster acceptance. These cases collectively suggest that while AI offers promising enhancements to indigenous health practices, the path forward requires careful, culturally aware development and deployment strategies.

**Community-Centric AI Development Strategies**

Community-centric AI development strategies in indigenous healthcare focus on creating systems that are by and for the community. Such strategies ensure that AI technologies are not just imposed but integrated in ways that respect and amplify local traditions and practices. Inclusiveness in the design, development, and deployment phases is crucial. This involves ongoing communication with community members and health practitioners to ascertain their needs and perspectives.

Strategic community involvement can lead to AI solutions that are more adaptable and responsive to specific health contexts. For instance, development teams might include local healers and language experts to ensure the AI interfaces and outputs are culturally consonant and linguistically appropriate. Regular feedback loops help refine these technologies to serve community-specific requirements better.

Moreover, community-centric approaches prioritize training locals to manage and operate AI systems, fostering technological self-sufficiency. By empowering communities with the knowledge to maintain and advance these systems, the longevity and efficacy of AI applications are significantly enhanced. Equally, this approach safeguards indigenous autonomy over their healthcare processes and data, aligning technological progress with traditional values and needs.

## Importance of Protecting Sacred Knowledge in AI Solutions

The integration of artificial intelligence in healthcare necessitates a cautious approach when it comes to sacred and traditional knowledge. This wisdom, often transmitted orally or through practice rather than written text, holds significant cultural and spiritual value for indigenous communities. Its incorporation into AI systems must be handled with the utmost respect and care to prevent misuse or misinterpretation.

As AI ventures into new realms, the risk of commodification of this knowledge becomes real. Without appropriate safeguards, sacred practices could be exploited for commercial gain, stripping them of their cultural significance and sovereignty. It is essential that these technologies are developed under strict ethical guidelines that ensure the protection of indigenous knowledge, making sure it is shared responsibly and with consent.

Finally, AI solutions must be constructed not only to preserve but also to celebrate this traditional knowledge. They should function as a bridge that reinforces indigenous practices rather than undermining them, fostering an environment where modern technology and ancient wisdom enhance each other, ensuring sustainability and respect across generations.

## Perspectives on Data Sovereignty and AI

Data sovereignty concerns emphasize control over data collection, storage, and utilization, particularly vital in indigenous contexts where data involves sensitive cultural knowledge. AI systems, when designed without input from these communities, risk violating data sovereignty by misappropriating or misinterpreting indigenous data, leading to inappropriate use in healthcare solutions.

Recognizing the significance of data sovereignty in AI involves integrating mechanisms that ensure data is managed according to the cultural, ethical, and legal expectations of indigenous populations. This means creating AI systems that not only respect but actively enforce the governance rules set by indigenous communities. Involvement of indigenous data stewards can help navigate the complexities associated with cultural data, ensuring AI applications adhere to sovereignty principles.

The future of culturally informed AI in medicine rests on frameworks that support data sovereignty comprehensively. Such frameworks align AI development with traditional knowledge protection goals, facilitating trust and cooperation between technology developers and indigenous communities. Establishing clear protocols for data handling in AI can bridge modern health technologies with ancient wisdom, fostering a mutually respectful integration.

## Indigenous Innovations in AI for Health

Indigenous communities are pioneering unique applications of AI in healthcare, reflecting their distinct cultural practices and perspectives. A notable innovation involves AI systems that integrate traditional herbal knowledge with modern diagnostics to offer personalized treatments. These systems are culturally sensitive, designed in consultation with elder healers, ensuring that ancestral wisdom is aptly interpreted and utilized.

Another breakthrough is the development of AI-powered mobile apps that facilitate remote consultations and follow-ups in indigenous languages. Such innovations are particularly crucial in areas where access to conventional health facilities is limited. These apps not only deliver medical advice but also guide users in applying local medicinal practices safely alongside prescribed treatments.

These examples underscore the potential of AI to transform healthcare in indigenous settings. By blending sophisticated technology with deeply rooted healing traditions, these innovations enhance healthcare accessibility and effectiveness, promising a future where technology truly serves the community's health needs.

## AI as a Tool for Preservation and Validation of Traditional Knowledge

Artificial intelligence offers transformative potential in preserving and validating the extensive repository of traditional knowledge inherent within indigenous communities. By leveraging AI, this ancient wisdom can be digitized and systematically analyzed, ensuring its longevity and accessibility for future generations. This process not only safeguards cultural heritage but also supports its empirical validation, potentially integrating it into broader medicinal practices.

However, the incorporation of AI in this domain requires cautious orchestration to avoid the misrepresentation or misuse of deeply rooted cultural knowledge. Collaborative frameworks involving indigenous knowledge keepers and AI technologists are crucial for creating respectful and accurate AI models. These partnerships facilitate the design of algorithms that comprehend the context and nuances of traditional practices, thereby ensuring their accurate interpretation and application.

Ultimately, AI could serve not just as a technological tool but as a bridge connecting ancient remedies and modern healthcare. The challenge lies in balancing technological advancement with cultural integrity, aiming to enhance healthcare outcomes while honoring and preserving indigenous wisdom.

## Balancing Modern Technology with Ancient Healing Practices

The nexus of modern technology and ancient healing practices represents a delicate equilibrium, essential for the respectful integration of AI in medicine. AI systems, when designed to incorporate traditional healing knowledge, must strike a balance between the precision of modern diagnostics and the wisdom of centuries-old practices. This orchestration seeks not just to facilitate medical interventions but also to preserve and respect ancient cultural legacies.

Developers and practitioners collaborate closely to ensure that AI technologies align with the philosophies underlying traditional healing. Such collaborative efforts are crucial in developing AI tools that comprehend and replicate the complexities of holistic therapies. The challenge lies in encoding this soft knowledge, rich in spiritual and communal nuances, into algorithms capable of operating within the rigid frameworks of contemporary technology without losing its essence.

Ultimately, the successful integration of AI into traditional healing practices hinges on a synergy that respects and enhances both domains. As AI ventures into these uncharted waters, it must do so with a commitment to cultural sensitivity and a deep appreciation of the heritage it seeks to serve, ensuring mutual enhancement and sustainability.

## The Role of AI in Supporting Community Health Initiatives

Artificial Intelligence (AI) continues to evolve as an invaluable tool in community health, particularly within indigenous populations where traditional practices and holistic approaches are prominent. By implementing AI, these communities can enhance their health monitoring and intervention strategies, allowing for more personalized and timely medical care.

AI systems can analyze vast amounts of health data at unprecedented speeds, providing insights that help identify trends and potential outbreaks within communities. This capability is particularly critical in areas where resources are scarce, and the standard health infrastructure may not be robust. For indigenous and holistic practitioners, AI offers a platform to integrate traditional knowledge with modern medical practices, ensuring culturally sensitive and appropriate healthcare solutions.

Moreover, AI-driven initiatives can empower communities by providing them with tools for self-management of health, reinforcing the community's role in preventive care. Community-driven AI applications foster greater engagement and ownership, crucial for the sustained success of health initiatives. Such tools also ensure that the solutions are not only practical but also respectful and inclusive of the community's wisdom and values.

## Practitioners' Views on AI's Impact on Diagnostic and Treatment Processes

Indigenous health practitioners are discerning yet optimistic about the role of AI in transforming diagnostic and treatment processes. These practitioners emphasize the necessity for AI to be calibrated to understand and respect diverse medical paradigms, including traditional and holistic healing methods. By integrating such knowledge, AI can offer more nuanced and culturally relevant medical advice, thus enhancing the credibility and effectiveness of health interventions within these communities.

However, disparities arise concerning AI's practical application, with some practitioners reporting concerns over the potential for AI to overlook or misinterpret traditional diagnostic methods, which could lead to inappropriate treatment recommendations. This underscores the critical need for developing AI systems in close collaboration with indigenous health experts to ensure these technologies are inclusive and accurately informed.

Despite challenges, many are hopeful about AI's potential to streamline healthcare delivery, especially in remote areas, making it faster and more accessible. Such advancements are particularly significant in settings where conventional medical resources are scarce, thereby directly benefiting underserved populations.

## Challenges of Integrating AI in Remote and Rural Healthcare

Integrating AI into remote and rural healthcare, particularly within indigenous communities, presents unique challenges. One major hurdle is the lack of reliable internet connectivity and infrastructure, which is critical for AI operations. Without robust digital frameworks, the potential of AI to provide accessible medical diagnostics and treatment is significantly hampered.

Moreover, there is a widespread scarcity of technical expertise in these areas. Training local health practitioners on AI tools is essential, yet the resources for such education are often insufficient. This gap undermines the efficiency and adoption of AI-driven healthcare solutions.

Additionally, cultural resistance and skepticism towards technology can impede the acceptance of AI systems. Ensuring that AI respects and integrates traditional healing practices is paramount yet achieving this requires sensitive and inclusive design choices that do not always align easily with advanced technological solutions.

Lastly, funding limitations pose a constant challenge. Investment in AI technology often competes with immediate, basic healthcare needs, making prioritization difficult for community leaders and policymakers.

## AI Training Programs Tailored for Indigenous Health Workers

Crafting AI training programs specifically for indigenous health workers is an essential step towards harmonizing traditional knowledge with modern healthcare technology. These programs are designed not only to equip practitioners with the necessary skills to utilize AI tools but also to ensure that these tools are culturally congruent and respectful of indigenous healing practices.

The curriculum is developed in collaboration with indigenous health experts and AI technologists, focusing on multidisciplinary approaches that cover both technical skills and cultural sensibilities. Training emphasizes the ethical use of AI, highlighting the preservation of community values and the protection of sacred knowledge within digital frameworks.

Moreover, these programs aim to foster a community of practice that supports ongoing learning and adaptation of AI in healthcare. By empowering health workers with AI competencies, we bridge the gap between ancient traditions and contemporary medical practices, enhancing healthcare delivery in culturally sensitive ways that respect and integrate indigenous wisdom.

## Opportunities for AI to Enhance Holistic Therapies

The integration of AI into holistic therapies opens transformative avenues for enhancing health delivery systems, especially within indigenous communities where traditional healing practices are deeply revered. By leveraging AI, these therapies can gain precision and personalization, making them more effective and widely accessible. AI can extend the reach of holistic health practitioners by analyzing patterns from wellness data that capture the nuances of individual health scenarios and success rates of various natural remedies.

Moreover, AI can facilitate the creation of tailored therapeutic plans that integrate with local medicinal practices, thereby increasing the efficacy and acceptance of treatments. The ability of AI to process and interpret vast arrays of data can also lead to discoveries of new health applications for traditional herbs and practices, enriching the holistic medical field.

Overall, AI stands to not only respect but also amplify the effectiveness of holistic therapies, ensuring these age-old practices evolve seamlessly with technological advancements while maintaining their cultural essence and proven health benefits.

## AI and the Future of Integrative Health Practices

The integration of AI into integrative health practices symbolizes a forward-thinking merger of technology with age-old holistic and indigenous healing methods. This promising future could see AI enhancing individualized treatment plans that incorporate both modern medical science and traditional healing wisdom. Innovative AI systems could analyze in-depth health data from both technological and traditional insights to recommend personalized wellness strategies.

Moreover, this integration promises to foster a new level of patient-centered care, where treatments are not only responsive but also preventative. AI's predictive analytics could foresee potential health issues based on historical data, lifestyle, and environmental factors, enabling proactive interventions that dovetail seamlessly with natural and community-based remedies.

Challenges remain in this visionary future, particularly in ensuring AI systems are designed with an inherent respect for cultural nuances and sacred practices. Continuous collaboration between AI developers, indigenous health practitioners, and holistic healers will be crucial to creating technologically advanced, yet culturally sensitive health solutions that truly honor and integrate the full spectrum of healing knowledge.

**Bridging Western Medicine and Indigenous Healing through AI**

Merging Western medicine with indigenous healing through AI presents a promising frontier in healthcare. The synthesis of advanced technology and age-old healing wisdom can generate comprehensive treatment models that respect cultural legacies while enhancing efficacy. AI's capability to assimilate vast arrays of traditional medicine insights with contemporary medical science allows the creation of personalized health strategies that honor patient diversity across various cultural spectrums.

This integration does not merely aim to incorporate indigenous practices as complementary alternatives; instead, it envisions a coequal incorporation where both Western and traditional methods inform treatment protocols equally. This requires the rigorous development of AI systems that are finely attuned to the subtleties of indigenous knowledge, ensuring these systems are both respectful and effective in their application.

Challenges in this integration include reconciling methodological differences and ensuring mutual respect among practitioners from diverse medical backgrounds. However, continuous collaboration and dialogue between AI developers, Western doctors, and indigenous healers are vital. Engagement through shared platforms helps build a healthcare ecosystem that genuinely reflects global diversity and interspersed knowledge systems.

**Concluding Remarks on Indigenous and Holistic Practitioners' Perspectives on AI**

Throughout this exploration of AI's interaction with indigenous and holistic medicine, it becomes evident that while the challenges are substantial, the opportunities for transformative healthcare are profound. AI presents a unique platform to amplify traditional knowledge, blending ancient wisdom with modern technology to provide personalized and effective health solutions.

Indigenous and holistic practitioners have highlighted the necessity for AI systems that not only integrate but also respect and prioritize traditional healing methods. This respect must be woven into the fabric of AI development, ensuring these technologies enhance, rather than eclipse, indigenous practices. The collaboration between AI developers and traditional health practitioners is crucial, where both parties engage deeply with mutual respect and learning.

As we look forward, AI in healthcare must continue to be a tool for empowering patients and preserving cultural heritage in medicine. Balancing modern technological advances with the rich, often understated value of traditional healing practices promises a healthier, more inclusive future for all.

**Summary**

The chapter explores the intricate interplay between artificial intelligence (AI) and the traditional medical practices of indigenous and holistic practitioners, highlighting both the potential benefits and the significant challenges associated with integrating these systems. Initial sections emphasize the importance of respecting and understanding the depth of indigenous knowledge, which encompasses a holistic view of health that connects mind, body, spirit, and environment, profoundly differing from the conventional, compartmentalized approach in modern medicine. This perspective encourages a more inclusive and culturally sensitive approach to AI development in healthcare, which could substantially enhance its effectiveness and acceptance across diverse cultural contexts. The narrative articulates that inclusivity not only involves integrating diverse medical philosophies into AI but also necessitates engaging directly with indigenous communities in the creation process to ensure the technologies developed are both culturally relevant and respectful of traditional wisdom. Utilizing AI with a culturally adjusted approach in indigenous settings is fraught with challenges, including significant technical barriers such as the digital divide, which limits access to necessary technologies, and cultural gaps that make it challenging to translate holistic and spiritual health practices into data formats that AI can utilize.

Additionally, ethical concerns are paramount, involving the risk of misappropriating sacred indigenous knowledge and the need to maintain data sovereignty. The chapter also explores practical case studies where AI has been successfully integrated with traditional practices, suggesting a potential for AI to augment indigenous healthcare systems respectfully. However, crucial to this success is the ongoing, respectful dialogue between technology developers and native practitioners, ensuring AI tools are designed thoughtfully to support, rather than supplant, traditional healing methods. Overall, the chapter advocates for an AI development approach that is not only technologically innovative but also deeply respectful and integrative of the ancient wisdom of holistic and indigenous medicinal practices, promoting a healthcare future that is both advanced and culturally rich.

## References

[1] Barker, Adam J., et al. "Ethics in Indigenous Research: An annotated bibliography." Indigenous Studies Portal Research Tool, University of Saskatchewan Library. 2006..
https://iportal.usask.ca/docs/Ethics%20in%20Indigenous%20Research.pdf
[2] Prussing, Erica, et al. 'Critical reflections on the use of AI and machine learning in global health.' The Lancet Digital Health, vol. 3, no. 6, 2021, pp. e384-e392..
https://www.thelancet.com/journals/landig/article/PIIS2589-7500(21)00066-1/fulltext
[3] Crawford, Kate. 'The trouble with bias: Allocative versus representational harms in machine learning.' SIGACCESS Accessibility and Computing, no. 121, 2017.. https://dl.acm.org/doi/10.1145/3178851.3178877
[4] Taylor, Linnet, et al. "Data justice and data sovereignty: Toward convergence?" Information Communication and Society, vol. 22, no. 7, 2019, pp. 1014-1023..
https://www.tandfonline.com/doi/full/10.1080/1369118X.2019.1573916
[5] Waldram, James B. 'The efficacy of traditional medicine: Current theoretical and methodological issues.' Medical Anthropology Quarterly, vol. 15, no. 4, 2001, pp. 603-625..
https://anthrosource.onlinelibrary.wiley.com/doi/abs/10.1525/maq.2001.15.4.603

## Case Study: Integrating AI in Traditional Navajo Healing Practices

In the heart of the Navajo Nation, a groundbreaking project was initiated to explore the integration of artificial intelligence (AI) within traditional Navajo healing practices. The case centers on a collaboration between Navajo healers, AI developers, and medical anthropologists aimed at creating an AI system to assist in diagnosing and managing diabetes, a prevalent health issue among the Navajo people.

The project began with extensive consultations, during which healers shared insights into their holistic approach to health, encompassing herbal remedies, spiritual healing, and community wellness. This knowledge was crucial in developing an AI model that respects and incorporates these traditional practices. Challenges arose when translating these non-linear and qualitative healing methods into quantitative data that AI systems could process. This required innovative data modeling and frequent adjustments to the AI algorithms to reflect the cultural nuances accurately.

Once developed, the AI tool was piloted in several community health centers. It was designed to provide recommendations based on both conventional medical treatments and Navajo healing practices, thus offering a dual perspective on health management. The tool also included a language component, recognizing and responding in the Navajo language to make it more accessible and culturally relevant.

The initial results were promising, with improvements in patient engagement and management of diabetes symptoms observed. However, there were significant lessons learned. Some community members expressed concerns about the AI tool misrepresenting or oversimplifying their cultural practices. This feedback led to further adaptations of the AI system, ensuring a more respectful and accurate integration of Navajo traditional medicine.

## Case Study: AI-Enhanced Healthcare Services in Remote Australian Aboriginal Communities

In the vast, remote areas of Australia's Northern Territory, healthcare delivery to Aboriginal communities presents unique challenges, including geographical isolation and cultural nuances. A novel project was launched to integrate artificial intelligence (AI) into healthcare services, aiming to improve access and cultural responsiveness. The project involved cooperation between local Aboriginal health practitioners, AI technicians, and cultural consultants who worked together to develop an AI system tailored for the community's specific needs.

The initial phase involved extensive community engagement, where the needs and preferences of the Aboriginal people were gathered. This information was crucial in shaping the AI system which was designed to recognize and incorporate traditional Aboriginal healing practices alongside modern medicine. Recognizing the value of traditional knowledge, the AI system included a database of herbal remedies and indigenous healing techniques inputted by the community elders themselves.

The AI system utilized natural language processing capabilities to communicate effectively in the local Aboriginal languages, enhancing usability for patients and practitioners. It also included diagnostic tools that combined conventional medical diagnostics with indicators used in traditional healing, providing a more comprehensive view of patient health.

However, the implementation phase revealed several challenges. The AI system required constant internet connectivity, which was unreliable in remote locations. Furthermore, some community members were skeptical about trusting a digital system with their health data due to fears of cultural misappropriation and data privacy.

To address these issues, the project team enhanced offline functionalities of the AI system and conducted regular community workshops to build trust and educate about the benefits and safeguards of the AI system. Although initial mistrust and technological challenges posed significant hurdles, ongoing adjustments and community-informed practices gradually led to higher acceptance rates. The case illustrates the complexities and potential of integrating AI into healthcare in culturally diverse settings, needing continuous dialogue, adaptation, and respect for local knowledge systems.

## Case Study: Revitalizing Traditional Quechua Healthcare with AI in Rural Peru

In the rural highlands of Peru, where the Quechua communities predominantly reside, access to healthcare is often limited by geographical and socio-economic barriers. A collaborative initiative was undertaken to introduce AI technology into traditional Quechua medicine, aimed at enhancing both the reach and the efficacy of healthcare practices rooted in centuries of indigenous knowledge.

The project began with a series of community meetings and workshops to understand deeply the Quechua's traditional health practices, which include the use of medicinal plants, spiritual cleansing rituals, and community-based healing ceremonies. The AI development team, made up of healthcare professionals, AI experts, and Quechua healers, embarked on creating a culturally sensitive AI tool designed to support the diagnostics of common diseases affecting the community, such as altitude sickness, gastrointestinal disorders, and respiratory conditions.

The AI system was developed to analyze symptoms and suggest treatments, drawing from both modern medical science and Quechua healing practices. One innovative feature was its ability to interpret local dialects, allowing patients to describe their symptoms in their native language, enhancing the user experience and ensuring better diagnostic accuracy.

However, the deployment of the AI tool faced several challenges. Initial resistance from the local healers, who feared that the AI might replace their traditional roles, was significant. To address this, the project emphasized AI as a supportive tool rather than a replacement. Moreover, intermittent internet connectivity in rural areas posed technical challenges, necessitating adaptations to enable offline functionalities.

The impact, after continued refinements and community-based participations, began to show promising results. Health practitioners reported a more streamlined process in diagnosing and managing diseases, with AI providing quick insights that were cross-referenced with traditional practices. The community's trust grew as they witnessed how AI respected and integrated their ancestral knowledge, not only offering modern health solutions but also revitalizing traditional practices that are the cornerstone of Quechua identity.

### Case Study: Implementing AI in Maori Health Strategies in New Zealand

In New Zealand, an innovative project was initiated to integrate artificial intelligence (AI) into Māori healthcare practices, focusing on addressing prevalent health issues such as cardiovascular disease and diabetes within the Māori community. The initiative aimed to blend traditional Maori healing practices, known as Rongoā, with modern AI-driven diagnostic tools, creating a culturally adaptive health management system.

The project commenced with collaborative workshops involving Maori healers, AI specialists, and healthcare professionals. These workshops served as a platform to communicate the nuances of Maori health perspectives, which are deeply embedded in spiritual, environmental, and community well-being. AI developers gained insights into the holistic Maori approach, which emphasizes the balance between the physical, spiritual, and familial health, crucial for the algorithm's cultural adaptability.

A specific challenge was the incorporation of non-quantifiable indicators used by Maori healers, such as family health history and environmental factors, into the AI system. Advanced data analytics techniques were utilized to model these holistic indicators, enhancing the AI's predictive accuracy. The system was designed not only to recognize physical symptoms but also to provide recommendations that align with Rongoā practices, such as herbal remedies and physical therapies.

During the pilot implementation, the AI system was integrated into a local health center serving the Maori community. Initial feedback highlighted areas for improvement, particularly in ensuring the AI system's language and recommendations resonated more deeply with Maori cultural expressions. This led to further refinements, with a greater emphasis on language inclusion and the system's ability to render culturally relevant health advice.

Throughout the project, maintaining the integrity and respect for Maori knowledge was paramount. Despite technical challenges, such as data integration and managing patient privacy concerns, the community's active participation provided continual guidance and validation, helping the AI system evolve into a tool that genuinely supports Maori health practices while leveraging the benefits of modern technology.

### Case Study: AI in Cherokee Herbal Medicine Practice Enhancement

In the cultural heritage of the Cherokee community, herbal medicine serves as a cornerstone of healthcare, reflecting a profound connection with nature and ancestral wisdom. The introduction of AI into this traditional practice aimed to augment the preservation and application of herbal knowledge, adapting to contemporary needs while respecting cultural heritage. The project, conducted in collaboration with Cherokee herbalists, AI developers, and ethnobotanists, focused on creating an AI system capable of identifying and suggesting herbal treatments based on traditional uses and modern medical research.

The development process began with thorough documentation and digitization of ancient herbal recipes and healing techniques, gathered from community elders and historical transcripts. AI developers worked closely with Cherokee practitioners to ensure that the algorithms could accurately understand and utilize this complex information. Cultural sensitivity was paramount, and the AI was designed to suggest treatments that align with both Cherokee tradition and clinical effectiveness.

During the pilot phase, the AI system was deployed in several community health clinics. It featured an interface that provided practitioners with information on herbal medicine interactions, potential side effects, and historical usage data. The AI also incorporated a learning module to adapt and improve its recommendations based on practitioner feedback and patient outcomes.

However, challenges arose during implementation. Some community members were hesitant to trust an AI system with their medicinal traditions, fearing misappropriation or misunderstanding of their cultural practices. Additionally, discrepancies between AI recommendations and practitioners' empirical knowledge caused initial resistance.

To address these issues, further modifications were made to the AI system to enhance its learning capabilities and ensure more transparent incorporation of practitioner insights. Continuous workshops and community meetings helped to foster trust and collaborative dialogue, gradually acclimating the community to the AI system's role and benefits. By integrating modern technology with traditional knowledge, the project not only conserved an essential aspect of Cherokee heritage but also enhanced the accessibility and effectiveness of herbal medicine practices.

## Case Study: Culturally Informed AI Platforms in Cree Community Healthcare

In a pioneering initiative in northern Canada, the Cree community has partnered with AI developers and healthcare professionals to develop a culturally informed AI platform designed to address mental health and wellness. This case study examines the collaboration that involves integrating Cree traditional healing practices with advanced AI technology to enhance mental health services. This initiative is particularly critical given the high incidence of mental health issues in many Indigenous communities, compounded by barriers such as geographical isolation and cultural misunderstandings with mainstream healthcare services.

The project began with a series of community workshops designed to understand Cree healing practices, which encompass spiritual rituals, community counseling, and traditional remedies. These practices are deeply embedded in the Cree worldview and emphasize healing from a community and spiritual perspective. The AI development team, which included cultural anthropologists, worked closely with Cree healers to ensure the platform would respect and integrate these practices alongside evidence-based medical approaches.

The AI system was designed to diagnose symptoms of mental distress and suggest interventions that incorporate both Cree and medical approaches. It featured language processing abilities to interact in the Cree language, enhancing accessibility and comfort for users. However, significant challenges surfaced during the implementation phase. The AI's recommendations sometimes clashed with the approaches of Cree practitioners, leading to debates about the validity of AI-generated advice. Additionally, concerns about data privacy and the potential misuse of cultural knowledge were significant hurdles.

To address these issues, the project team adjusted the AI algorithms to include more input from Cree healers during the diagnosis and treatment recommendation phases. Regular community feedback sessions were established, enabling the ongoing refinement of the AI system. Through these adaptive measures, the project not only facilitated improved engagement with mental health services but also set a precedent for the respectful incorporation of traditional knowledge in technological solutions.

## Case Study: Incorporation of AI in Enhancing Lakota Healing Practices for Behavioral Health

In the expansive Sioux reservations, particularly within the Lakota communities, behavioral health issues such as depression and anxiety have long been treated through a combination of community-supported rituals, herbal medicine, and spiritual counseling. Recognizing the rising incidence of these conditions, particularly among young people, a unique initiative was proposed to integrate Artificial Intelligence (AI) into traditional healing frameworks. The aim was to enhance the reach and effectiveness of treatments while respecting crucial cultural sensitivities.

The collaboration began with a series of dialogue sessions among Lakota healers, AI technology experts, and behavioral health specialists. These meetings aimed to map out the indigenous knowledge related to mental and emotional well-being and identify how AI could support these traditional practices without supplanting them. One of the primary challenges was the development of an AI model that could understand and incorporate Lakota language nuances and the non-linear, holistic approach to health that is a hallmark of Lakota traditions.

An AI system was subsequently developed to act as an assistive tool for Lakota healers. The system featured machine learning algorithms trained on anonymized data about herbal remedies and their impacts, patterns of emotional distress described in the Lakota language, and outcomes of various spiritual practices. Notably, the system included a user interface in both English and Lakota to ensure usability and acceptance.

Despite the promising integration, the initial deployment faced resistance. Concerns were raised about the AI interpreting the spiritual components of healing too mechanically, potentially leading to inappropriate suggestions that could undermine the healers' credibility. To address these issues, continuous feedback loops were established, allowing healers to adjust and validate the AI's recommendations before they were provided to patients.

As refinements continued, there was a measurable improvement in community engagement and treatment outcomes. AI began to be seen not just as a technological tool, but as a supportive bridge that enhanced the efficacy of traditional practices while fostering a deeper understanding of behavioral health within the Lakota context.

### Case Study: AI-driven Revitalization of Wendat Traditional Health Practices

In the region of Quebec, Canada, an innovative AI initiative was launched aimed at revitalizing and integrating Wendat (Huron) traditional health practices with modern healthcare technologies. This initiative represents a collaboration between Wendat health practitioners, AI researchers, and cultural anthropologists. The project's goal was to develop an AI system that not only aids in the effective diagnosis and management of chronic diseases prevalent in the community but also nurtures and preserves the rich heritage of Wendat medicinal practices.

The project commenced with a series of workshops and immersive sessions where Wendat healers shared their knowledge on medicinal herbs, healing rituals, and the cultural narratives that guide their practices. This knowledge was crucial for the AI team, which aimed to develop a system that is culturally sensitive and aligned with Wendat healing traditions. One of the primary challenges faced was the translation of orally transmitted knowledge. Additional challenges were qualitative healing methods translated into a format that AI algorithms could efficiently process. This challenge necessitated the creation of innovative data encoding schemes that preserved the integrity and context of traditional knowledge.

As the AI platform was developed, it incorporated features such as natural language processing to recognize and interpret the Wendat language, and machine learning algorithms designed to suggest health interventions that align with both medical and traditional Wendat practices. However, the integration phase underscored significant challenges, including resistance from the community elders, who were skeptical about the capacity of a digital system to understand and respect their ancestral knowledge.

To address these concerns, continuous feedback mechanisms were established, allowing for the ongoing refinement of the AI system based on direct input from the Wendat healers. Regular community engagement forums were also held to ensure transparency and cultivate trust. As the project evolved, it demonstrated promising results in enhancing healthcare delivery by providing insights that were deeply rooted in Wendat traditional medicine while leveraging advanced diagnostic technologies. Yet, the journey was riddled with learning curves, particularly in balancing technological innovation with deep-seated cultural values.

## Review Questions

**1. A 45-year-old woman with a history of type 2 diabetes and hypertension is experiencing persistent migraine headaches. She has tried various Western medications without significant relief and is interested in exploring holistic approaches, particularly based on her Indigenous heritage that embraces natural remedies. Considering her medical history and interest, which of the following would be the most appropriate recommendation?**

A) Start a rigorous physical exercise regimen immediately

B) Introduce a daily routine of meditation and incorporate herbal remedies like ginger tea

C) Immediately cease all Western medications, as they might be ineffective

D) Increase the dosage of her current Western medications, as they might be subtherapeutic

**Answer: B**

Explanation: Considering the patient's Indigenous background and interest in natural remedies, along with her chronic health conditions, the most culturally sensitive and potentially beneficial approach would be to introduce her to a daily routine of meditation. Meditation has been scientifically shown to help manage pain and stress, which could be contributory factors in her migraines. Adding herbal remedies like ginger tea can be beneficial, as it's known for its anti-inflammatory properties, which can help alleviate migraine symptoms. This approach respects her cultural beliefs and integrates her interest in holistic practices without disregarding the significance of her existing health conditions.

**2. A Native American patient with chronic back pain, interested in integrating traditional healing practices into their treatment plan, approaches a clinic that utilizes AI-based health assessments. The AI system recommends only pharmacological treatments. What could be a culturally sensitive addition to the AI's recommendation to respect the patient's desire for traditional healing methods?**

A) Recommend ignoring the AI's advice and only following traditional practices

B) Include recommendations for traditional Native American healing rituals, such as healing ceremonies and the use of medicinal herbs

C) Advise the patient that traditional methods are scientifically unproven and should be avoided

D) Suggest increasing the dosage of prescribed painkillers

**Answer: B**

Explanation: For a Native American patient wishing to incorporate traditional practices into their treatment, it would be culturally sensitive and beneficial to adjust the AI's recommendations to include conventional healing rituals and medicinal herbs recognized in Native American communities for treating pain. This integrated approach enables patients to honor their cultural practices while still benefiting from the advancements of modern medicine. Studies show that combining traditional and Western medicine can improve treatment adherence and satisfaction, especially in communities with strong ties to their cultural heritage.

**3. An AI system for diagnosing diabetes in an Indigenous community overlooks traditional dietary habits and herbal medicines that are part of the community's practices. How should the AI be adjusted to provide culturally appropriate care?**

A) Program the AI to recognize and suggest alternative local traditional diets and herbal remedies in its management suggestions

B) Remove the option for inputting dietary habits as they are irrelevant to the AI's diagnostic accuracy

C) Exclusively promote Western dietary adjustments and pharmacological treatments recommended by the AI

D) Advise the community to abandon traditional practices in favor of Western medicine

**Answer: A**

Explanation: Adjusting the AI to recognize and incorporate local traditional diets and herbal remedies can significantly enhance its usefulness and acceptability in an Indigenous community. By including these culturally specific elements, the AI respects and upholds the community's traditional knowledge and practices, which can lead to better patient engagement, adherence, and overall health outcomes. Integrating traditional and modern practices is vital for providing care that is sensitive to cultural needs and preferences, and it helps build trust and cooperation between healthcare providers and community members.

**Frameworks for Evaluating and Improving AI in Medicine**

**Defining Evaluation Frameworks for Medical AI**

Establishing robust frameworks for evaluating medical AI is pivotal to ensuring its efficacy and safety in healthcare settings. These frameworks serve as the blueprint for assessing AI systems at various stages of their lifecycle, from development to deployment. A comprehensive evaluation framework typically encompasses both technical and ethical standards, requiring a multifaceted approach to validate the technology's reliability, accuracy, and fairness.

The first step in defining these frameworks involves setting clear, measurable criteria that align with clinical goals and patient safety standards. This includes precision in diagnostic procedures, effectiveness in treatment recommendations, and the integration of patient data privacy. Additionally, the frameworks must account for the dynamic nature of medical environments, adapting to new medical evidence and technological advancements.

Moreover, a critical aspect of these frameworks is their inclusivity. They must address potential biases and ensure AI tools are equally effective across diverse patient demographics, including those represented in traditional, indigenous, and holistic medicine. This inclusivity enhances the credibility and acceptance of AI applications in healthcare, fostering trust among practitioners and patients alike.

**Criteria for Effective AI Performance Assessments**

Establishing criteria for effective AI performance assessments in medicine is critical to ensure the technology's impact benefits all facets of healthcare. These criteria should encompass a broad range of factors that gauge not only the functionality and efficiency of AI systems but also their fairness and inclusivity, particularly when integrating traditional, indigenous, and holistic healing methods.

Firstly, accuracy and predictive quality are fundamental, as AI must correctly interpret medical data and predict outcomes with high reliability. Alongside, its adaptability to diverse medical cases is crucial, ensuring that AI performs consistently across varied patient demographics, including those treated with non-conventional methods. Furthermore, transparency in AI processes allows healthcare providers to understand and trust AI decisions, which is vital for its integration into clinical settings.

Lastly, ethical considerations form a cornerstone of assessment criteria. AI systems must be scrutinized for biases, especially those against non-Western forms of medicine, and rectifications must be made to support equitable healthcare services. Regular updates and checks should monitor these criteria to maintain AI's relevance and efficacy in dynamic medical landscapes.

## Role of Clinical Trials in AI Validation

Clinical trials have long stood as the gold standard for validating medical treatments, ensuring efficacy and safety before public deployment. Similarly, the validation of AI in medicine demands rigorous testing through clinical trials to ascertain its operational integrity and therapeutic value. These trials assess AI tools in real-world clinical settings, evaluating not only their precision but also their adaptability to diverse medical complexities and patient needs.

However, conducting AI-focused clinical trials introduces unique challenges. Unlike drug trials, AI systems learn and evolve, creating variables that must be tightly controlled to maintain the trial's integrity. It is crucial that trial designs are robust enough to account for AI's dynamic nature, ensuring consistent and reliable results across different stages of AI learning.

Moreover, clinical trials for AI must also reflect ethical considerations, particularly in the realm of patient data privacy and the potential for unintended biases. Incorporating traditional, indigenous, and holistic healing perspectives into these trials can provide critical insights into how AI may perform in varied cultural and medical contexts. This multidimensional approach not only enriches the validation process but ensures a broader, inclusive base of AI applications in healthcare.

## Standards for AI Accuracy and Reliability Testing

In the realm of medical AI, setting standards for accuracy and reliability is crucial for fostering trust and effectiveness in healthcare applications. These standards must provide a scaffolding for AI tools to deliver consistent and verifiable results that clinicians can rely on, particularly when these tools intersect with traditional, indigenous, and holistic healing practices.

Accuracy involves the AI's ability to produce results that align closely with verified medical outcomes, while reliability pertains to the consistent performance of AI applications under varied conditions and patient populations. Each of these standards must be rigorously defined and adhered to, ensuring that AI systems are robust against the diverse and dynamic nature of medical practice. This includes calibrating AI with large, diverse datasets that reflect a wide array of health conditions and treatments.

Moreover, considerations for continuous monitoring and updating of these standards are essential, reflecting new advancements in medical knowledge and technology. By implementing comprehensive testing protocols and periodic re-evaluations, medical AI can adapt to evolving healthcare landscapes, maintaining high standards of accuracy and reliability.

**Integrating Real-World Data into AI Testing**

Incorporating real-world data into AI testing is important in fostering algorithms that perform effectively across a myriad of clinical environments. Traditional statistical models in medicine often operate under controlled, idealized conditions, which can potentially skew AI performance when applied to actual patient care scenarios. By embedding real-world data, AI systems can be attuned to the nuances, complexities, and varied presentations of diseases as they occur in diverse populations.

The integration process involves sourcing data from multiple healthcare settings, including remote and underserved areas where traditional and indigenous practices are prevalent. This practice ensures that AI systems recognize and appropriately incorporate holistic treatments into their outcomes. Moreover, real-world data facilitates the identification and mitigation of biases that may be ingrained in clinical algorithms, promoting equitable and inclusive healthcare solutions.

Additionally, the ongoing infusion of fresh, real-world data helps in refining AI algorithms. This enables continuous learning and adaptation, which are crucial for maintaining relevance and accuracy as new medical insights and treatment methodologies emerge. Through this, AI systems remain dynamic and responsive, mirroring the ever-evolving landscape of global healthcare.

**Ethical Considerations in AI Evaluation**

Ethical considerations in the evaluation of AI in medicine encompass a broad spectrum of issues, central to which is the imperative to uphold moral integrity and protect patient welfare. AI systems, when integrated into healthcare, must embody ethical principles not only in their operation but also during their testing and validation phases. The commitment to ethics involves rigorously addressing potential biases that AI might harbor, ensuring that these technologies do not inadvertently perpetuate existing disparities in healthcare access and outcomes.

Moreover, the ethical evaluation of AI tools should enforce transparency and accountability, enabling clinicians and patients to understand and scrutinize the AI decision-making process. This transparency is pivotal not only for building trust but also for facilitating informed consent, where patients are aware of the AI-driven components of their care.

Lastly, ethical AI evaluations must consider the implications of data privacy and security, ensuring that patient data utilized during AI development and testing is handled with the utmost confidentiality and respect for patient autonomy. Incorporating these ethical principles steadfastly supports the development of AI technologies that are not only clinically efficient but also morally sound and culturally sensitive.

**Establishing Benchmarks for AI in Healthcare**

Benchmarks for AI in healthcare serve as vital metrics to measure the efficiency, effectiveness, and equity of AI applications in healthcare. These benchmarks are essentially targeted standards designed to evaluate various dimensions of AI performance, including clinical accuracy and cultural competence, particularly in incorporating traditional and holistic medical practices. They provide clear, quantifiable targets that AI systems must achieve before being fully integrated into healthcare settings.

The development of these benchmarks involves collaboration among technologists, healthcare professionals, and representatives from diverse medical traditions. Ensuring that benchmarks address the broad spectrum of medical practices is crucial. They must reflect the values and efficacy of various health systems, providing AI with a robust, inclusive framework to operate within. This inclusivity is key to mitigating bias and enhancing the effectiveness of AI across all types of medical interventions.

Ultimately, benchmarks guide continuous improvement and adaptation of AI technologies. They are regularly reviewed and updated to reflect advancements in medical science and technology, ensuring AI applications remain aligned with changing healthcare demands and maintain high standards of patient care.

## Continuous Improvement Processes for AI Algorithms

The pursuit of excellence in AI-driven medical solutions requires an ongoing commitment to refining and enhancing AI algorithms. This continuous improvement process is based on systematic reviews, iterative updates, and ongoing learning loops that incorporate new information and feedback from medical practice.

One critical aspect involves the collection and analysis of performance data. This data not only informs us about current efficacy but also highlights areas that require modification. Adjustments might include algorithmic tuning to accommodate new patient data or emerging medical protocols. Regularly scheduled reviews ensure that these tools evolve in sync with medical advancements and patient needs, thereby maintaining their relevance and utility.

Additionally, stakeholder engagement is essential. Feedback from healthcare professionals and patients contributes to a more nuanced understanding of AI applications in clinical settings. This collaborative approach enriches AI systems, aligning them more closely with the humans they serve, thereby elevating both the precision of care and the trust in technological solutions.

## Feedback Mechanisms for Enhancing AI in Medicine

Effective feedback mechanisms are pivotal in the realm of medical AI, ensuring that systems not only meet current healthcare standards but also continually adapt to the evolving medical landscape. Feedback loops facilitate this by capturing insights from actual AI usage in clinical environments, including both healthcare professionals' and patients' perspectives. These inputs are critical for identifying discrepancies in AI performance and areas where the integration of traditional, indigenous, and holistic healing may be overlooked or underrepresented.

Incorporating structured feedback channels enables ongoing dialogue between technology developers and end-users. This collaborative framework is essential for fine-tuning AI tools, ensuring they are responsive to real-world conditions and diverse medical practices. Additionally, feedback mechanisms help in assessing the ethical implications of AI applications, which is crucial for maintaining trust and integrity in AI-driven healthcare solutions.

Ultimately, robust feedback systems play a crucial role in the sustainability of AI technologies in medicine. They ensure that AI tools not only comply with high standards but also remain culturally competent and inclusive, respecting a broad spectrum of healing traditions and practices. This ongoing process of feedback and refinement is vital for the progressive integration of AI into global healthcare systems.

## Incorporating Patient Outcomes into AI Evaluations

Incorporating patient outcomes into AI evaluations is a critical step towards ensuring that AI-driven medical technologies align with patient-centered care objectives. This process involves the systematic measurement of AI impacts on patients' health status, recovery patterns, and overall well-being, which is essential for gauging the effectiveness and safety of AI applications in real-world settings.

Patient outcomes provide tangible evidence of AI utility and effectiveness, helping to refine algorithms based on actual therapeutic results rather than purely theoretical data. By tracking recovery times, patient satisfaction, and recurrence rates, developers can adjust AI models to better meet patient needs and optimize clinical workflows. This feedback loop not only enhances algorithmic accuracy but also bolsters patient trust in AI-assisted treatments.

Furthermore, using patient outcomes as a metric for AI evaluation supports transparent reporting and accountability in healthcare. It ensures that AI tools are scrutinized under the lens of patient impact, promoting the development of technologies that genuinely enhance the health outcomes of diverse populations. This focus on patient-centric measures enriches the AI evaluation process, fostering innovations that are both technologically advanced and empathetically delivered.

## Interdisciplinary Approaches to AI Testing

Interdisciplinary approaches to AI testing in medicine harness the collective expertise from various fields to enhance the integrity and applicability of AI technologies. This fusion of knowledge from computer science, healthcare, ethics, and even social sciences fosters a holistic evaluation of AI systems. By engaging experts from diverse disciplines, testing processes address a broader range of potential issues, from technical performance to ethical implications and social impact.

Incorporating perspectives from traditional and indigenous medical practitioners can significantly enrich AI systems. This integration ensures that AI tools are not only technically competent but also culturally sensitive and inclusive. Such interdisciplinary collaborations create a feedback-rich environment that can quickly identify and correct biases, enhancing the reliability of AI in diverse healthcare scenarios.

Furthermore, engaging ethicists and patient advocacy groups in testing rounds ensures that AI systems uphold high ethical standards and prioritize patient welfare. This cooperative framework is crucial for developing AI technologies that are both innovative and deeply aligned with human values.

## AI Audits: Methods and Importance

AI audits are essential in ensuring the integrity and effectiveness of AI applications in healthcare. Through a combination of systematic reviews and compliance checks, these audits assess whether AI systems adhere to established medical standards and ethical guidelines. They primarily aim to identify and mitigate any biases that might influence outcomes, particularly those affecting underrepresented groups in healthcare, fostering a fairer deployment of AI technologies.

The methodology of AI audits involves both retrospective and prospective analyses. Retrospective audits review past AI decisions and outcomes to detect patterns of possible bias or error, while prospective audits are designed to ensure new systems perform as intended before full-scale implementation proactively. This layered approach helps maintain continuous oversight over AI systems, crucial for adapting to evolving medical trends and technologies.

Moreover, the significance of AI audits extends beyond mere regulatory compliance. They serve as a trust-building mechanism, reassuring patients and healthcare providers about the reliability and safety of AI-driven solutions. An effective audit not only highlights areas for improvement but also validates the positive impacts of AI, ensuring progressive and responsible healthcare innovation.

## Mapping AI Capabilities to Medical Needs

Mapping AI capabilities to medical needs requires a nuanced understanding of the diverse spectrum encompassing both modern and traditional medical practices. This alignment ensures that AI technologies not only address prevalent medical challenges but are also attuned to the specificities of individual patient profiles and cultural sensitivities. Effective mapping hinges on developing comprehensive datasets that represent the full range of human health conditions, including those traditionally handled by indigenous and holistic practices.

Engagement with healthcare practitioners from various disciplines is vital. Their insights help inform the design and adjustment of AI systems to meet a wide array of medical needs, integrating seamlessly into multifaceted healthcare environments. This collaborative approach helps bridge the gap between technological possibilities and practical healthcare applications, ensuring AI solutions are both innovative and applicable.

Moreover, continuous revisiting of these mappings is essential as medical needs evolve and new treatment modalities emerge. Regular updates, supported by ongoing research and feedback loops from clinical settings, empower AI systems to adapt dynamically, thereby enhancing their relevance and effectiveness over time. This process not only optimizes clinical outcomes but also boosts patient trust in AI-driven healthcare solutions.

## Adapting AI Evaluation Frameworks According to Specialty

The adaptation of AI evaluation frameworks to specific medical specialties is crucial for enhancing the precision and applicability of AI technologies in diverse healthcare fields. Specializations such as oncology, pediatrics, and geriatrics present unique challenges and requirements, demanding tailored AI solutions that accurately address the specific conditions and treatment modalities inherent to each discipline.

For instance, AI tools designed for oncology must be evaluated on their ability to discern subtle variations in imaging that are crucial for early cancer detection. Similarly, in pediatrics, AI systems should be assessed for their sensitivity and accuracy in interpreting symptoms that manifest differently in children compared to adults. This specialization-specific adaptation ensures that AI evaluations are not only technically sound but also clinically relevant.

Furthermore, by customizing evaluation frameworks, developers can better align AI tools with specialty-specific protocols and ethical standards, enhancing patient safety and care quality. Continuous dialogue between AI developers and specialty practitioners is crucial for refining these frameworks, ensuring they remain responsive to advancements in medical science and practice.

## Role of AI Ethics Boards in Evaluation Processes

AI Ethics Boards play a pivotal role in the evaluation processes of medical AI, ensuring that the development and implementation of AI technologies adhere to high ethical standards. These boards comprise diverse stakeholders, including ethicists, practitioners, and patient advocates, who scrutinize AI systems for their moral integrity and social impact.

Their responsibilities include reviewing AI algorithms to detect and mitigate biases, particularly those that could disproportionately affect marginalized communities. By setting ethical benchmarks and monitoring adherence, Ethics Boards facilitate responsible AI innovation that respects patient dignity and promotes fairness in healthcare outcomes.

Additionally, these boards evaluate the transparency of AI operations, advocating for clear communication of AI decision-making processes to patients and healthcare providers. This transparency is crucial for building trust and facilitating informed consent. The aim is to foster AI systems that not only excel in technical performance but also advance equitable and empathetic medical practices.

**Adherence to Regulatory Standards in AI Development**

Adherence to regulatory standards in AI development is paramount for ensuring that medical AI systems are safe, effective, and ethically sound. Regulations, often instituted by healthcare authorities and governmental bodies, provide a framework that guides the development, testing, and deployment of AI technologies. These standards are designed to safeguard patient data privacy, ensure accuracy in AI diagnostics and treatments, and promote fairness by mitigating biases that might otherwise harm vulnerable populations.

Incorporating these regulatory standards from the earliest stages of AI development facilitates compliance and enhances the integration of AI tools into clinical settings. It additionally serves as a preventive measure against potential legal and ethical issues that might arise post-deployment. Developers must regularly communicate with regulatory bodies to stay updated with the latest guidelines, reflecting the dynamic nature of both technology and healthcare requirements.

Fundamentally, adherence to these standards not only supports the ethical deployment of AI but also bolsters public trust in AI-driven healthcare solutions. By aligning AI development with stringent regulatory frameworks, we ensure that these technologies contribute positively to healthcare outcomes and uphold the highest standards of medical practice.

**Techniques for AI Bias Identification and Reduction**

Identifying and mitigating AI bias is crucial in developing equitable medical AI systems. Techniques involve both algorithmic adjustments and comprehensive analysis of training data. Initially, the development phase includes bias audits, leveraging statistical methods to uncover inherent biases in AI algorithms. These audits scrutinize algorithmic decision patterns against diverse datasets to ensure no demographic is disadvantaged.

Subsequently, incorporating synthetic data or underrepresented data subsets enhances the model's performance across varied patient demographics. This technique helps balance dataset representation and improve the algorithm's accuracy and fairness. Furthermore, continual learning systems are employed to adapt AI models in real-time, adjusting to new data inputs and evolving demographic distributions, which mitigates the accrual of bias over time.

Lastly, collaboration with interdisciplinary teams, including ethicists and community representatives, ensures diverse perspectives are considered in algorithm development. This multifaceted approach not only identifies biases but also implements robust strategies for their reduction, fostering trust and inclusivity in AI-driven medical services.

**Harnessing AI Meta-Analyses for Comprehensive Reviews**

Meta-analyses in the realm of medical AI represent a pivotal strategy for synthesizing results from multiple AI studies, offering a comprehensive overview of their effectiveness and safety. By aggregating and analyzing data across various AI-driven projects, researchers can discern patterns and determine the generalizability of findings, which is crucial in assessing AI's reliability in diverse medical contexts.

These meta-analyses also play a key role in identifying outlier results and commonalities in AI performance, enriching the process of refining AI systems. This holistic approach ensures that evaluations are not based on isolated studies but reflect broader operational insights, facilitating more informed decisions in AI applications and development.

Furthermore, the rigorous methodologies employed in meta-analyses foster deeper understanding of AI capabilities and limitations. By meticulously examining large datasets, researchers uncover nuances that might be overlooked in smaller studies, thereby contributing to the creation of more robust and equitable AI solutions in healthcare.

## Utilizing AI in Clinical Decision Support Systems

Integrating AI into clinical decision support systems (CDSS) revolutionizes medical diagnostics and treatment plans by providing healthcare professionals with incredibly sophisticated tools. These systems analyze large volumes of medical data, allowing for precise assessments that can suggest personalized treatment options.

To ensure these AI-driven CDSS are effective, robust evaluation frameworks are essential. Evaluations must measure how these tools influence decision-making processes and patient outcomes, focusing on accuracy, usability, and integration into existing clinical workflows. For instance, an AI system designed for diagnostics must align with the precise needs of emergency care settings, where rapid and accurate decision-making is critical.

Moreover, continuous feedback from clinical users is crucial for improving AI functionality in CDSS. By incorporating real-time data from clinical environments, AI systems can be fine-tuned to meet the practical demands of healthcare providers better, ensuring they remain relevant and effective in diverse clinical situations.

Ultimately, the goal is to develop AI-supported CDSS that not only enhance clinical efficiency but also uphold the highest standards of patient care, seamlessly integrating with the complex fabric of medical practice.

## Challenges in Standardizing AI Evaluations

Standardizing the evaluation of AI in medicine presents myriad challenges, primarily due to the diversity of medical specializations and the complexity of individual patient cases. Each medical domain requires bespoke AI solutions tailored to its unique diagnostic and therapeutic needs, complicating the creation of a uniform evaluation standard.

Additionally, the rapid evolution of AI technology itself poses a significant hurdle. As AI systems continuously improve, maintaining consistent evaluation criteria becomes a moving target, requiring constant updates to assessment protocols. This dynamic nature of AI capabilities demands flexible yet rigorous evaluation frameworks that can adapt without compromising the reliability or relevance of the assessment criteria.

Moreover, the ethical considerations involved in AI evaluations add another layer of complexity. Ensuring that AI evaluations are not only technically effective but also ethically sound and free of biases necessitates a multi-faceted approach, involving stakeholders from diverse backgrounds to encompass all ethical dimensions.

## Future Technologies Impacting AI Evaluations

The landscape of AI evaluation in medicine is poised to undergo transformative changes with the advent of emerging technologies. Quantum computing, for instance, offers unprecedented processing power, facilitating more complex data analysis that could drastically refine AI testing models. This could lead to faster, more accurate assessments of AI systems, significantly shortening development cycles and enhancing patient care sooner.

Furthermore, advancements in blockchain technology could introduce new levels of transparency and security to AI evaluations. By securely logging each step of the AI evaluation process on a decentralized platform, stakeholders can ensure that all modifications and updates are traceable and tamper-proof. This might bolster trust in AI applications and foster broader acceptance within the medical community.

Additionally, the integration of augmented and virtual reality into AI assessments could revolutionize how results are visualized and interpreted. Through immersive simulations, medical professionals could gain deeper insights into how AI applications perform in complex, real-world scenarios. Such technologies not only promise to enrich the evaluative processes but also enhance collaboration across multidisciplinary teams, ultimately leading to more sophisticated and fine-tuned AI solutions in healthcare.

## Scalability and Reproducibility in AI Tests

Scalability and reproducibility are crucial criteria in the realm of AI testing for medical applications. As AI technologies play increasingly pivotal roles in healthcare, the ability to scale solutions to different setting sizes and patient demographics without a loss in performance or accuracy becomes paramount. Scalability involves expanding AI systems to handle larger datasets or more complex diagnostic scenarios without degrading the system's operational efficiency or outcome accuracy.

Reproducibility, on the other hand, ensures that AI-driven diagnostics and treatments can consistently produce the same results under similar conditions across various healthcare environments. This element is vital for maintaining trust in AI applications, affirming that they are reliable regardless of geographical or institutional variations. Ensuring reproducibility involves rigorous validation techniques and repeated testing across a broad range of scenarios.

Lastly, overcoming the challenges of scalability and reproducibility involves developing robust frameworks that can adapt to advancements in technology while maintaining high standards of care. Techniques such as automated testing and the use of synthetic data can help achieve consistent performance, ensuring that AI applications are both scalable and reproducible in diverse medical settings.

## Innovative Tools for AI Performance Monitoring

The evolution of AI in healthcare necessitates innovative tools for performance monitoring, pivotal for maintaining strict quality and reliability standards. Innovations such as real-time analytics dashboards enable continual observation of AI systems, providing immediate feedback on performance anomalies and facilitating rapid adjustments. These tools are paramount for agile responses in a field where patient outcomes directly hinge on AI precision.

Further advancements stem from predictive analytics, which anticipate potential failures or inaccuracies before they occur. By integrating predictive mechanisms, healthcare facilities can refine AI algorithms preemptively, thereby safeguarding against errors that could impact clinical decisions and patient health. This proactive approach marks a significant shift from traditional reactive methods, positioning AI systems ahead of possible challenges.

Moreover, the integration of machine learning techniques into monitoring tools enables dynamic learning from operational data. This constant adaptation enhances the AI's decision-making capabilities, ensuring the technology evolves in line with medical advancements and the evolving needs of patients.

Ultimately, these innovative monitoring tools empower healthcare professionals to trust in AI applications, ensuring these systems function optimally and ethically within the clinical environment.

## Case Studies of AI Improvement Cycles in Healthcare

In examining AI improvement cycles, multiple case studies across various clinical environments have demonstrated significant progress in healthcare delivery. One notable instance involves a large urban hospital integrating AI in its cardiovascular unit. Initially, AI algorithms faced accuracy issues, leading to unreliable risk assessments for heart disease. Through an iterative cycle of feedback and algorithm refinement, the system gradually enhanced its precision and reliability, ultimately reducing misdiagnosis rates significantly.

Another case saw the development of an AI-driven oncology treatment adviser at a cancer research center. Despite promising early outcomes, the AI struggled with tailoring precise treatment protocols for rare cancers. Continuous cycles of evaluations with real-world patient data allowed developers to refine the model significantly, ensuring treatments were better customized and thus more effective.

These examples illustrate the importance of continually adapting AI systems through ongoing evaluation and feedback, as this is crucial for meeting the dynamic needs of medical practitioners and patients. This highlights the importance of continuous improvement throughout the AI lifecycle, ultimately ensuring optimal outcomes in healthcare.

## Summary

The chapter, 'Frameworks for Evaluating and Improving AI in Medicine', offers a comprehensive exploration of methodologies essential for assessing and enhancing artificial intelligence (AI) within the healthcare sector. It underscores the need for robust evaluation frameworks defined through clear, measurable criteria that align with clinical goals, emphasizing the importance of accuracy, effectiveness, fairness, and inclusivity. These frameworks must be adaptable to the dynamic nature of medical environments and technological advancements, while ensuring that AI systems are free from biases and uniformly effective across diverse patient demographics. The chapter delves deeper into specific criteria for AI performance assessments, highlighting the necessity of precision, predictive quality, adaptability, ethical considerations, and transparency in AI operations to ensure seamless integration into medical practices. Clinical trials are depicted as crucial in validating AI through stringent testing in real-world clinical settings, adapting to the complexities of diverse medical conditions and ethical standards. Furthermore, the text discusses the establishment of accuracy and reliability standards, the integration of real-world data, and the continuous improvement of AI algorithms. Additionally, the role of Ethics Boards in maintaining ethical integrity in AI applications and the adherence to regulatory standards in AI development are central themes. The necessity of interdisciplinary approaches and rigorous AI audits to ensure compliance with medical and ethical guidelines is emphasized. By mapping AI capabilities to medical needs and adapting evaluation frameworks according to medical specialties, the chapter proposes an operational blueprint to ensure the effectiveness, reliability, and ethical soundness of AI tools. It concludes with insightful discussions on upcoming technologies that could impact AI evaluation, challenges in standardizing AI evaluations, and the pivotal roles of scalability, reproducibility, and innovative tools in AI performance monitoring, which foster robust, efficient, and fair AI systems in healthcare.

## References

[1] Jiang F., Jiang Y., Zhi H., et al.. https://www.ncbi.nlm.nih.gov/pmc/articles/PMC5962261/
[2] He J., Baxter S. L., Xu J., et al.. https://www.nature.com/articles/s41746-019-0191-0
[3] Char D. S., Shah N. H., Magnus D..

https://www.sciencedirect.com/science/article/pii/S0140673618312626
[4] Esteva A., Robicquet A., Ramsundar B., et al.. https://www.nature.com/articles/s41591-019-0656-7

## Case Study: Enhancing Patient Outcomes with AI-Integrated Oncology Treatments

A major metropolitan hospital recently embarked on a transformative project integrating Artificial Intelligence (AI) into its oncology department to enhance treatment precision and patient care. The hospital partnered with a leading AI technology firm to develop an AI system capable of assisting oncologists in diagnosing, planning treatment, and monitoring patient responses to various cancer therapies.

The first phase involved the AI system's training using thousands of anonymized patient records, clinical trial data, and real-time diagnostic information to create predictive models for cancer progression and treatment outcomes. Oncologists and AI specialists worked closely, examining the AI's predictive accuracy in breast, lung, and colorectal cancers, initially chosen due to their high incidence rates.

During the implementation, several challenges became apparent. The AI system sometimes produced recommendations that contradicted the oncologists' clinical judgments, leading to critical reviews of its decision-making processes. Moreover, discrepancies in treatment results highlighted potential biases in the AI system against certain demographics, necessitating an immediate and robust methodological review.

Addressing these issues involved refinements to the AI's algorithms and the inclusion of more diverse data sets, particularly incorporating underrepresented groups in clinical datasets to improve fairness and accuracy in AI predictions. The hospital also established an Ethics Oversight Committee to regularly review AI decisions and maintain continuous alignment with ethical medical standards.

This ongoing evaluation and adjustment process underscores the necessity of incorporating strong feedback mechanisms, continuous AI training with new data, and robust ethical considerations in treatment planning. By acknowledging and addressing these initial setbacks, the hospital's AI-integrated oncology treatments gradually improved, demonstrating enhanced accuracy and patient satisfaction in subsequent months, leading to better patient outcomes and increased trust in AI-assisted healthcare.

## Case Study: Implementing AI in Emergency Medicine: Challenges and Solutions

In this detailed case study, we explore the challenges and solutions associated with implementing Artificial Intelligence (AI) in emergency medicine at a large urban hospital, specifically focusing on the application of AI in improving rapid diagnostic processes and treatment decisions. The hospital aimed to reduce wait times and enhance diagnostic accuracy, leveraging AI to assist in triaging and initial patient assessments. The AI system was designed to analyze symptoms, medical history, and vital signs to prioritize patients based on the urgency of their conditions.

The initial integration phase involved the collaboration between AI developers, medical staff, and IT departments to customize an AI tool that could interface seamlessly with existing electronic health records (EHRs). During the pilot testing, the AI demonstrated a promising ability to swiftly analyze and prioritize patient cases. However, issues arose when the AI's recommendations occasionally conflicted with those of the senior medical staff, raising concerns about its decision-making process.

Further investigation revealed two primary challenges: the AI's limited ability to interpret nuanced patient expressions and behaviors, and occasional discrepancies in data interpretation between the AI and human doctors. Such challenges underscore the necessity for an adaptive AI system, equipped to learn from real-time feedback and improve over time.

Addressing these challenges involved refining AI algorithms with a broader set of patient interaction data, enhancing their learning algorithms to understand the subtleties of emergency medical care better. Ethics oversight was intensified, ensuring all AI-driven diagnostics adhered to established medical guidelines, and regular multidisciplinary meetings were instituted to evaluate AI performance and integration.

As solutions were implemented, the hospital observed significant improvements in patient triage efficiency, resulting in reduced waiting times and increased satisfaction among both patients and staff. This case study exemplifies the dynamic process of integrating AI into critical healthcare settings, involving continuous refinement and collaboration across various departments to enhance the efficacy and reliability of AI systems in emergency medical services.

**Case Study: Adapting AI for Pediatric Asthma Management: A Multidisciplinary Approach**

A regional children's hospital embarked on an innovative project to integrate Artificial Intelligence (AI) into its pediatric asthma care unit. Asthma, being one of the most common chronic diseases in children, presents considerable challenges in monitoring and management. The hospital aimed to utilize AI to personalize treatment plans based on individual patient profiles and dynamically adjust treatments in response to environmental triggers.

The project began with a developmental phase, during which an AI model was trained on a vast dataset comprising longitudinal patient health records, environmental data, and outcomes from various treatment protocols. A team comprising pediatricians, AI developers, and data scientists collaborated to ensure that the AI system could effectively interpret pediatric-specific data, such as variability in symptom presentation across different ages and developmental stages.

Initial deployment highlighted several challenges. One significant issue was the AI's integration with real-time environmental data sensors, which were critical in predicting asthma triggers. Discrepancies in data consistency and accuracy resulted in unreliable predictions of asthma flare-ups. Another challenge involved ensuring the AI's recommendations complied with the nuanced needs of ongoing pediatric treatments that often affect other medical conditions.

To address these issues, the hospital initiated a series of iterative improvements. Firstly, improving the AI's algorithm to process inconsistencies in environmental data better. Second, pediatricians held workshops with developers to refine the AI's decision-making algorithms, aligning them with the complexities of pediatric care. Ethical considerations were paramount, with a focus on ensuring patient data privacy and obtaining informed consent from guardians.

As the AI system's reliability improved, the hospital observed a reduction in emergency treatments for asthma attacks and an increase in maintaining optimal patient health through proactive management strategies. This case illustrates the importance of continual feedback loops and multidisciplinary collaboration in the effective integration of AI into specialized pediatric healthcare.

**Case Study: AI-Driven Approaches in Geriatric Healthcare: Integrating AI to Manage Chronic Diseases in Elderly Populations**

In this detailed exploration, we dive into the transformative power of Artificial Intelligence (AI) in geriatric healthcare at a specialized care facility dedicated to elderly patients. The primary focus was on chronic disease management, particularly addressing the complications of diabetes and heart disease, which are prevalent in older adults. The facility partnered with a technology provider to develop an AI system aimed at predictive health monitoring and personalized care plans.

The initial phase involved training the AI with extensive historical health records, treatment outcomes, and continuous health monitoring data. This training aimed to enable the AI to predict exacerbations, suggest proactive interventions, and optimize treatment plans. The interdisciplinary team, comprising geriatric specialists, data scientists, and AI experts, faced the vital task of ensuring that the AI's suggestions were not only medically sound but also tailored to the unique physiological characteristics of the elderly.

However, several challenges were encountered. The AI initially struggled with over-predicting risks, causing unnecessary alarms and patient anxiety. Furthermore, the integration of AI-generated recommendations into traditional care routines was met with resistance from some veteran healthcare providers who trusted established methods more.

Addressing these issues, the project team enhanced the AI algorithms by refining the predictive models and incorporating feedback from clinical staff into the learning loop. Additionally, extensive training sessions were conducted for healthcare providers, highlighting the AI's reliability and the empirical reasoning behind its recommendations. The project also implemented a robust ethics review process to safeguard patient autonomy and consent, which are particularly significant given the vulnerability of the geriatric population.

As the system progressively integrated into daily operations, it became evident that the AI could significantly streamline care processes. The facility reported reductions in emergency hospitalizations and improved patient engagement with their health management. This scenario exemplifies the careful balance required between innovative AI solutions and the existing healthcare ecosystem in managing chronic diseases in sensitive populations such as the elderly.

**Case Study: Integrating AI in Rural Healthcare: Optimizing Maternal and Child Health Services**

In an ambitious endeavor, a health organization collaborated with AI developers to enhance maternal and child healthcare services in remote rural areas, where access to specialists and advanced medical facilities is often limited. Key goals were to improve prenatal and postnatal care delivery and diminish child mortality rates using intelligent AI-driven solutions.

Phase one of the project included the development of an AI system trained on extensive datasets, including thousands of health records, outcome studies, and regional health statistics. Special emphasis was placed on teaching the AI to recognize and predict complications during pregnancy and childbirth that are prevalent in the targeted rural regions. The system was designed to provide support to local healthcare workers by offering tailored care plans and recommendations for action in emergency situations, bridging the gap where specialist consulting is scarce.

However, several hurdles emerged as the deployment proceeded. One major challenge was the AI's initial inability to adapt to the diverse and sometimes incomplete medical records typically found in rural settings, where documentation practices could be inconsistent. Moreover, integrating AI recommendations into existing healthcare protocols proved difficult, as local professionals expressed skepticism about the AI's advice, favoring traditional practices.

To address these issues, the team introduced comprehensive adjustments. AI algorithms were refined to better handle variations in data quality and completeness, and simulation training was provided to healthcare staff to enhance their confidence in using the system's advice. To further ease the integration, AI outputs were tailored to complement traditional practices, showing respect for and adaptation to local medical norms.

Regular feedback sessions were established, creating a two-way learning process between AI developers and rural healthcare providers. As the AI system matured, its acceptance grew, shown by a marked improvement in patient outcomes and increased utilization of AI-driven recommendations. With ongoing evaluation and community engagement, the project underscored the importance of culturally and contextually sensitive AI applications in enhancing healthcare services in low-resource settings.

**Case Study: AI Optimization of Neurodegenerative Disease Treatment in Multinational Clinical Settings**

In a groundbreaking initiative, a multinational consortium of healthcare providers and AI developers collaborated on employing Artificial Intelligence to optimize treatment protocols for neurodegenerative diseases like Alzheimer's and Parkinson's. The project, spread across healthcare facilities in the US, Europe, and Asia, aimed to harness AI's analytical prowess to personalize treatment for variably progressing illnesses and improve patient outcomes on a global scale.

Phase one centered on the rigorous compilation of data—an extensive merge of localized clinical studies, patient health records, and ongoing treatment results. These were not just volumes of data, but diverse arrays reflecting multiple ethnicities, progression stages, and treated symptoms. The AI system employed deep learning to analyze these data shadows, identifying patterns that eluded conventional methods and suggesting nuanced treatment modifications.

As the implementation spread among differently equipped healthcare settings, disparities in AI efficacy became apparent. In some locations, AI-driven suggestions led to marked improvements in patient responsiveness to treatment, while in others, the outcomes were not as encouraging, highlighting inconsistencies possibly due to variances in regional medical practices and data quality.

Addressing these disparities involved a dual approach: refining AI algorithms to enhance understanding of complex health datasets and initiating a training program for local healthcare providers to better interpret AI-driven data. This stage was crucial for the standardization of data input and interpretation methods across border-diverse clinical settings.

Simultaneously, ethical considerations were overseen by an International Ethics Committee, assuring that patient data security and AI decisions adhered to both local and international regulations. As data flowed in and the algorithm refined, iterative feedback loops from all participating regions led to increasingly sophisticated AI models. Healthcare systems observed gradual but significant reduction in the variability in patient outcomes, affirming AI's role in standardizing excellence in care across disparate medical landscapes.

**Case Study: Revolutionizing Stroke Rehabilitation with AI-driven Adaptive Therapies**

A leading neuro-rehabilitation center embarked on an innovative journey to integrate Artificial Intelligence (AI) into its stroke rehabilitation program, aiming to revolutionize treatment protocols and improve recovery outcomes for patients. This initiative involved the development of an AI system designed to personalize and adapt physical therapy regimens based on patient-specific progress and responses.

The development phase commenced with the collection of extensive patient data, including motor function assessments, cognitive evaluations, and daily therapy outcomes. This data was then utilized to train a sophisticated AI model capable of analyzing patient recovery patterns and predicting optimal therapy adjustments. Initial trials of the AI system demonstrated promising results, with noticeable improvements in patient recovery speeds and therapy engagement.

However, the integration faced significant hurdles. The AI system occasionally recommended therapy intensities that exceeded patient capacities, resulting in fatigue without additional recovery benefits. Additionally, the varied technological literacy among rehabilitation staff posed challenges in effectively utilizing the AI system, sometimes leading to erroneous data inputs and misinterpretations of AI suggestions.

Addressing these challenges required a multifaceted approach. First, the AI algorithms were recalibrated to better align with realistic human physical limits and recovery trajectories. Training sessions were then implemented for staff, focusing on the operation and rationale of the AI system to ensure accurate usage and interpretation. Furthermore, to ensure the ethical use of AI, patient consent processes were enhanced, and an Ethics Oversight Panel was established to review changes to AI-driven therapies for appropriateness and safety regularly.

As the AI system evolved through continuous learning and adaptation, it became a pivotal component of the rehabilitation program. Patients received more tailored therapy regimens that dynamically adjusted to their day-to-day progress, resulting in faster and more sustainable recovery outcomes. This adaptive approach not only enhanced patient recovery but also allowed therapists to allocate more time to severe cases, optimizing resource utilization and care delivery across the center.

### Case Study: Navigating AI Integration in Chronic Pain Management: A Multisite Clinical Study

A prominent healthcare system initiated a multisite clinical study to incorporate Artificial Intelligence (AI) into chronic pain management across several of its facilities. This ambitious project aimed to personalize pain management strategies by predicting patient responses to various treatments using AI-driven analytics, thereby improving patient quality of life and reducing reliance on opioid prescriptions.

The initial phase involved aggregating and anonymizing extensive patient data on pain levels, treatment histories, demographic details, and psychosocial factors. Special attention was paid to assembling diverse data sets to avoid biases that could affect AI's treatment recommendations. AI developers, data scientists, and pain management specialists collaborated intensively to design AI models that could interpret this complex, multidimensional data.

As the AI models were deployed, they faced the challenge of accurately interpreting the subjective nature of pain, which varied significantly across patients. Early trials revealed that the AI's pain threshold predictions did not consistently align with patient-reported outcomes, leading to some inappropriate treatment recommendations. Furthermore, integration issues arose as existing clinical workflows were disrupted by the new AI tools, resulting in delays and initial resistance among clinical staff.

To address these challenges, the project team implemented a series of iterative enhancements. The AI algorithms were continually refined with incoming patient data to improve accuracy. Training sessions were organized to familiarize clinicians and staff with the AI systems, explaining the technology's capabilities and limitations. Ethical considerations were prioritized, with a focus on maintaining patient privacy and ensuring that the AI's recommendations did not introduce new biases into treatment decisions.

Over time, as the AI models became more sophisticated and staff more adept at interpreting AI aids, the project observed a significant improvement in treatment outcomes. Pain management became more tailored to individual needs, reducing unnecessary medication while optimizing therapeutic interventions. The case illustrates the importance of flexible, iterative processes in integrating AI into healthcare, addressing both technological and human factors to enhance patient care.

### Review Questions

**1. A 55-year-old female patient with a history of chronic lower back pain and anxiety attends an integrative health center after experiencing limited relief from conventional NSAID therapy. She receives a combination of traditional Thai massage and Reiki during her visit. After several weeks, she reports significant improvement in both pain and anxiety levels. What is the most likely explanation for her improved condition?**

A) The placebo effect was solely responsible for her improvement.

B) The integrative approach effectively addressed both physiological and psychological aspects of her conditions.

C) NSAIDs took longer to show effects, which coincided with the timing of the massage and Reiki.

D) There was no actual improvement; the patient's reporting was biased.

**Answer: B**

Explanation: The integrative approach to the patient's treatment, which included both traditional Thai massage and Reiki, likely offered a holistic remedy that addressed not only the physical aspect of pain but also psychological factors associated with anxiety. Traditional Thai Yoga Therapy can help alleviate physical pain through Puja (Prayer), manual manipulation (Marma Chikitsa), improve circulation, and relieve muscle tension. Reiki, a form of energy healing, might have contributed to reducing stress and promoting a sense of mental well-being. This case illustrates how combining physical and energy therapies can provide a comprehensive treatment solution, improving overall patient outcomes.

**2. In a Native American community's clinic, a new AI system is introduced to improve healthcare delivery. The AI is programmed to recommend treatments based on widely accepted clinical guidelines. However, the community members express dissatisfaction with the AI's recommendations, citing a lack of consideration for their traditional healing practices. How should the clinic's administration respond to ensure the AI system serves the community effectively?**

A) Ignore the community's feedback as the AI recommendations are based on proven medical guidelines.

B) Turn off the AI system and revert to traditional healing practices exclusively.

C) Adjust the AI system to incorporate traditional healing practices into its database and offer culturally sensitive recommendations.

D) Educate the community about the benefits of conventional medicine to reduce reliance on traditional practices.

**Answer: C**

Explanation: To effectively serve the community and respect their cultural practices, the clinic's administration should adjust the AI system to incorporate traditional healing practices into its recommendations. This involvement should include dialogues with community healers and knowledge holders to gather accurate data about traditional practices and their effectiveness. By integrating this knowledge into the AI system, the clinic can ensure that the technology respects and reflects the community's healthcare preferences, enhancing trust and compliance with treatment protocols. Educating the AI about local customs and traditional medicine can make it a supportive tool rather than a replacement for culturally rooted practices.

**3. A research team uses AI to analyze a database of clinical outcomes for patients using various herbal supplements. They find that patients taking St. John's Wort show a statistically significant improvement in symptoms of mild depression compared to those who don't. How should this information be utilized to influence future healthcare AI development and patient care strategies?**

A) The findings should be ignored as they do not align with traditional pharmaceutical approaches.

B) AI developers should integrate these findings into AI systems to suggest St. John's Wort for similar patients.

C) Only traditional herbalists should use this information; AI should focus on pharmaceutical recommendations.

D) Due to legal and ethical concerns, the findings should be kept confidential and not used in patient care.

**Answer: B**

Explanation: The statistically significant improvement in patients using St. John's Wort suggests that the herbal supplement may be beneficial for treating mild depression. Integrating these findings into healthcare AI systems could help personalize treatment options for patients suffering from similar symptoms, offering them an effective alternative to conventional pharmaceuticals. This approach aligns with the principles of evidence-based practice and personalized medicine, allowing patients access to a broader range of validated treatment options. Accordingly, AI developers should work to update existing systems to reflect this new data, thereby enhancing the AI's capability to support healthcare providers in delivering patient-centered care that includes both modern and traditional therapeutic options.

**4. An AI system in an urban hospital frequently recommends advanced biomedicine treatment options for diabetes management. However, a significant portion of the patient population prefers using integrated approaches involving traditional remedies. What adjustments should be made to the AI system to better accommodate the needs and preferences of this patient population?**

A) Program the AI to strictly discourage the use of traditional remedies as they are not evidence-based.

B) Remove the AI system completely and allow physicians to decide without technological assistance.

C) Update the AI system to include information and guidelines on evidence-based traditional remedies, allowing for an integrative care approach.

D) Enforce the AI's existing recommendations more strictly to phase out the use of traditional remedies.

**Answer: C**

Explanation: To better accommodate the patient population's preferences for an integrated approach to diabetes management, the AI system should be updated to include evidence-based traditional remedies alongside biomedical treatments. This adjustment will enable the AI to offer comprehensive treatment options that respect patient preferences and cultural values, potentially increasing satisfaction and adherence to treatment plans. By incorporating a broader spectrum of validated medical practices, the AI can truly support personalized and culturally sensitive care. Such an integrative approach not only showcases the flexibility and adaptability of AI in healthcare but also promotes respect for diverse medical traditions and patient autonomy in treatment decisions.

**Policies to Support Equitable AI Applications in Health**

**Defining Equitable AI in Healthcare**

Defining Equitable AI in Healthcare necessitates a framework that promotes fairness, inclusivity, and equal access to technological advancements. Equitable AI must effectively address and adapt to the diverse healthcare needs of various demographic groups, ensuring that no community is disenfranchised by AI implementations.

The concept encompasses developing algorithms that are unbiased and transparent, prioritizing the eradication of historical disparities in medical treatment. This includes incorporating data from a broad spectrum of populations to avoid skewing AI decisions that could perpetuate healthcare inequities. Moreover, equitable AI should facilitate healthcare delivery in a way that respects and integrates both traditional and contemporary medical practices, enhancing rather than replacing the human element in healthcare.

Ultimately, creating an equitable AI environment in the healthcare sector requires rigorous and continuous oversight to maintain its alignment with ethical standards. Policymakers must ensure these technologies benefit all individuals equally, particularly those from marginalized and underserved communities, thus supporting a holistic approach to health equity.

## Regulatory Frameworks Governing AI in Health

The development of regulatory frameworks for AI in health is pivotal to ensuring that these technologies are used safely and ethically. Governments and international bodies must collaborate to establish standards that safeguard patient rights while promoting innovation. This involves setting clear guidelines on data privacy, algorithm transparency, and the ethical use of AI-generated insights.

Moreover, the regulatory environment must be flexible enough to adapt to rapid technological changes without stifling progress. This can be achieved by establishing dynamic regulations that are regularly updated in accordance with the latest scientific evidence and evolving societal expectations. Public consultations and expert panels play a critical role in this process, ensuring that diverse perspectives inform the development of these frameworks.

Lastly, the enforcement of these regulations requires robust mechanisms. This includes the creation of specialized agencies to monitor AI applications in healthcare, conduct audits, and enforce compliance with relevant laws and regulations. Effective regulation not only enhances public trust in AI health technologies but also ensures that innovations contribute positively to patient care and health outcomes. However, we will stress repeatedly that any regulations for AI model development must not inadvertently also act to curtail or restrict the literal practices of indigenous traditional medicine and religious therapeutics as practiced by the native communities themselves.

## Creating Inclusive AI Policies: Scope and Ambitions

Creating inclusive AI policies in healthcare demands a multi-faceted approach centered on a comprehensive scope and ambitious goals. This involves framing policies not only to correct existing imbalances but also to design systems that are supportive of all patient groups preemptively. To successfully implement this, policymakers must commit to a thorough audit of AI systems, ensuring they cater effectively to diverse ethnic, economic, and regional demographics without inherent biases.

Ambitions here must be visionary yet actionable, aiming for the integration of AI tools that uplift rather than inadvertently sideline traditional, indigenous, and holistic practices. Inclusivity means developing mechanisms that evaluate AI outcomes through the prism of equity, reinforcing the importance of diverse data inputs that reflect the multifarious nature of human health.

Finally, the scope of these policies should adaptively expand with technology advances, adhering to ethical standards that evolve and respond to new challenges and insights. This proactive stance ensures that AI healthcare policies remain relevant and equitable, aligning technological progress with the highest standards of care and inclusivity.

**Guidelines for Ethical AI Implementation in Healthcare**

Establishing guidelines for the ethical implementation of AI in healthcare is crucial to ensuring that AI technologies enhance medical practice without compromising ethical standards. These guidelines must emphasize transparency in AI operations, ensuring that algorithms are explainable and their decision-making processes are accessible to both practitioners and patients.

Moreover, ethical AI must prioritize patient confidentiality and data security, particularly given the susceptibility of healthcare data to breaches. Developers must design AI systems that uphold patient autonomy by incorporating consent protocols directly into the AI user interface, thereby safeguarding individuals' control over their medical data.

In addition, fairness must be a central tenet, requiring that AI tools undergo rigorous protocols to mitigate bias. Regular audits should be mandated to evaluate AI systems continuously for unintended biases that may perpetuate healthcare disparities.

Ultimately, the integration of ethical AI in healthcare requires a collaborative approach, involving stakeholders from diverse backgrounds to ensure the broadest perspectives in guiding AI development.

**Policy Recommendations for AI Data Management**

To uphold the principles of equity in healthcare AI, data management policies must prioritize transparency, security, and inclusiveness. First, transparency in data handling and algorithmic decision-making processes must be ensured. This includes clear documentation of data sources, the methodologies employed in training AI systems, and the rationale behind algorithmic decisions. Patients and providers should have understandable access to this information, promoting trust and accountability.

Secondly, maintaining robust data security is imperative. Policies should mandate strict protocols for data encryption, secure data storage, and regular audits to prevent breaches that could compromise patient privacy and confidentiality. Such measures safeguard sensitive health information, reinforcing the reliability of AI systems.

Finally, inclusivity in data collection processes is crucial. Policies should require AI systems to be trained on diverse datasets that reflect the broad spectrum of patient demographics. This prevents biases against underrepresented groups and ensures AI-driven decisions benefit all patients equally, thereby supporting a universally equitable healthcare system.

**Legal Protections for Patients in AI-Driven Healthcare**

In the ever-evolving landscape of AI-driven healthcare, the legal protections for patients serve as crucial safeguards. These laws must ensure that AI technologies do not infringe upon patient rights, particularly in terms of privacy, consent, and access to transparent information about AI-driven decisions and their impacts. Legislation must clearly delineate the responsibilities of AI providers in safeguarding personal health information against misuse or breaches.

Furthermore, patients must have the right to contest and seek redress for decisions made by AI that may adversely affect their healthcare outcomes. This includes implementing mechanisms that enable patients to gain insight into the rationale behind AI decisions, consistent with the principles of informed consent. Such frameworks should also accommodate the specific needs of vulnerable populations to prevent exacerbating existing healthcare disparities.

To this end, proactive legal frameworks are vital. They should not only react to emerging technological advancements but also anticipate future developments, ensuring that patient protections evolve in tandem with the advancement of AI capabilities. Continuous dialogue between legal experts, technologists, and patient advocacy groups is essential to shaping these laws, ensuring they are comprehensive and uphold the dignity and rights of all patients in a digitized healthcare environment.

## Standards for Transparency and Accountability in Health AI

Elevating standards for transparency and accountability in health AI is pivotal as these technologies become more entrenched in our medical systems. This must begin with the clear articulation of how AI models function and the decisions they inform. Detailed documentation and open access to AI processes safeguard practitioners' and patients' rights to transparent understanding, facilitating informed consent in therapy and treatment choices.

Accountability structures should encompass regular external and internal audits, assessing systems for bias and accuracy while ensuring adherence to ethical norms. This promotes continuous improvement in AI reliability and sensitivity towards diverse patient needs. Moreover, the accountability framework should clearly outline consequences for non-compliance, ensuring that stakeholders uphold the highest ethical standards.

Furthermore, transparency is not merely about access to information, but also about understanding its implications. Clear communication strategies should therefore be employed to demystify AI technologies for all stakeholders, which supports equity in healthcare outcomes. This transparency extends to stakeholders' involvement in shaping the systems that impact their care, affirming their role in driving ethical AI development.

## International Cooperation on AI Health Regulations

Addressing the complexities of AI in healthcare demands robust international cooperation to harmonize regulations across borders. This global approach ensures that AI technologies are deployed safely and equitably, considering the diverse ethical, cultural, and regulatory landscapes. International forums and agencies can facilitate the sharing of best practices and the development of universal standards that accommodate varying health systems while preventing disparities.

Effective international cooperation necessitates the establishment of interoperable frameworks that facilitate seamless data exchange and regulatory alignment. Collaboration in research and policy development can accelerate the adaptation of AI technologies that respect universal human rights and ethical standards. Moreover, such cooperation fosters resilience against global health challenges by synchronizing responses and allocating resources effectively.

Policymakers must also prioritize diplomacy and global governance in AI, cultivating an environment of mutual trust and accountability. Strategic partnerships among nations will not only streamline regulatory processes but also enhance the collective capability to oversee AI advancements, ensuring they contribute positively to global health outcomes.

## Incorporating Stakeholder Voices in AI Policy Making

Incorporating diverse stakeholder voices into AI policymaking is vital for crafting equitable healthcare solutions. Engaging with patients, practitioners, ethicists, and community leaders ensures a comprehensive understanding of the unique needs and potential impacts of AI. This inclusive approach fosters policies that are not only technically sound but also socially sensitive and ethically aligned with the welfare of all community segments.

Regularly scheduled forums and consultative panels can facilitate this integration, allowing stakeholders to express concerns and offer insights that may otherwise be overlooked in the technocratic sphere. Such platforms should be designed to capture a broad spectrum of perspectives, particularly from underrepresented groups whose needs and views might differ significantly from the mainstream.

Incorporating these voices through transparent, structured processes enhances trust in AI technologies. Policymakers must commit to not only hearing these voices but actively responding to them, ensuring that AI health policies are continuously revised to reflect the evolving public consensus and ethical considerations in healthcare.

## Balancing Innovation with Consumer Protection in AI Health

In the rapidly evolving domain of AI in healthcare, a paramount challenge is striking an optimal balance between fostering innovation and ensuring robust consumer protection. Innovations in AI technologies promise to revolutionize healthcare delivery, offering unprecedented diagnostic and therapeutic capabilities. However, without adequate consumer safeguards, these advances could risk patient privacy, autonomy, and trust.

Crafting legislation that supports cutting-edge AI research while instituting stringent protections for users is crucial. This involves creating legal frameworks that encourage transparency in AI development and implementation processes. Correspondingly, robust oversight mechanisms must be in place to monitor AI applications, ensuring they adhere to ethical standards that prioritize patient well-being and respect for the patient's cultural beliefs. Policies should also facilitate consumer education on AI health products, empowering patients to make informed decisions.

Moreover, consumer protection in AI health must be dynamic, adaptable to the swift pace of technological changes. This requires ongoing governmental and stakeholder engagement to continually assess and refine these frameworks, ensuring they stay relevant in protecting consumers against the potential risks associated with AI innovations.

## Enforcement Mechanisms for AI Health Regulations

The effectiveness of AI health regulations hinges on robust enforcement mechanisms. These frameworks must be equipped to not only monitor compliance but also to enforce regulations proactively across various jurisdictions. This entails establishing clear, enforceable penalties for violations that can act as a deterrent against the misuse of AI in healthcare.

Key to this process is the creation of specialized oversight bodies empowered to audit, review, and sanction entities that fail to adhere to established AI health standards. These bodies should have multidisciplinary teams, including experts in law, ethics, technology, and healthcare, to ensure a holistic approach to enforcement.

Moreover, there should be a mechanism for regular updates and refinement of enforcement strategies to keep pace with technological advancements. This dynamic approach enables adaptation to new challenges and scenarios in AI applications for health, ensuring long-term compliance and protection of patient rights.

Collectively, these enforcement mechanisms form the backbone of a trustworthy AI-driven healthcare system, aligning technological innovations with ethical medical practices and legal standards.

## Public Health Strategies to Utilize AI Equitably

Public health strategies that utilize AI equitably require meticulously designed frameworks that consider both technological capabilities and societal needs. To ensure the efficient allocation of healthcare resources, AI tools must be configured to address the specific health indicators and environmental factors unique to each population segment. This involves developing programs that are culturally sensitive and accessible to underserved communities, thereby reducing health disparities.

Central to this equitable utilization is the establishment of AI systems that support preventive healthcare. By leveraging predictive analytics, public health officials can identify at-risk populations and deploy interventions proactively, before the onset of more severe health issues. Such strategic use of AI not only optimizes resources but promotes a preventative health culture, shifting the focus from treatment to prevention.

Moreover, transparency in AI-driven public health strategies empowers citizens, enhancing trust and participation. Reporting the outcomes of AI integrations and maintaining open channels for public feedback are crucial for ongoing adaptation to community needs. Additionally, these strategies must evolve in response to technological advancements and changing public health dynamics, ensuring their sustained relevance and effectiveness.

## AI Certification Processes: Criteria and Best Practices

Establishing criteria and best practices for AI certification in healthcare is crucial to ensuring the safety, reliability, and ethical deployment of AI technologies. Certifications must assess AI systems for accuracy, fairness, and compliance with legal and moral standards, forming a fundamental piece of the regulatory puzzle. These certifications must consider diverse data sets to prevent bias and ensure equitable healthcare outcomes across different demographics.

Best practices in AI certification should include rigorous testing phases, both pre-market and post-deployment, to evaluate performance and impact continuously. Additionally, there should be a clear pathway for re-evaluation and certification renewal to accommodate ongoing technological advancements and evolving clinical needs. Input from multidisciplinary teams comprising AI experts, healthcare professionals, ethicists, and patient representatives can enrich the certification process, ensuring a holistic approach.

Moreover, certification bodies need to operate with transparency, publishing their criteria and audit results. This transparency fosters trust among healthcare providers, patients, and policymakers, promoting the broader adoption and integration of AI in healthcare systems.

## Addressing Disparities in AI Access and Effectiveness

Addressing disparities in AI access and effectiveness is pivotal to ensuring equitable healthcare solutions. Challenges stem from a complex interplay of socio-economic factors, geographical limitations, and variable tech infrastructure, which often disproportionately affects marginalized communities. Enhanced policies must prioritize accessibility and tailor AI tools to meet the diverse health needs and contexts of individuals.

To bridge these gaps, initiatives must incorporate extensive community engagement to understand specific barriers to AI adoption and effectiveness. This approach ensures that solutions are not just theoretically effective but practical and beneficial at the grassroots level. Tailored educational programs for both users and providers are essential in fostering an inclusive AI healthcare environment.

Furthermore, investment in infrastructure is crucial to rectify inequities in AI effectiveness. Equipping underserved areas with the necessary tech resources and training enables a more uniform distribution of AI benefits. Regular impact assessments will help policymakers understand progress and pivot strategies as needed, ensuring the sustained relevance of AI tools across all populations.

## Developing Policies for AI in Emergency Health Services

The critical nature of emergency health services demands stringent and responsive policies for AI applications. Rapid decision-making, often under considerable pressure, is a hallmark of these scenarios, where AI can significantly impact outcomes. Therefore, policy frameworks must prioritize real-time data analysis capabilities while ensuring these technologies are robustly tested for reliability and accuracy in high-stakes environments.

It is also essential to address the ethical implications of AI in emergency health settings. Policies should clearly outline guidelines for prioritizing care, managing sensitive data, and upholding patient rights during automated interactions. These guidelines must uphold ethical standards and patient consent, especially in life-threatening situations where AI's role is critical.

Furthermore, integrating AI into emergency health services requires collaboration across regulatory bodies, healthcare providers, and technology developers to foster innovations that enhance rather than complicate care delivery. Regular policy reviews and updates are crucial as AI technology evolves, ensuring that emergency health services can leverage AI effectively without compromising patient safety or care quality.

## AI in Health Insurance: Regulation and Fairness

Regulating AI in health insurance necessitates a careful balance between innovation and fairness. As AI technologies increasingly pervade the health insurance sector, they must be thoroughly scrutinized to ensure they do not perpetuate or exacerbate existing biases or inequalities. Regulatory frameworks should demand transparency in the AI algorithms used for setting premiums and making coverage decisions, ensuring that they are both understandable and justifiable to policyholders.

Fairness in AI-driven health insurance also requires rigorous testing for biases related to race, gender, socioeconomic status, and other demographic factors. This is crucial for preventing discriminatory practices that could affect the accessibility and affordability of insurance. Additionally, continuous monitoring and regular audits by independent bodies can help maintain fairness and rectify any discrepancies or unfair practices that may arise over time.

Ultimately, policy recommendations should aim to protect consumers by ensuring that AI applications in health insurance align with the core values of equity and justice. This includes establishing legal protections for consumers and creating an environment where technological advancements benefit all segments of society equally.

## Strategic Planning for AI in Public Health Administration

Strategic planning for AI in public health administration is essential to harnessing the full potential of technology while ensuring it serves the broad public health goals. This requires a comprehensive understanding of both the capabilities of AI and the unique needs of public health sectors. Strategic plans should outline clear objectives for AI integration, such as improving disease surveillance systems and optimizing resource allocation across health services.

To succeed, these strategies must incorporate robust risk management protocols to address potential AI failures or ethical concerns, ensuring that AI solutions are reliable and protect public health data integrity. Collaboration among health administrators, AI technologists, and public policymakers is crucial to anticipate future challenges and opportunities.

Moreover, strategic planning must also include continuous training for public health officials on the latest AI tools and practices. This empowers them to make informed decisions and tailor AI solutions effectively to meet evolving public health needs, ultimately leading to enhanced health outcomes and reduced disparities.

## Crafting policies for AI use in mental health services

The integration of AI in mental health services necessitates nuanced policies that address both the potential benefits and inherent challenges of technology application. As mental health issues vary greatly in their manifestations and impacts, AI-driven solutions must be adaptable to diverse psychological conditions while maintaining high ethical standards. Policymaking in this area must prioritize patient confidentiality, informed consent, and the sensitivity of personal data.

Key to this is designing policies that ensure AI tools in mental health are transparent and accountable. They should foster an environment where decisions made by AI can be understood and challenged by both practitioners and patients. Regulatory frameworks must also consider how AI could perpetuate existing health disparities or introduce new biases, setting strict guidelines on algorithm fairness and efficacy.

Moreover, collaborations with mental health professionals, ethicists, and AI technologists are crucial for developing dynamic policies that support continuous improvement and the ethical use of AI. Input from mental health advocacy groups will further guide the development of empathetic and inclusive AI policies, ensuring that technological advances benefit all segments of the population equitably.

## Ensuring Equity in AI Algorithms through Policy Frameworks

Ensuring equity in AI algorithms requires rigorous policy frameworks that address inherent biases and promote fairness across diverse demographics. To achieve this, policymakers must establish clear guidelines that focus on the ethical design and ongoing assessment of AI systems in healthcare. These frameworks should address the needs of diverse patient groups, particularly those who have been historically marginalized or underrepresented in medical research.

Effective policy frameworks must establish standards for data diversity and algorithmic transparency to ensure accountability and transparency. Diverse datasets enhance the representativeness of AI models, thereby reducing skewed outcomes. Additionally, transparent operations facilitate easier monitoring and accountability, which are crucial for maintaining trust in AI-driven health systems. Policies should encourage open sharing of methodology and results, enabling independent reviews and adjustments as necessary.

Moreover, inclusionary policies should mandate stakeholder involvement in the development and evaluation stages. Collaboration with healthcare professionals, ethicists, and patients will ensure that AI technologies are aligned with broader societal values and patient care standards, ultimately sustaining equity in healthcare AI.

**Government-led Initiatives to Support Fair AI Use**

In response to the growing influence of AI in healthcare, government-led initiatives have become pivotal in ensuring that artificial intelligence is utilized fairly and ethically. By spearheading programs that focus on equitable AI development and implementation, governments can directly address potential biases and ensure that all societal segments benefit from the advancements in AI.

Key to these initiatives is the creation of comprehensive guidelines that mandate fairness in AI algorithms and the equitable distribution of AI benefits. Governments often facilitate workshops and forums that bring together AI developers, healthcare professionals, and representatives from the public. These platforms not only foster dialogue but also promote mutual understanding and cooperation among diverse stakeholders.

Furthermore, these initiatives typically include funding for research into AI ethics, support for technology trials in diverse settings, and the development of educational resources to raise awareness about the capabilities and limitations of AI. Ultimately, the goal is to cultivate an AI-enhanced healthcare environment that upholds justice and inclusivity, continuously adapting to emerging technologies and challenges.

**AI Auditing: Methods and Policy Support**

AI auditing in healthcare emerges as a critical mechanism to safeguard ethical standards and uphold public trust in AI applications. Proper auditing techniques ensure that AI systems perform as intended without causing harm or exhibiting biased outcomes. It involves systematic reviews and the validation of algorithms against established ethical benchmarks and operational requirements.

Policy support enhances these efforts by providing a framework for continuous oversight and updating audit processes in line with technological advances. Governments and regulatory bodies play a pivotal role by setting industry-wide standards for audit procedures, including frequency, scope, and methodology. These policies enhance the transparency and accountability of AI systems, which are needed for maintaining public confidence in health AI.

Furthermore, policy-driven support is crucial for training and equipping auditors with the necessary skills to tackle new AI challenges. Collaboration with AI developers during the auditing phase can facilitate real-time feedback and immediate corrections, thereby enhancing the overall efficiency and safety of AI health applications.

**Educating Policymakers on AI Capabilities and Challenges**

Educating policymakers on the capabilities and challenges of AI is paramount for crafting informed and effective healthcare policies. As AI continues to reshape various aspects of healthcare, understanding its potential and limitations helps policymakers endorse regulations that foster innovation while ensuring safety and ethics. Educational initiatives should start with comprehensive overviews of AI's role in diagnostic processes, treatment personalization, and operational efficiencies.

Moreover, special emphasis must be placed on elucidating the challenges associated with AI, such as data bias and the need for transparency. Policymakers equipped with this knowledge are better prepared to question and understand the implications of AI deployments in medical settings. Workshops, seminars, and collaboration with AI experts and ethicists can bridge knowledge gaps.

Ultimately, a well-informed legislative body is crucial for creating laws that safeguard patient rights and promote equitable AI applications. Such proactive educational efforts ensure that policy adjustments keep pace with technological advancements, underpinning a health system that leverages AI responsibly and justly.

**Impact Assessment of AI Policies in Healthcare**

Assessing the impact of AI policies in healthcare is pivotal to ensuring these regulations effectively elevate care quality without exacerbating disparities. This process involves a comprehensive evaluation of how AI applications, governed by these policies, perform in real-world settings. Impact assessments help identify unforeseen consequences and areas that require adjustment, thereby fostering policies that evolve in response to technological advancements and changing healthcare needs.

Key aspects of these assessments include analyzing the accessibility and outcomes of AI-driven interventions across diverse populations. This ensures that AI benefits do not disproportionately favor one group over another. By measuring such disparities, policymakers can refine AI guidelines to promote inclusivity and fairness.

Moreover, impact assessments provide the feedback essential for continuous policy improvement. They serve as a bridge between the practical applications of AI in healthcare and the theoretical aspirations outlined in policy documents. Regularly scheduled reviews, driven by data and stakeholder feedback, underline a commitment to dynamically adapting healthcare ecosystems in response to AI's evolving role.

**Future Projections: Adapting Policies to AI Advancements in Health**

The future landscape of AI in healthcare brims with potential, driving the need for adaptive policies that both anticipate and respond to rapid technological progress. As AI capabilities expand, so too must the frameworks be guiding their application in medical scenarios. These future-oriented policies must seamlessly integrate with existing health regulations while remaining flexible enough to accommodate innovations such as predictive analytics and personalized medicine.

Key to this evolution is foreseeing AI's trajectory, identifying emerging capabilities early and assessing their implications for healthcare delivery and ethics. This foresight will enable policymakers to devise regulations that not only protect patients but also foster an environment conducive to breakthroughs in AI-driven care. Such proactive measures are crucial for maintaining a balance between innovation and patient safety.

Moreover, the policy adaptations will require ongoing collaboration with technology developers, healthcare providers, and patients to ensure that advancements in AI are leveraged responsibly. Through continuous dialogue and regular assessments, healthcare systems can remain aligned with both technological advancements and evolving societal values, ensuring that every step forward is a step toward greater equity and effectiveness in healthcare.

## Summary

The chapter outlines comprehensive strategies to ensure equitable AI implementation in healthcare, focusing on creating inclusive, ethical, and transparent AI systems that address diverse healthcare needs without perpetuating existing disparities. The framework begins by defining equitable AI in healthcare, emphasizing the need for algorithms that are unbiased and incorporate diverse datasets to cater to all demographic groups. This leads to the development of regulatory frameworks that ensure the safe and ethical use of AI technologies, alongside dynamic regulations that are adaptable to rapid technological changes. Establishing ethical guidelines is crucial, particularly in terms of transparency in AI operations and safeguarding patient data and autonomy. The chapter also discusses the importance of AI certification processes that assess fairness and compliance with ethical standards to maintain trust and reliability in healthcare AI applications. Policy recommendations emphasize the importance of maintaining robust data management and enforcing strict legal protections to uphold patient rights in AI-driven healthcare. Additionally, the role of international cooperation is emphasized to harmonize AI health regulations globally, ensuring equitable benefits from AI worldwide. Incorporation of diverse stakeholder voices i.e., traditional and indigenous peoples themselves, in policymaking is advocated to craft socially sensitive and technically sound healthcare solutions. Moreover, the strategic use of public health AI and continuous education of policymakers on AI capabilities are crucial for informed policy creation. Ensuring rigorous enforcement mechanisms for AI regulations and regular AI auditing are highlighted to sustain compliance and efficacy in health AI applications. Lastly, the chapter addresses the necessity of future-oriented policies that adapt to ongoing AI advancements, ensuring policies evolve in response to technological and ethical demands to maintain equity in AI-enhanced healthcare systems.

## References

[1] Artificial Intelligence in Healthcare: Anticipating Challenges and Opportunities. https://www.jmir.org/2020/4/e17287/
[2] Defining Ethics in Artificial Intelligence: A Road Map. https://link.springer.com/article/10.1007/s11948-019-00175-1
[3] Guidelines for Artificial Intelligence in Healthcare: Focusing on Ethical and Inclusive Practices. https://academic.oup.com/jamia/article/26/8/773/5575441
[4] Equity in Digital Health: Creating AI Systems for Fair and Just Healthcare Distribution. https://www.nejm.org/doi/full/10.1056/NEJMp1909086
[5] Healthcare Regulation for AI Technologies: Balancing Innovation with Patient Safety. https://www.sciencedirect.com/science/article/pii/S2589750020300366
[6] International Strategies to Address Ethical Challenges of AI in Healthcare. https://www.healthaffairs.org/doi/abs/10.1377/hlthaff.2019.01518
[7] Patient-Centric AI: Ensuring Transparency and Fairness in Medical AI Systems. https://ieeexplore.ieee.org/document/9216085/
[8] Stakeholder Engagement for Inclusive AI Policy Development. https://www.frontiersin.org/articles/10.3389/fpubh.2020.567526/full

## Case Study: Integrating AI in Rural Healthcare: Challenges and Strategies

The integration of Artificial Intelligence (AI) in healthcare has been heralded as a significant breakthrough, particularly in improving treatment outcomes and operational efficiencies. However, its deployment in rural settings presents unique challenges, characterized by limited technological infrastructure, scarce medical resources, and a dispersed population. This case study examines the scenario in the rural district of Hillview, where, despite significant health disparities, recent initiatives aim to leverage AI to transform local healthcare systems.

Hillview's healthcare officials initiated an AI program to enhance diagnostic accuracy and patient management. The primary challenges included erratic internet connectivity, a lack of local AI expertise, and hesitancy among healthcare workers and patients regarding the use of AI technology. To address connectivity, the project partnered with a telecommunications firm to bolster the local internet infrastructure, facilitating reliable AI operations. AI experts organized training workshops to enhance the proficiency of local healthcare workers in utilizing AI tools and integrating these technologies into their everyday medical practices.

However, acceptance among locals was slow. Many were skeptical about replacing traditional healthcare methods with AI-driven approaches. To counteract this, community engagement programs were introduced, explaining the benefits of AI in local languages and demonstrating its role in enhancing, rather than replacing, traditional healthcare. Regular town hall meetings were set up, allowing the community to voice concerns and obtain clarifications directly from AI specialists and healthcare administrators.

These strategic steps fostered a more inclusive atmosphere for AI adoption in Hillview's healthcare services. Yet, continuous monitoring and adaptive strategies were necessary to maintain alignment with community needs and technological advancements. This ongoing dialogue ensured that AI implementation was both ethical and practical, addressing the healthcare disparities inherent in rural settings while adapting to emerging challenges and opportunities in AI technology.

### Case Study: Equitable AI Deployment in Urban Public Hospitals

The concept of equitable AI in healthcare extends beyond theoretical frameworks into practical, impactful implementations. This case study examines the implementation of AI technologies in public hospitals in Metroville, a metropolitan center renowned for its diverse population and pronounced socio-economic disparities. The aim was to utilize AI to streamline operational efficiencies and enhance clinical outcomes across all demographics, with a particular focus on historically underserved communities.

Metroville's health department collaborated with AI developers and local community organizations to develop AI systems that could address specific health inequities. The primary focus areas were Emergency Departments (EDs) and outpatient services, where the patient influx was notably higher and more diverse. AI-driven triage systems were introduced to efficiently prioritize patient care, thereby significantly reducing wait times.

However, the implementation faced initial resistance from medical staff, primarily due to concerns about job displacement and the reliability of AI in making life-critical decisions. To address these issues, extensive training programs and AI-assisted simulation workshops were set up. These programs not only helped staff understand the AI tools but also demonstrated that AI would work as an aid, not a replacement.

An essential aspect of this project was maintaining transparency with the patients. Information kiosks and digital platforms were established, providing patients with access to understandable information about how AI was being used in their care processes. In line with equitable principles, these resources were made available in multiple languages and formats to accommodate varying levels of health literacy.

While the deployment initially aimed to improve operational efficiency and facilitate faster clinical care, an unexpected benefit was the enhancement in patient data management. AI systems enabled better tracking of health trends across different demographics, leading to more personalized and preventive healthcare strategies. Continuous feedback mechanisms were established, allowing the ongoing improvement of AI systems based on staff and patient feedback, ensuring that these innovations were appropriately aligned with the actual needs of Metroville's population.

### Case Study: Advancing AI in Pediatric Care: Tackling Ethical and Regulatory Challenges

The deployment of Artificial Intelligence (AI) in pediatric healthcare settings presents unique challenges and opportunities, particularly in terms of ethical standards and regulatory compliance. This case study examines the initiatives at the Children's Hospital in Centerville, which have integrated AI systems to enhance diagnosis accuracy and treatment efficacy for various pediatric conditions, including rare genetic disorders.

Children's Hospital faced several challenges initially, most notably the ethical concerns related to consent and data privacy. Since the patients were minors, obtaining informed consent required careful handling to ensure that parents and guardians fully understood the implications of AI-based diagnoses and treatments. Furthermore, the sensitive nature of pediatric medical data raised significant concerns about security and confidentiality, necessitating stringent data protection measures.

To address these ethical concerns, the hospital established a multi-disciplinary ethics committee comprising healthcare professionals, bioethicists, legal experts, and parent representatives. This committee was tasked with overseeing AI implementations and ensuring that all procedures aligned with ethical guidelines and legal requirements. Additionally, the hospital organized educational sessions for parents, elucidating the role of AI in healthcare and the measures taken to protect their children's data.

Regulatory hurdles also posed significant challenges. The hospital had to navigate a complex landscape of health regulations, which varied significantly from one jurisdiction to another, complicating the deployment of AI systems designed to be used across different states or regions. To comply with these varied regulations, the hospital partnered with legal experts to create a compliance framework that adapted to the specific regulatory requirements of each area in which it operated.

The implementation of AI at Children's Hospital not only enhanced diagnostic and treatment capacities but also provided invaluable data that contributed to a better understanding of pediatric illnesses. This AI integration, underpinned by strong ethical standards and rigorous regulatory compliance, illustrated the potential of AI to transform pediatric healthcare when aligned with meticulous ethical consideration and adherence to regulations.

## Case Study: Innovative AI Approaches to Mental Health in Underserved Communities

The use of Artificial Intelligence (AI) in mental health services promises revolutionary changes, especially in addressing the needs of underserved communities. This case study explores the innovative application of AI in psychiatric and psychological services in the economically disadvantaged region of Southtown, where residents suffer disproportionately from mental health issues and have historically lacked adequate mental health services.

Southtown's health authorities collaborated with AI technology companies to develop and implement AI-driven tools specifically tailored to address the community's mental health needs. These tools included AI-powered diagnostic systems, virtual therapy assistants, and mobile apps for self-management of mental health conditions. One particular innovation was an AI-driven predictive analytics system that identified individuals at high risk of mental health crises, enabling proactive interventions.

However, the introduction of AI technologies faced several challenges, including data privacy concerns, a lack of trust in technology among the local population, and the digital divide that limited access to AI tools. To overcome these hurdles, Southtown's project team initiated comprehensive community engagement programs. These programs provided education on the benefits and safety of AI tools through workshops, community meetings, and collaboration with local influencers and health workers who spoke the community languages.

Moreover, to tackle the digital divide, the project included providing subsidized smartphones and internet services to low-income residents, ensuring that everyone could access the AI mental health tools. The local health workers were also trained to assist residents in using these technologies, and continual feedback loops were incorporated to adapt AI tools based on community needs and responses.

The ongoing efforts in Southtown are a testament to how AI can transform mental health services when its deployment is thoughtfully connected with the community it aims to serve. This case exemplifies how integrating technology with a deep understanding of community dynamics and challenges can lead to meaningful improvements in public health, particularly in mental health, inclusivity, and access.

## Case Study: AI-Enhanced Geriatric Care: Bridging Gaps and Ensuring Equity

The growing integration of Artificial Intelligence (AI) into geriatric medicine presents a promising frontier for addressing the complex healthcare needs of the elderly. In Greenbrooke, an area characterized by a high population of aging adults, the local hospital introduced an AI-powered health management system to enhance care delivery and mitigate typical healthcare inequalities affecting older adults. This case study examines the ethical implementation and community-driven adaptation of AI technologies in geriatric care at Greenbrooke Senior Health Center.

Implementations began with the integration of AI tools designed to monitor health patterns, manage chronic conditions, and provide predictive analytics for preventative care. A particular challenge faced was ensuring the AI system was transparent and fair, given the fundamental demographic differences in morbidity rates and technological literacy among the elderly. To address this, the Center's IT team collaborated with AI specialists to tailor user interfaces that were intuitive and simple for elderly patients to use. They conducted extensive testing with focus groups to ensure the product's adaptability and inclusiveness.

Additionally, the ethical implications of AI in this sensitive sector require rigorous oversight mechanisms. A bespoke ethical committee was formed, featuring geriatricians, AI ethics experts, local government representatives, and patient families, tasked with ensuring AI usage protected patient dignity and privacy while aligning with care standards. Moreover, the committee maintained public transparency through quarterly community meetings, where it discussed the impacts of AI and gathered feedback directly from the elderly and their caregivers.

The introduction of AI into geriatric care at Greenbrooke was a nuanced process that required striking a balance between innovation and compassionate care. The Center successfully enhanced healthcare delivery through this technology by making the benefits of AI accessible and equitable. They achieved this by prioritizing patient-centric usability in AI solutions, ensuring comprehensive ethical oversight, and fostering community engagement, which increased trust and acceptance of AI in elderly healthcare provision.

### Case Study: AI-Driven Approaches to Chronic Disease Management in Resource-Limited Settings

The challenge of managing chronic diseases in resource-limited settings is profound, often exacerbated by inadequate healthcare infrastructure, a shortage of medical professionals, and limited patient education. This case study explores the implementation of AI-driven solutions in the rural community of Eastville, which faces significant challenges due to its isolated location and economic constraints. Eastville, with high rates of diabetes and hypertension, became the focal point for a pilot AI program aimed at transforming chronic disease management through technology.

The program introduced a mobile health (mHealth) platform leveraging AI to monitor patient symptoms, manage treatment adherence, and predict potential health risks. Local healthcare workers were provided with smartphones equipped with the mHealth app, which was designed to collect real-time data on patient vitals and medication adherence. AI algorithms analyzed this data to provide personalized feedback and alerts to both healthcare providers and patients.

Initially, the implementation faced several hurdles. The primary concern was the digital literacy of both healthcare workers and patients, many of whom were unfamiliar with smartphones and their use. To address this, the program coordinators conducted extensive training sessions, and ongoing support was made available through a dedicated helpline. Another significant challenge was ensuring consistent data privacy and security, which is critical for fostering trust in the new system.

Despite these challenges, the AI-driven mHealth platform began to show promising outcomes. Improved medication adherence rates were observed, and healthcare workers were able to intervene proactively when patients exhibited signs of deteriorating health, resulting in a reduction in emergency hospital visits. Patients reported feeling more empowered and involved in their healthcare processes.

To scale this success, continuous evaluation and adaptation of the AI algorithms are necessary to better meet the needs of the Eastville population. These efforts include enhancing AI capabilities to handle more complex health scenarios and incorporating more comprehensive training for all users. Enhanced community engagement and the integration of AI-driven data insights into broader health policy planning are also critical steps moving forward.

**Case Study: AI for Cardiovascular Health: Navigating Ethical Terrains and Public Policy**

In the bustling urban landscape of Tech City, healthcare providers and policymakers faced an impactful challenge: addressing the rising incidence of cardiovascular diseases (CVD) using AI technologies. The city embarked on a pioneering project to integrate AI in cardiac care, aiming not only to advance treatment protocols but also to test a model that could potentially revolutionize healthcare policy, focusing on equitable AI applications in health systems.

The first phase involved deploying AI in local hospitals to assist in diagnosing and predicting cardiovascular events, primarily based on machine learning algorithms that analyzed vast datasets from diverse populations within the city. Early results showed promise with improved diagnosis accuracy and personalized treatment plans leading to better patient outcomes. However, the implementation journey was met with rigorous ethical debates concerning patient consent, data privacy, and algorithmic bias.

Acknowledging these issues, Tech City's health department collaborated with ethical committees to create a transparent operational framework. Efforts concentrated on developing comprehensive consent forms, enhancing data security measures, and implementing ongoing AI monitoring to mitigate biases. The AI systems were regularly audited by an independent body, ensuring compliance with ethical standards and adapting to feedback from both healthcare professionals and patients.

Simultaneously, public health advocates pushed for policies that would support the sustained integration of AI across all healthcare sectors in Tech City. These policies were crafted to promote AI literacy amongst medical staff and the public to foster an environment of trust and acceptance. Crucial to this policy was the provision of resources to underserved areas, ensuring equitable access to AI-enhanced cardiovascular care, which historically lagged in these communities.

Over time, this integrative approach saw a marked reduction in CVD-related hospital admissions and an increase in early detection rates. The case of Tech City showcased the potential of AI in transforming health practices through ethical application and informed policymaking, highlighting the importance of maintaining a balance between innovation and patient-centered care in the advancing digital age.

## Case Study: Implementing AI in Multicultural Urban Health Centers: Approaches and Ethical Considerations

In the diverse urban area of Cityscape, the introduction of Artificial Intelligence (AI) in public healthcare centers was aimed at enhancing health service delivery to a multicultural population. This case study delves into the strategic deployment of AI technologies in Cityscape's health centers, focusing on linguistic and cultural barriers, ethical implications, and the ultimate impact on healthcare accessibility and efficiency.

Cityscape Health Authority initiated the AI-powered project with the primary goals of improving diagnostic accuracy, personalizing patient care, and managing a vast array of health data derived from a culturally and linguistically varied patient base. Key AI applications included multilingual chatbots for patient interaction, predictive analytics for disease outbreak prediction, and AI-driven diagnostic tools that adapted to culturally specific health issues.

The project faced considerable challenges, particularly in designing AI systems that were culturally sensitive and free of algorithmic bias. To tackle these, the development team incorporated diverse datasets that reflected the ethnic mosaic of Cityscape. Furthermore, the project employed cultural consultants and linguists to adapt the AI interfaces and communication protocols, ensuring all patient interactions were culturally relevant and linguistically appropriate.

Ethical considerations were at the forefront of the project. The stakeholder committee, consisting of ethicists, technologists, healthcare professionals, and patient representatives, was established to oversee the ethical deployment of AI technologies. This committee was tasked with ensuring patient privacy, securing informed consent, and maintaining transparency in AI decision-making processes. Public forums and feedback systems were set up to gauge community response and adapt AI systems accordingly.

Despite the initial hurdles, the AI initiative in Cityscape Health Centers gradually improved service efficacy. Patient wait times decreased, satisfaction levels rose, and healthcare providers noted better resource management and reduced error rates in diagnostics. However, the project highlighted the need for continuous adaptation and rigorous oversight to preserve ethical standards and respond effectively to the dynamic needs of a multicultural urban populace.

## Review Questions

**1. While consulting with a 73-year-old moderately active male patient, Dr. Smith, a cardiologist, notices that the patient has been relying solely on AI-driven online consultations for managing his hypertension and heart conditions due to previous dissatisfaction with in-person healthcare experiences related to cultural insensitivity. The patient, who is Native American, expresses that while the AI provides accurate medicine dosages and health monitoring, it fails to integrate his cultural practices and traditional healing methods, which he values significantly. Based on this scenario, what should Dr. Smith's approach be to provide care that respects the patient's cultural values while ensuring medical safety?**

A) Continue solely with AI recommendations, disregarding the patient's cultural practices

B) Integrate the patient's cultural practices and traditional healing methods into his healthcare plan

C) Dismiss the patient's traditional methods as superstition and enforce only modern medical treatments

D) Refer the patient to a specialist who only practices Western medicine

**Answer: B**

Explanation: Dr. Smith should opt for an integrative approach that respects the patient's cultural background and personal preferences while ensuring medical safety. Integrating cultural practices into healthcare treatments can significantly enhance patient satisfaction and adherence to the treatment plans. Dr. Smith can collaborate with cultural liaisons or Indigenous health specialists who understand the patient's heritage and medical needs. This approach not only fosters trust but also aligns with holistic care principles, emphasizing treating the 'whole' person, which includes their cultural and spiritual health. Ignoring or dismissing the patient's traditional healing methods could lead to a lack of trust and non-adherence, potentially worsening his health outcomes.

**2. A 56-year-old woman with chronic low back pain is using an AI-driven therapeutic app recommended by her physiotherapist. The AI suggests daily routines based on biometric feedback, which generally improves her condition. However, she prefers integrating some traditional Thai massage techniques she learned from her mother, which she finds equally effective. What strategy should the healthcare provider adopt to enhance the AI's recommendations with the patient's preferred traditional methods?**

A) Discourage the use of traditional Thai massage as it is not part of the AI's recommendations

B) Find a way to incorporate feedback about the effects of Thai massage into the AI system

C) Completely replace AI recommendations with traditional methods

D) Ignore the patient's preference as AI provides more scientifically validated recommendations

**Answer: B**

Explanation: The healthcare provider should consider incorporating the patient's feedback about the effects of traditional Thai massage into the AI treatment planning system. This approach respects the patient's cultural and personal preferences, enhances the personalized care plan, and may potentially improve patient satisfaction and treatment efficacy. The inclusion of patient-derived data can also help in refining AI algorithms to be more responsive to diverse therapeutic practices. Failing to acknowledge or disregard traditional methods that a patient finds beneficial can lead to dissatisfaction and non-compliance with prescribed treatment regimens.

**3. During a clinical trial, an AI system is used to assign patients to different treatment groups based on algorithmic predictions. However, concerns arise regarding the cultural appropriateness of the treatments for Indigenous participants, which might affect their participation and outcomes. What should the trial coordinators consider to ensure fairness and respect toward cultural diversity?**

A) A. Continue the trial without modifications to maintain consistency

B) B. Adjust the AI algorithm to accommodate cultural considerations and treatment preferences

C) C. Exclude Indigenous participants from the trial to avoid complications

D) D. Focus solely on biomedical outcomes, ignoring cultural impacts

**Answer: B**

Explanation: Trial coordinators should adjust the AI algorithm to accommodate cultural considerations and participants' treatment preferences. This adjustment ensures that the treatment strategies are culturally appropriate and respectful, potentially enhancing participation rates and the effectiveness of the interventions for Indigenous participants. Modifying AI algorithms to be culturally sensitive can help generate more accurate and applicable scientific data, foster trust among Indigenous communities, and maintain ethical standards in research. Excluding Indigenous participants or ignoring cultural impacts would undermine the diversity and relevance of the study, possibly skewing results and reducing the applicability of the research findings.

## Fostering Cultural Competence in AI Models

### Defining Cultural Competence in AI

Cultural competence in AI refers to the ability of artificial intelligence systems to understand, respect, and effectively interact within diverse cultural contexts they serve. It involves programming AI to perceive and respond to variances in cultural beliefs, practices, and communication styles in a respectful and understanding manner.

This competence is critical in medicine as it ensures AI tools provide inclusive and equitable care. For instance, an AI diagnostic tool must interpret symptoms and recommend treatments considering cultural determinants of health, such as dietary habits or traditional healing practices. Achieving this requires a nuanced embedding of cultural intelligence in the AI's algorithms.

To establish such models, it's essential to involve data from a broad spectrum of cultures during the training phase. This inclusivity enables the AI to handle diverse health beliefs organically rather than merely applying a standardized, possibly culturally blind, medical model to all.

## Importance of Diversity in AI Training Data

Diversity in AI training data is pivotal for fostering cultural competence in medical AI applications. By incorporating a wide array of data representing various cultural, ethnic, and demographic backgrounds, AI can become more accurate and less biased in its function. This ensures that medical AI tools do not favor one group over another and can effectively serve a global population with diverse healthcare beliefs and practices.

Lack of diversity in training datasets leads to AI solutions that are narrowly tailored and potentially unsafe. For instance, AI trained predominantly on data from specific demographics may misinterpret symptoms and recommend inappropriate treatments for individuals from other demographics. Ensuring diversity in AI training data includes not only ethnic and cultural variations but also different languages, genders, and age groups, enhancing the AI's ability to make informed and sensitive medical decisions.

To achieve this, collaboration with diverse groups during the data collection phase is crucial. It is also essential to continuously evaluate and update AI systems as more diverse data becomes available. This ongoing process helps mitigate existing biases and adapt to the evolving cultural landscape, ultimately improving patient outcomes globally.

## Best Practices for Ensuring Representation Across Cultures

To ensure AI models are culturally competent, certain best practices must be observed. Firstly, involving a diverse group of stakeholders from various cultural backgrounds in the development process is crucial. These stakeholders can provide unique insights into how different cultures might interpret AI actions and suggestions, enabling the creation of more inclusive systems.

Secondly, conducting thorough cultural audits of AI training data can identify gaps in representation. This involves assessing the cultural dimensions covered by the data and actively seeking sources that fill missing aspects. This proactive approach ensures the AI does not perpetuate existing cultural biases but rather appreciates and integrates a broad spectrum of human experience.

Moreover, implementing continuous feedback loops with culturally diverse users can enhance AI cultural competence over time. User feedback is vital for adjusting AI algorithms to reflect cultural sensitivities accurately and for addressing any unintended biases or oversights in initial models.

## Cultural Bias in AI: Identification and Mitigation

Identifying and mitigating cultural biases in AI is pivotal for fostering culturally competent systems. This process begins with a robust analysis of AI algorithms, seeking out biases that might skew diagnostic or therapeutic outcomes based on cultural parameters. Tools such as fairness metrics and bias audits can highlight skewed outputs, allowing developers to recalibrate AI systems accordingly.

Once identified, efforts to mitigate these biases include refining AI models with diverse datasets that mirror the real-world spectrum of cultural experiences. This is complemented by employing cultural experts who guide the infusion of cultural knowledge into AI training phases. These efforts aim to create AI systems that do not inadvertently favor or overlook any group, ensuring equitable treatment across cultures.

Moreover, ongoing monitoring is essential to sustain bias mitigation. AI systems evolve, and so do cultural contexts, making continuous adaptation a necessity. Implemented comparison studies and periodic algorithm updates help maintain the relevancy and integrity of AI applications in diverse cultural landscapes.

## Tailoring AI to Meet Global Cultural Sensitivities

Tailoring AI to meet global cultural sensitivities requires a multifaceted approach, integrating sensitivity and awareness into the very fabric of technology. To achieve this, AI systems must be designed with a deep understanding of the varied cultural contexts in which they operate. This begins with a comprehensive cultural analysis, ensuring the AI not only recognizes but also respects and adapts to diverse cultural norms and practices.

Developers must prioritize embedding cultural flexibility in AI architectures, allowing systems to adjust outputs based on cultural data inputs. For example, an AI health advisor should adjust its dietary recommendations to reflect regional cuisines and eating habits associated with cultural identity. Moreover, AI interfaces designed to interact with users should adjust their communication style to be more culturally congruent, employing locally familiar idioms and expressions.

Ultimately, the success of culturally sensitive AI hinges on ongoing collaboration with cultural scholars and community feedback. Such iterative refinements enhance AI's relevance and efficacy across different cultural environments, fostering a more inclusive global digital ecosystem.

## Ethics of Cultural Inclusivity in AI Development

The ethical underpinnings of cultural inclusivity in AI development pivot around the principles of fairness, respect, and justice. In an AI-enhanced medical landscape, moral imperatives demand that cultural barriers do not preclude access to innovative treatments or management approaches, thereby ensuring that every individual's cultural context and health identities are valued and addressed equitably.

A central ethical challenge is the deployment of AI systems that may inadvertently prioritize or marginalize populations due to incomplete cultural understanding. Ethical AI development must, therefore, incorporate diverse cultural insights from the onset, not merely as an afterthought but as foundational components of design and execution. This involves deep engagement with cultural experts and adherence to inclusive design principles that resonate with global ethical standards.

Another ethical consideration is the need for accountability mechanisms in AI systems to track and analyze biases. Transparent reporting and rectification processes, when cultural oversights occur, are crucial. They uphold not only user trust but also fortify the moral integrity of AI development. It's not just about creating tools; it's about crafting socially responsible technologies that understand and adapt to the diversity of human experiences.

## Creating Culturally Adaptive AI Models

Developing culturally adaptive AI models involves creating systems that dynamically adjust to multicultural inputs, recognizing the nuances that define diverse user contexts. This requires a sophisticated understanding of cultural frameworks and sensitivities, which can be encoded into AI through advanced algorithms and machine learning techniques. Importantly, these models must be designed to learn from ongoing interactions, continuously refining their cultural acumen.

A central strategy in this approach includes the implementation of adaptive learning systems that adjust their operations based on cultural feedback. By analyzing interactions across multiple cultural settings, AI can identify patterns and make nuanced adjustments to its protocols. This approach not only enhances user experience but also ensures that AI applications remain relevant and sensitive across different cultural landscapes.

Ultimately, the success of culturally adaptive AI depends on its ability to integrate and evolve in response to feedback. Incorporating robust feedback mechanisms enables AI systems not only to function within a cultural context but also to grow within it, fostering lasting user engagement and trust.

**Training AI to Recognize Cultural Signifiers**

Training artificial intelligence (AI) to recognize cultural signifiers is a crucial step towards building culturally competent systems. This training involves teaching AI to identify and interpret significant indicators within various cultural contexts, such as language nuances, social norms, or symbolic representations. Successfully integrating this capability requires a multifaceted approach that includes the collection and analysis of culturally rich datasets.

Developers must employ sophisticated machine learning techniques that can discern subtle cultural cues embedded in data. This might involve analyzing text for region-specific idioms or speech patterns in voice recognition systems. Similarly, visual AI systems need the capability to recognize culturally specific non-verbal cues or symbolic imagery, which vary widely between cultures.

Further, simulating real-world cultural interactions in a controlled environment allows AI models to learn from live data, making them more adept at handling diverse cultural scenarios. This training ensures that AI applications not only perform their tasks efficiently but also do so in a manner that is culturally informed and sensitive, promoting global applicability and acceptance.

**Incorporating Multilingual Support in AI**

Multilingual support in AI is crucial for mitigating cultural barriers and improving accessibility in global healthcare settings. By integrating multiple languages, AI can serve a broader demographic, respecting linguistic diversity and reducing misunderstandings in medical instructions and advice.

The implementation of multilingual capabilities involves complex natural language processing techniques and comprehensive linguistic databases that cover a range of dialects and colloquialisms. This ensures that AI systems can understand and generate communication in various languages with high accuracy. These systems must be continuously updated and refined based on user interactions to adapt to evolving language use and include medical terminology specific to different cultures.

Engaging native speakers in the development process helps fine-tune the linguistic accuracy of AI applications. This collaborative approach not only enhances the system's functionality but also fosters trust among users by providing culturally respectful and linguistically appropriate services. Ultimately, multilingual support empowers patients by providing accessible, understandable, and culturally relevant medical information.

**Engaging with Cultural Experts During AI Design**

Engaging cultural experts in AI design is crucial for developing systems that genuinely comprehend and respect diverse cultural norms and values. These experts bring deep insights into societal nuances, ensuring AI systems are not only technically proficient but culturally attuned. Their involvement enables AI to move beyond handling surface-level data, addressing the underlying cultural dynamics that influence user interaction and response.

Involving cultural experts ensures that AI technologies do not inadvertently propagate cultural stereotypes or biases. For example, by consulting with linguists and cultural historians, developers can create AI systems that accurately interpret and respond to local dialects and historical contexts. This collaboration fosters an AI development environment where ethical considerations and cultural nuances are integrated from the outset, not added as afterthoughts.

Furthermore, cultural experts can guide AI behavior to align with local customs and practices, which is indispensable in fields like medicine where cultural sensitivity is paramount. Regular interaction with these experts during the design process ensures ongoing refinement of AI capabilities, making them more dynamic and contextually aware.

## Utilizing Anthropological Insights in AI Algorithms

Anthropological insights provide a profound advantage in advancing AI's cultural competence, particularly in the medical domain. By embedding anthropological research into AI algorithms, developers can harness a deeper understanding of cultural behaviors, health practices, and societal norms that define different communities. This integration helps in designing AI systems that are not only technically sophisticated but also culturally resonant.

To implement this, anthropologists collaborate with AI developers to translate ethnographic data into discernible patterns that AI can learn and apply. For instance, local health remedies, ritualistic practices, and community health narratives are converted into data formats conducive to machine learning, allowing AI to recognize and propose solutions that are culturally appropriate.

This interdisciplinary approach bridges the gap between technological innovation and cultural understanding, ensuring AI systems advocate for inclusivity and respect for diversity in healthcare contexts. Leveraging these insights leads to AI applications that are genuinely attuned to the cultural fabric of the user base, promoting better health outcomes and enhanced trust in AI-driven medical services.

## Challenges and Solutions in Cultural Adaptation of AI

Adapting AI to different cultural contexts presents significant challenges. Firstly, data scarcity in underrepresented cultures can skew AI behavior, reinforcing dominant cultural norms and sidelining minority ones. Additionally, cultural nuances are dynamic and multifaceted, making them difficult to capture comprehensively in datasets and algorithms.

Solutions to these challenges begin with diversifying data sources to include a broader spectrum of cultural inputs. Collaborating with cultural anthropologists and sociologists can enhance the depth of data, ensuring AI systems gain a more nuanced understanding of diverse cultures. Furthermore, the implementation of continuous learning mechanisms allows AI to adapt to cultural shifts over time, maintaining relevance and sensitivity.

To effectively manage these solutions, a robust framework for regularly evaluating and updating AI systems is crucial. This ensures that cultural adaptations are not only implemented but also refined based on feedback and changing cultural landscapes, thereby promoting consistent alignment with global cultural diversity.

## Case Studies of Culturally Competent AI Systems

Examining case studies of culturally competent AI systems reveals profound insights into successful implementations. One notable example is the AI-driven telemedicine platform in India, which integrates Ayurvedic medicine practices alongside conventional medical advice. Here, AI algorithms have been trained to understand regional health beliefs and treatment preferences, thereby significantly enhancing patient satisfaction and adherence to prescribed health regimens.

Another case is found in North America, where an AI system was developed to support indigenous populations. This system leverages traditional healing knowledge, documented and inputted by cultural scholars, to provide culturally resonant health assessments. It proves especially effective in communities with strong ties to ancestral practices, enhancing the trust and receptiveness towards modern healthcare solutions.

These examples underscore the tangible benefits of embedding cultural awareness into AI. By respecting and incorporating traditional knowledge, such systems not only promote inclusivity but also enhance the efficacy of medical interventions across diverse populations.

### Partnerships for Diverse Data Collection

Forming partnerships for diverse data collection is critical in building culturally competent AI systems. Collaborative endeavors with academic institutions, healthcare providers worldwide, and community organizations enable the collection of diverse and extensive datasets that reflect different cultures. These alliances ensure that AI algorithms are trained on a broad spectrum of health paradigms, encompassing both mainstream and alternative medical practices.

Key to these partnerships is active engagement with communities that are often underrepresented in medical research. By involving these groups in the data collection process, AI developers can gain authentic insights into traditional and indigenous healing practices, which are often overlooked in conventional datasets. Moreover, this involvement promotes transparency and trust, pillars crucial to the ethical development of AI technologies.

Such collaborative networks also facilitate the sharing of best practices and innovations across borders, enhancing the reliability and applicability of AI in medicine. As AI continues to enter diverse markets, partnerships focused on diversifying data sources become not only beneficial but also essential for the accurate interpretation and respectful integration of cultural knowledge in healthcare solutions.

### Evaluating AI Cultural Competence Effectiveness

Evaluating the effectiveness of AI's cultural competence is pivotal for ensuring these technologies perform equitably across diverse cultural landscapes. This evaluation process must be systemic, involving both quantitative metrics and qualitative feedback from users affected by the AI's decision-making. Metrics can include the accuracy of cultural recognition and the ability to tailor responses to specific cultural contexts.

Qualitative assessments, conversely, provide deeper insights into the user experience, highlighting areas where AI may misinterpret or overlook cultural nuances. These evaluations should be continuous, allowing for the dynamic evolution of AI systems in response to shifting cultural norms and practices. Regular updates and adjustments ensure that AI remains relevant and sensitive to the diverse cultures it serves.

Ultimately, the effective evaluation of AI's cultural competence not only enhances technology but also fosters greater trust and acceptance among users. By regularly assessing and refining AI, developers can build systems that genuinely respect and uphold cultural diversity, a crucial aspect in global applications.

**Feedback Mechanisms for Cultural Appropriateness**

Feedback mechanisms are vital for assessing and refining AI's cultural appropriateness. These systems collect insights directly from end-users, facilitating ongoing improvements to ensure AI sensitivity to diverse cultural contexts. User feedback, gathered through surveys, focus groups, or interactive online platforms, allows developers to pinpoint areas where AI may misinterpret or inadequately address cultural nuances.

Incorporating these feedback mechanisms into the development process enables a participatory approach, ensuring that the voices of those directly affected by AI technologies are heard and valued. This can lead to the adjustment of algorithms to better reflect cultural understandings and preferences. For example, feedback on AI's handling of traditional healing practices can guide developers in refining AI models to be more inclusive and respectful of non-Western medical approaches.

Moreover, continuous feedback loops help in maintaining a dynamic AI system that evolves alongside cultural shifts. Establishing robust channels for user input and genuinely integrating this feedback reinforces AI's role as a supportive tool in culturally diverse settings, enhancing trust and efficacy in its applications.

**Cultural Competence Training for AI Developers**

Cultural competence training for AI developers is pivotal in crafting algorithms that understand and respect diverse cultural dimensions. It involves enriched educational programs that extend beyond mere coding skills to include in-depth explorations of sociology, anthropology, and cultural studies. These programs are designed to sensitize developers to the subtleties of various sociocultural environments, ensuring that the technologies they create are versatile and culturally sensitive.

Such training equips developers to consider a wide array of cultural narratives and values during the design process, which is essential for minimizing the risk of cultural bias in AI applications. Workshops and seminars can be instrumental, featuring experts from diverse disciplines who convey the importance of incorporating holistic cultural understanding into AI development.

Ultimately, by fostering a workforce that's not only technically proficient but also culturally aware, we can anticipate the development of AI systems that perform ethically across multiple cultural contexts. Regular updates and professional development courses in cultural competence should be mandatory, ensuring that the knowledge base of AI developers evolves in tandem with global cultural shifts.

**Standardizing Cultural Competence Across AI Applications**

Standardizing cultural competence across AI applications requires a coherent framework that ensures uniform sensitivity and adaptability towards diverse cultural contexts. Such standardization aims not just to implement a one-size-fits-all approach; rather, it seeks to establish a set of guidelines that foster respect and efficiency in cultural integration, adaptable to specific requirements. Establishing such standards involves multidisciplinary collaboration to encapsulate a wide range of cultural dimensions, which are crucial for the successful operation of AI globally.

Regulatory bodies and international standards organizations play a pivotal role in this process. They devise clear policies and frameworks, ensuring AI developers adhere to ethical and cultural accuracy. Such regulations should include best practices for handling cultural data, model training, and guidelines for real-time adaptation, providing a clear pathway towards universally respectful AI systems.

Moreover, industry-wide adoption of these standards will promote consistency and foster trust among users. As AI technology traverses across borders, a standardized approach ensures that cultural competence remains central, enhancing the inclusivity and effectiveness of AI solutions in diverse global environments.

## Role of Governments in Promoting Culturally Competent AI

Governments could play a pivotal and positive role in shaping the landscape of culturally competent AI by enacting policies that prioritize cultural diversity within technological advancements. Recognizing the profound impact of AI on public services and societal operations, governments can drive the adoption of inclusive practices through regulation and funding incentives aimed at enhancing cultural competence in AI development.

Legislative frameworks can mandate that AI systems deployed in public sectors, such as healthcare and education, undergo rigorous testing to ensure they adequately reflect and respect cultural diversity. Such regulations help in minimizing cultural biases, ensuring that AI solutions are equitable and accessible to all citizens. Moreover, public funding can be strategically allocated to research and development projects that focus on integrating cultural knowledge into AI, fostering innovations that resonate with global cultural nuances.

In addition, governments can spearhead international collaborations to standardize cultural competence in AI globally. By leading such initiatives, they not only set the bar for cultural appropriateness but also promote a unified approach towards a culturally aware AI future. These efforts collectively serve to align technological advances with the broader societal values of inclusion and respect.

## Legal and Ethical Aspects of Cultural Competence in AI

Navigating the legal and ethical aspects of cultural competence in artificial intelligence is critical. Legal frameworks need to establish clear guidelines on the use of culturally diverse data, ensuring AI systems do not perpetuate biases or infringe on cultural rights. This involves implementing laws that mandate transparency in AI algorithms and the sources of their training data, thereby preventing discriminatory practices.

Ethically, developers must commit to responsible AI by incorporating diverse cultural perspectives during the design and deployment stages. Ethical AI means actively avoiding the erasure of minority cultural expressions and ensuring that AI systems respect cultural identifiers. This ethical commitment should be reflected in corporate policies and the overarching mission statements of organizations involved in AI development.

Moreover, legal accountability frameworks must be established to address any misuse or harm resulting from culturally incompetent AI applications. These frameworks should facilitate remedial measures, ensuring that damages can be rectified and that there are clear avenues for legal recourse for affected individuals.

By addressing these legal and ethical dimensions, AI development can progress towards more just and culturally aware implementations, ultimately fostering trust and broad acceptance across various cultural groups.

## Cultural Misinterpretations by AI and Rectifications

Artificial Intelligence, when not attuned to diverse cultural landscapes, can inadvertently perpetuate cultural misinterpretations. These errors can stem from skewed training data, underlying biases in the algorithm's design, or a lack of cultural insight among the developers. Misinterpretations might manifest as inappropriate translations, misrecognition of cultural symbols, or misaligned medical advisories that overlook indigenous healing practices.

Recognizing these missteps is crucial. AI systems should include mechanisms to identify and rectify errors swiftly. Initiatives could involve real-time monitoring for anomalies in AI responses and setting up dedicated teams to adjust the algorithms based on culturally sensitive feedback. Collaboration with cultural experts and continuous learning modules for AI systems can ensure these rectifications are not merely superficial but are deeply ingrained improvements.

Ultimately, sincere rectification efforts entail a commitment from AI developers to continually understand and integrate a wide array of cultural norms and values. This ongoing process not only enriches AI's interaction within diverse settings but also reinforces trust and reliability in AI applications across different cultural spectrums.

## Future Directions in Enhancing AI's Cultural Competence

As AI continues to evolve, enhancing cultural competence remains a crucial pathway. Future directions will likely leverage advanced computational methods and deeper integration of cultural datasets to create more nuanced and culturally aware AI systems. Emergent technologies, such as machine learning interpretability and ethical AI frameworks, will play pivotal roles in this development, ensuring that AI systems are not only practical but also culturally respectful.

In parallel, collaboration between AI developers, cultural scholars, and global communities will enhance mutual understanding and foster more inclusive AI designs. Initiatives might include international cultural competence hackathons or global AI ethics symposiums, aimed at cross-pollinating AI technology with diverse cultural insights. Such collaborative efforts can lead to breakthrough innovations in AI, personalized to cater to the cultural specifics of different regions.

Moreover, predictive analytics could serve to anticipate cultural impacts of AI applications, enabling proactive adjustments before deployment. Combining these approaches will ensure the future of AI not only embraces technological advancements but also deeply values and integrates the cultural diversity inherent in global societies.

## Developing AI With Cultural Empathy

Developing AI with cultural empathy involves creating systems that inherently understand and respect the nuances of different cultural backgrounds. This concept extends beyond mere data input to encompass a profound grasp of emotional and social context, which is essential for AI to act in a culturally sensitive manner. To achieve this, AI models must be trained on diverse datasets that include a broad spectrum of cultural norms, values, and expressions.

Crucially, the process necessitates an immersive collaboration between technologists and cultural experts to ensure AI systems interpret and respond sensitively. Insights from anthropology, sociology, and cultural studies can inform AI in accurately recognizing and valuing diverse cultural elements. Such collaboration results in AI that can genuinely empathize, adapting interactions to be more personal and culturally informed.

Furthermore, incorporating feedback mechanisms allows AI to learn from its experiences, continuously refining its cultural sensitivity. This dynamic learning process enables AI systems to evolve over time, aligning them more closely with the complexities of human culture and providing a more empathetic and nuanced service.

**Public Perception and Trust in Culturally Competent AI**

Public perception and trust in AI systems significantly hinge on how these technologies manage and reflect cultural nuances. Culturally competent AI promises an inclusive approach, aiming to foster broad acceptance across diverse societal segments. However, trust develops only when the public sees consistent, visible efforts in AI applications that respect cultural diversity and operate without biases. This requires transparent communication about the AI's development processes and its ability to handle cultural complexities.

Engagement with the public through educational campaigns and open dialogues can help demystify AI capabilities and intentions, particularly in addressing sensitive cultural aspects. Success stories of culturally competent AI can also be showcased to highlight the benefits and reliability of such systems. These narratives not only build confidence but also demonstrate AI's potential in enhancing everyday interactions across varied cultural landscapes.

Ultimately, the trust in AI systems reflects their perceived fairness and effectiveness. Continual feedback loops and improvements, guided by public input and cultural expert reviews, ensure these systems remain aligned with evolving cultural expectations and retain public trust over time.

## Summary

The chapter 'Fostering Cultural Competence in AI Models' explores how artificial intelligence (AI) can be programmed to respect, understand, and engage with diverse cultural contexts effectively. The emphasis is on embedding cultural intelligence into AI algorithms, particularly in the medical field, to ensure equitable healthcare delivery. Different strategies outlined include enhancing diversity in training data, engaging cultural experts during the AI design process, and continuously refining AI systems based on feedback from culturally diverse user groups.

Defining cultural competence in AI involves programming AI to recognize differences in cultural beliefs, practices, and communication styles. It demands sensitivity to factors such as dietary habits or traditional healing methods, reflecting these variations in AI diagnostic tools and treatment recommendations. This chapter highlights the importance of diverse data in AI training, emphasizing how a homogeneous dataset can lead to biased AI outputs that may be unsafe for underrepresented groups.

Ethical dimensions are highlighted, emphasizing that AI should be developed with cultural insights from the outset, rather than retrofitting them later. Ensuring diversity involves incorporating different languages, genders, and ages, which enhances AI's capability in providing accurate and relevant medical advice. Cultural audits, stakeholder involvement, and ongoing adaptations of AI systems are recommended to maintain their effectiveness and relevance.

The text also discusses legal and ethical challenges, stressing the importance of government roles in regulating AI and mandating inclusivity. It calls for standardization in cultural competence across AI applications through international collaborations and guidelines. Finally, case studies illustrate the successful implementation of culturally competent AI, showing tangible benefits in AI-driven healthcare platforms in India and support for indigenous populations in North America.

In summary, establishing culturally competent AI necessitates deliberate efforts in training AI to recognize and adapt to cultural signifiers, with active participation from diverse cultural experts during the development and iterative refinement processes. This ensures that AI systems are both technically proficient and culturally attuned, fostering global inclusivity and trust.

## References

[1] P. Natarajan, J. Tsang, and L. Zhou, 'Embedding Cultural Competence in Artificial Intelligence Systems', Journal of AI Technology and Cultural Adaptivity. https://journalofaitc.com/embedding-cultural-competence
[2] J. O'Donnell and S. Gupta, 'Multidisciplinary Approaches to Integrating Cultural Insights in AI Development', Global AI Journal. https://globalaijournal.com/multidisciplinary-approaches
[3] H. Chu and F. Meng, 'Legal Frameworks for Culturally Competent AI', Law and AI Review. https://lawandaireview.com/legal-frameworks-for-ai
[4] R. Singh, T. Mei, and N. Kumar, 'Case Studies on Culturally Competent AI Implementations in Healthcare', International Journal of AI in Healthcare. https://ijaih.com/culturally-competent-ai

### Case Study: Cultural Competence in AI: The Case of HealthBot Inc.

HealthBot Inc., a leading developer of AI-driven healthcare applications, has recently ventured into creating an advanced diagnostic tool designed for a globally diverse user base. The tool, named 'DiaLog', was conceptualized to interpret symptoms and suggest potential health care recommendations. However, initial deployment revealed significant shortcomings in cultural sensitivity, leading to misinterpretations related to dietary habits and local medicinal practices. For instance, in East Asian communities, common dietary elements like seaweed were incorrectly flagged as potential health risks due to their high iodine content, which the AI failed to contextualize within the region's normal dietary patterns.

Recognizing these issues, HealthBot Inc. embarked on a transformative journey towards genuine cultural competence. The company initiated partnerships with cultural experts and conducted extensive field research to gather diverse health data directly from local communities across several continents. They incorporated this new, culturally rich data into DiaLog's algorithms to better understand and integrate various health beliefs and traditional practices. The revised version of DiaLog was equipped to offer advice considering, for example, traditional African herbal medicines or South Asian yoga practices as part of treatment plans.

Despite these improvements, challenges remained. The AI occasionally misconstrued the cultural significance of certain symptoms and the related therapeutic practices, leading to less effective or culturally insensitive advice. To address these continuous challenges, HealthBot Inc. established a real-time feedback mechanism, allowing users to report and discuss any cultural inaccuracy or insensitivity found in the AI's recommendations. This feedback was directly used to refine the algorithm, making DiaLog an evolving tool learning actively from its global user base.

The efforts of HealthBot Inc. illustrate the complexities and ongoing nature of integrating cultural competence in AI systems within healthcare. It underscores not only the technological challenges but also the ethical responsibility companies hold in providing equitable and sensitive care across diverse patient populations.

### Case Study: Integrating Cultural Sensitivity in AI: The Journey of TerraVoice Technologies

TerraVoice Technologies, an emerging tech company, developed an AI-powered multilingual customer support system, aiming to revolutionize customer interactions across different regions. Named 'GlobeSpeak', their system promised to bridge the communication gap between service providers and a culturally diverse user base. Initially, GlobeSpeak focused on major languages such as English, Spanish, and Mandarin, providing basic translation and interaction capabilities. However, as the system rolled out, it became apparent that linguistic capabilities alone were insufficient for true cultural competence.

Feedback from early users in regions such as the Middle East and North Africa highlighted that GlobeSpeak often misinterpreted local dialects and colloquialisms, leading to frustrating user experiences. Additionally, the system's lack of sensitivity to cultural contexts, such as greeting norms and politeness protocols, led to user alienation. For example, the AI's direct communication style, derived from Western conventions, was perceived as blunt or rude in cultures that value indirectness and formality in interactions.

Recognizing these shortcomings, TerraVoice embarked on a comprehensive overhaul of GlobeSpeak. They collaborated with linguistic and cultural experts from various regions to deepen the AI's understanding of local languages and cultural nuances. This involved not only refining the language models but also integrating cultural sensitivity into the AI's response mechanisms. Techniques included AI simulations with native speakers and cultural immersion workshops for the development team, focusing on key aspects like non-verbal cues and regional etiquette.

Moreover, TerraVoice established continuous improvement protocols, including a robust feedback system where users could submit reports on GlobeSpeak's cultural mishandlings. These insights were crucial for iterative updates, allowing the AI to adapt more dynamically to cultural expectations. As a result, GlobeSpeak transformed into not just a multilingual tool but a culturally adaptive interface, enhancing communication effectiveness and user satisfaction across diverse global markets.

## Case Study: Innovative Cultural Integration in MedAI Solutions

MedAI Solutions, a pioneering force in the integration of AI with healthcare services, recently endeavored to enhance the cultural competence of its medical diagnostic tool, 'CuraAI'. The initial version of CuraAI was proficient in diagnosing a broad spectrum of diseases, yet it struggled with cultural disparities in symptom presentation and treatment acceptance. This was starkly evident when CuraAI suggested treatments that were culturally unsuitable or misunderstood local health practices, such as recommending pharmaceutical solutions to populations that favor holistic or traditional remedies.

Understanding these limitations, MedAI Solutions committed to refining CuraAI to better respect and integrate the cultural nuances of its diverse user base. The team embarked on a collaborative initiative with cultural anthropologists and healthcare professionals from varied cultural backgrounds, aiming to construct a database enriched with culturally specific health data. They organized community interaction programs worldwide to gather firsthand insights into local health beliefs, dietary habits, and traditional healing practices. This data was meticulously integrated into CuraAI's algorithms to improve its diagnostic accuracy and treatment suggestions.

However, adapting AI to encompass such a wide array of cultures presented substantial challenges. For instance, integrating traditional Chinese medicine concepts with Western medical practices within the AI system raised issues in balancing differing medical ideologies and treatments. To address these and other complexities, MedAI Solutions developed a dynamic, learning AI model that continuously updates its database and algorithms based on real-time feedback and ongoing research findings.

To ensure ongoing accuracy and cultural relevance, MedAI Solutions implemented a structured feedback loop with end-users and healthcare providers. This loop enables the continuous refinement of the AI, ensuring that CuraAI adapts to the evolving cultural and medical landscapes. The AI now not only diagnoses but also suggests culturally resonant health management plans, improving patient adherence and satisfaction across the globe. The case of MedAI Solutions highlights the importance of continuous engagement with cultural diversity and adaptation in developing effective and respectful AI-driven healthcare solutions.

## Case Study: Enhancing Cultural Adaptation in AI: The Efforts of LinguisticAI Corp

LinguisticAI Corp, a pioneering developer of AI-driven linguistic tools, launched its latest product, 'PolyglotAI', designed to assist in language learning and translation across diverse cultural contexts. Initially, PolyglotAI supported major global languages, but users quickly reported issues with less common languages and dialects. Users noted that idiomatic expressions and regional slang were often literally translated, leading to awkward or, in some cases, offensive outputs. This was particularly pronounced in remote dialects of Southeast Asia and indigenous languages in South America, where linguistic nuances are deeply intertwined with cultural identity.

To address these challenges, LinguisticAI Corp partnered with linguistic anthropologists and local language experts to overhaul PolyglotAI's database. They engaged in extensive fieldwork, recording conversations and collecting linguistic data firsthand from a variety of locales, which helped capture the unique colloquialisms and idiomatic expressions specific to each culture. The development team then integrated machine learning algorithms that could better learn from and adapt to this richer, more varied linguistic data, ensuring that translations were not only linguistically accurate but also culturally pertinent and respectful.

However, adapting PolyglotAI to such diverse inputs also introduced complexities. The AI sometimes misinterpreted cultural context, resulting in translations that, although technically correct, were contextually inappropriate. To combat this, LinguisticAI implemented a cultural sensitivity filter, designed to review translations for potential cultural insensitivities. Moreover, they established an ongoing user feedback system that allowed users to flag problematic translations in real-time. These contributions were used to continually train the AI, thereby enhancing its ability to navigate cultural subtleties with greater ease.

Despite these efforts, the challenge of balancing cultural sensitivity with accurate translation remains. LinguisticAI continues to refine PolyglotAI through continuous updates and community engagement, striving for an AI that is not only multilingual but truly multicultural.

### Case Study: Cultural Nuance Navigator: Enhancing AI's Cultural Sensitivity at GlobalMedTech

GlobalMedTech, a leading innovator in the development of AI-enhanced healthcare technologies, embarked on creating a new AI system called 'Cultural Nuance Navigator' (CNN) designed to support healthcare professionals by providing culturally informed medical advice. Initially, CNN was successful in recognizing broadly diverse cultures but faltered in understanding nuanced local sensitivities, such as recognizing sub-cultural variations within larger demographic groups. For example, CNN initially misinterpreted symptom descriptions and dietary references from subpopulations within India, treating the cultural dietary habits and medical beliefs of these distinct groups as homogeneous. This confusion led to recommendations that were culturally inappropriate or ineffective.

To address these deficiencies, GlobalMedTech gathered a consortium of cultural experts, AI ethicists, and data scientists to refine CNN's capabilities. The team embarked on a project to integrate a more granular level of cultural data, including dialects, regional health practices, and local medicinal knowledge, into the existing AI framework. This process involved collecting ethnographic field data through partnerships with local health practitioners and patients to ensure the richness of the cultural information.

Despite these enhancements, challenges persisted. The newer version of CNN struggled to balance a vast array of cultural data without compromising the speed and efficiency of medical advice. GlobalMedTech then implemented a dynamic learning algorithm within CNN to prioritize data relevant to the patient's cultural context as indicated by initial interaction cues. Additionally, they introduced an iterative feedback loop that involved continuous input from both users and cultural advisors, enabling real-time updates to the system's cultural understanding.

This approach transformed CNN into a more adaptive tool capable of providing culturally nuanced medical advice. It also highlighted the complexities inherent in designing AI systems that effectively handle detailed cultural intricacies without oversimplification. The case of GlobalMedTech underlines the importance of continuous interaction with cultural data and community engagement in maintaining the relevance and effectiveness of culturally competent AI systems.

### Case Study: Navigating Cultural Challenges in AI: The AdaptDx Project

AdaptDx, a startup specializing in AI-driven adaptive learning tools, undertook a project to develop an educational platform that tailors learning experiences to students from diverse cultural backgrounds. The initial launch saw EduCulture AI, the platform, implemented in schools across several countries, providing personalized learning paths tailored to students' educational needs. However, it soon became apparent that the AI struggled with cultural nuances, misunderstanding regional educational norms, and failing to adapt to local pedagogical styles, which led to decreased engagement and learning effectiveness among users.

Recognizing the importance of cultural competence, AdaptDx initiated a comprehensive review of EduCulture AI's performance. They discovered that the AI system had been primarily trained on data from Western educational systems, which did not adequately represent the educational approaches and values of other regions. For instance, in some Asian countries, where rote memorization is often emphasized, the AI's focus on exploratory learning techniques was less effective and even counterintuitive to the students' and teachers' expectations.

To address these issues, AdaptDx partnered with cultural anthropologists and education experts from around the globe. They conducted workshops and immersive research within classrooms in different countries to gather in-depth insights into the local educational contexts. This ethnographic research was crucial in reshaping the AI's algorithms, allowing EduCulture AI to recognize and align with different educational methodologies and cultural expectations properly.

Additionally, AdaptDx developed a dynamic feedback system where educators and students could provide ongoing input about the AI's performance. This real-time feedback was used to make continuous adjustments to the AI, ensuring its adaptability and relevance across varied educational settings. As a result, EduCulture AI evolved into a culturally aware platform that respected and incorporated local educational values, enhancing student engagement and learning outcomes.

This case study illustrates the complexities involved in creating culturally adaptive AI systems and underscores the necessity of incorporating diverse cultural data and continuous community feedback in developing effective AI solutions.

### Case Study: Culturally Attuned AI in Elderly Care: The Personal Health Experience

PersonaHealth, an innovative technology company specializing in AI solutions for elderly care, faced significant cultural sensitivity challenges in their AI system, AgeCare AI. The system was designed to assist elderly individuals by providing daily reminders, social interaction prompts, and personalized healthcare advice. However, initial feedback indicated that AgeCare AI struggled with cultural nuances in its interactions, particularly in ethnically diverse regions. For instance, the system often failed to adjust its communication styles and health advice to accommodate cultural preferences and norms around aging and elderly care, which varied significantly across cultures.

In response to these issues, PersonaHealth took a proactive approach by integrating cultural competence into their technology. They formed partnerships with cultural experts and gerontologists from various cultural backgrounds to create a comprehensive database of cultural norms and health practices related to elderly care. This initiative included detailed ethnographic studies to understand the daily routines, dietary preferences, and health beliefs of elderly individuals from different cultures. The insights gained from these studies were then used to retrain AgeCare AI, focusing on culturally sensitive communication and tailored health management strategies.

However, the challenges did not end with the integration of new data. The updated AgeCare AI occasionally misinterpreted cultural cues, leading to inappropriate suggestions or interactions that could confuse or offend users. To refine their approach, PersonaHealth established a continuous feedback loop with users and caregivers, allowing them to report any issues or cultural insensitivity. This feedback was invaluable for making iterative improvements to AgeCare AI's algorithms, enhancing its cultural acuity.

PersonaHealth's journey in developing a culturally competent AI for elderly care highlights the importance of continuous engagement with cultural diversity and the need for AI systems to evolve dynamically with their user base. It also emphasizes the role of collaborative efforts in designing technologies that respect and adapt to the rich tapestry of human cultures, thereby improving the quality of care and interactions for elderly individuals across different cultural settings.

## Case Study: AI Globalization in Telehealth: The NuanceCare Initiative

NuanceCare, a rising star in the telehealth sector, recently unveiled its AI-powered platform designed to provide medical diagnostics and patient care recommendations to a global audience. Termed 'HealthScope AI', its vision was to eliminate geographical barriers and offer quick, culturally sensitive medical advice. Initially, HealthScope AI was deployed in North America, Europe, and parts of Asia. It successfully addressed common ailments but soon experienced a setback when it expanded into Middle Eastern and African markets, where it faltered in accurately interpreting local languages and respecting local health practices. For example, HealthScope AI, which is primarily trained on Western dietary norms, frequently misunderstands the nutritional discussions in Middle Eastern diets, often misclassifying common foods like dates and figs as potential health risks due to their sugar content, without recognizing their cultural and health significance.

To address these cultural competence gaps, NuanceCare collaborated with cultural experts and local healthcare providers from diverse regions to enhance the AI's understanding. This collaborative effort involved the collection of diverse health datasets, including typical regional diets, common genetic health issues, and prevalent local medicinal practices. These datasets were integrated into HealthScope AI's algorithms, which were revamped to not only translate but also interpret and suggest within the appropriate cultural contexts.

Despite these improvements, challenges persisted. HealthScope AI occasionally issued recommendations that aligned with generic medical practices but clashed with local health philosophies. For instance, recommending pharmaceutical interventions where holistic approaches were preferred. NuanceCare responded by establishing a dynamic feedback system that allowed patients and doctors to provide immediate feedback on AI advice, which was crucial for ongoing adjustments.

NuanceCare's journey sheds light on the complex nature of creating a globally competent AI telehealth platform. It highlights the need for continual data integration, the value of local partnerships, and the dynamic nature of cultural competence, which requires ongoing recalibration of AI systems to cater effectively to diverse populations.

## Review Questions

**1. In a remote community in India, a 53-year-old woman with a history of diabetes uses a combination of Ayurvedic medicines and Western medications to manage her condition. Lately, she has reported feeling unwell with increased fatigue and fluctuating blood sugar levels despite adherence to her medication regimen. Her family is concerned about the effects of combining different types of medicine. What could be the most likely cause of her symptoms?**

A) Adverse interactions between her Ayurvedic medications and Western medications.

B) Progression of her diabetes due to age.

C) Inadequate dose of Western medications.

D) Non-compliance with the prescribed treatment regimen.

**Answer: A**

Explanation: This patient's symptoms of increased fatigue and fluctuating blood sugar levels, despite adherence to medication, suggest the possibility of adverse interactions between her Ayurvedic medications and Western medications. Combining treatments from different medical systems without proper guidance can lead to interactions that modify the effects of the medications. It is crucial for patients using a combination of traditional and Western medicine to do so under the supervision of healthcare providers knowledgeable in both areas, to ensure the safety and effectiveness of the treatment regimen.

**2. A 45-year-old man from an indigenous tribe in the Amazon with a history of hypertension refuses conventional treatment and instead seeks healing through shamanic rituals involving spiritually based practices and herbal medicines. Despite the community's respect for these traditions, his blood pressure readings remain high. What should be the most appropriate approach for a healthcare provider?**

A) Disregard his cultural practices and prescribe antihypertensive medications only.

B) Incorporate his cultural practices into a holistic plan that includes monitoring and possible integration of conventional medicine if necessary.

C) Only support his decision to use traditional medicine without any interference.

D) Recommend immediate hospitalization, ignoring his cultural beliefs.

**Answer: B**

Explanation: The most appropriate approach for a healthcare provider in this scenario is to incorporate the patient's cultural practices into a holistic plan that respects his traditions while also ensuring his health is safeguarded. This can include monitoring his condition and discussing how conventional medicine might be used alongside his traditional practices to manage his hypertension effectively. It's essential to engage in a respectful dialogue, recognizing the cultural significance of his choices, to promote compliance and optimize treatment outcomes.

**Community-Driven Approaches to Healthy AI Practices**

**Defining Community-Driven AI in Healthcare**

Community-driven AI in healthcare represents a transformative approach where AI development is not only informed by but actively shaped by the communities it serves. This paradigm prioritizes input from diverse population groups, ensuring that healthcare solutions are not only technologically advanced but also culturally sensitive and relevant to the various needs of different groups.

The core of community-driven AI lies in its participatory framework. Communities are not passive recipients but active contributors in the AI lifecycle, from ideation to deployment. Such involvement ensures that AI tools address real-world issues accurately while respecting local knowledge and practices, including traditional, indigenous, and holistic healing methods.

Implementing community-driven AI involves integrating local health data and insights into AI algorithms, resulting in more personalized, effective, and equitable health outcomes. This model not only enhances service delivery but also fosters a sense of ownership and trust among community members, critical for the sustainable success of AI applications in medicine.

## Roles of Local Communities in Shaping AI Tools

Local communities play a crucial role in the development of culturally sensitive AI systems. Their involvement ensures that these tools resonate with the local customs, health practices, and the nuanced needs of the population they serve. By integrating community feedback and traditional knowledge into the AI design process, tools become more applicable and sensitive to the specific health profiles of each region.

This participatory approach also facilitates the creation of AI models that are not merely scientific but also respect and incorporate indigenous healing practices. Such integration can decrease health disparities by aligning modern healthcare technologies with long-established local practices. Community knowledge can guide AI in interpreting health data contextually, improving the accuracy and relevance of its applications in real-world scenarios.

Moreover, engaging local communities in AI development enhances trust and fosters broader acceptance of technological solutions. It ensures that AI tools are not just designed for communities but shaped by them, promoting transparency and accountability in AI deployments. This cooperative relationship not only empowers communities but also instills a sense of ownership, increasing the likelihood of successful AI integration in local healthcare infrastructures.

## Collaborative AI Development: Engaging Stakeholders

Successful collaborative AI development hinges on effectively engaging a diverse array of stakeholders. This engagement is not merely consultative; it is an immersive partnership where stakeholders from various sectors contribute actively to designing AI tools that address genuine healthcare needs. These stakeholders include healthcare professionals, technologists, patients, and representatives from underrepresented communities.

By involving stakeholders early in the development process, AI projects can benefit from multiple perspectives, enhancing the relevance and acceptability of the technology. Regular workshops and feedback sessions are instrumental in fine-tuning AI solutions in real-time, ensuring they align well with user expectations and ethical standards. Moreover, such participatory practices help in identifying potential biases in AI programming and propose inclusive algorithms that honor diverse healing traditions.

The cornerstone of collaborative AI development is transparency and continuous dialogue, ensuring all voices are heard and valued. This approach not only mitigates risks of cultural oversight but also strengthens the AI's capability to serve broad demographic spectrums with sensitivity and accuracy, thereby fostering trust and wider adoption.

## Case Studies of Community Input Transforming AI

Community involvement in AI development has catalyzed significant transformations in medical AI applications, as illustrated by various case studies. One remarkable example from rural India involved the integration of local health practices into an AI system for diagnosing common ailments. By incorporating feedback from indigenous healers, the AI tool was enhanced to recognize symptoms and suggest treatments that aligned with local traditions, vastly improving its acceptance and effectiveness.

Another case study in Brazil showcased the impact of community input on personalizing AI-driven nutritional advice. The AI system was programmed to consider local dietary habits and available resources, ensuring that the health recommendations were practical and culturally appropriate. This approach not only improved user compliance but also fostered a deeper trust in AI technologies within the community.

These examples demonstrate the profound influence of community engagement in AI development, underscoring the potential for culturally sensitive and inclusive AI solutions that truly meet the needs of the populations they serve, while fostering sustainable, trust-filled interactions between technology and tradition.

## Utilizing Public Feedback to Enhance AI Systems

Public feedback serves a critical role in the iterative refinement of AI systems in healthcare. By aggregating input from diverse users, developers can identify unforeseen usage issues or biases that may not surface during initial testing phases. This collective insight empowers AI to evolve in ways that are increasingly sensitive to the nuances of community health practices and cultural preferences.

Incorporating public feedback involves systematic collection, analysis, and integration of user experiences. These processes ensure that AI tools are not only technically proficient but also culturally resonant and user-friendly. Regularly updated feedback mechanisms, such as surveys, focus groups, and digital forums, allow continuous interaction between users and developers, fostering an environment where AI can be dynamically adapted to meet changing healthcare needs.

Ultimately, the involvement of the public in shaping AI tools leads to enhanced trust and efficacy. As AI systems implement changes based on community feedback, they become more aligned with user expectations and needs, thereby improving overall outcomes in healthcare practices and increasing the acceptance of AI-driven solutions.

## Community-Based Testing of AI Technologies

The concept of community-based testing of AI technologies pivots on real-world evaluations where local populations test AI tools tailored to their specific healthcare needs. This process validates AI solutions, ensuring they perform effectively within diverse environments and under various practical conditions. Such testing naturally extends the development lifecycle into the community sphere, fostering participation and ownership from those who are directly impacted by these technologies.

Conducting these tests in community settings not only uncovers unique insights into the cultural and environmental factors affecting AI performance but also highlights potential disparities in effectiveness across different demographics. It pushes developers to address these issues promptly, adapting AI systems to serve more equitably. This stage of testing is crucial for assessing how well AI integrates into the daily health practices of community members and adapts to their traditional healing methods.

Ultimately, community-based testing serves as a crucial feedback loop, providing developers with tangible data to refine AI tools before widespread deployment. It creates a foundation for trust and dependability in AI applications, ensuring the technologies are not only innovative but also genuinely beneficial and reliable for the community's use.

## Ethical Considerations in Community-AI Interactions

When integrating AI into community health initiatives, ethical considerations are paramount. The primary ethical concern involves ensuring that AI applications respect the cultural values and privacy of individuals. This involves designing AI systems that are transparent in their functions and intentions, clearly communicating what data is collected and how it will be used.

Moreover, there is a critical need to establish robust consent processes that are culturally sensitive and tailored to the specific needs of each individual. Communities must have the opportunity to opt in or out without coercion or manipulation. Ethical AI must also avoid exacerbating existing inequalities; therefore, it should be accessible and beneficial to all community segments, including marginalized groups.

Safeguarding against biases in AI that may lead to health disparities is another ethical priority. Continuous oversight and revisions should be implemented as communities evolve and new ethical challenges arise. Engaging ethicists and community representatives in ongoing AI development processes ensures that ethical considerations keep pace with technological advancements, thereby fostering stronger, trust-based relationships within the community.

## Training AI with Diverse, Community-Sourced Data

Leveraging diverse, community-sourced data in AI training is critical for developing systems that respect and understand varied healthcare practices. This approach prioritizes inclusivity, ensuring AI tools are not just technically sound but also culturally competent. By tapping into a wide range of community inputs, AI can better serve its users by reflecting a broader spectrum of experiences and medical traditions.

The process involves collecting data from different demographic segments, including underrepresented communities, to create a well-rounded dataset. Such data collection is conducted ethically, with clear consent and transparency regarding how the data will be utilized. The resulting AI models are enriched, providing outputs that are more accurate and culturally sensitive, which in turn boosts their acceptance and effectiveness within the community.

However, training AI with diverse data sets presents challenges, such as maintaining data quality and navigating privacy concerns. Addressing these effectively requires robust methodologies and ongoing community engagement to ensure that AI systems remain relevant, trustworthy, and equitable. Engaging community liaisons or cultural experts during data collection and algorithm training can bridge gaps between technology and traditional knowledge, ensuring ethical standards are upheld.

## Overcoming Challenges in Community-AI Collaboration

Community-AI collaborations, while vital for creating inclusive AI systems, encounter multifaceted challenges that require careful navigation. One significant hurdle is the potential for cultural misunderstandings, which can undermine the goals of AI projects. Effective communication and education across diverse groups help to bridge these gaps, ensuring that AI initiatives are sensitive to local cultural nuances and capable of genuinely benefiting the community.

Another challenge in community-AI partnerships lies in aligning diverse expectations and objectives. Community members might prioritize immediate healthcare improvements, while developers may focus on long-term data collection for AI refinement. Structured dialogue and transparent goal setting become crucial in synchronizing these expectations, fostering a collaborative environment where all stakeholders see their needs and contributions valued.

Lastly, technical disparities present substantial barriers. Not all communities possess the technological infrastructure or literacy required for optimal AI integration. Developing targeted training programs and adapting technologies to fit local contexts are essential strategies for empowering communities and harnessing AI's full potential, thereby truly democratizing health technology innovations.

## Success Metrics for Community-Driven AI Initiatives

Defining success in community-driven AI initiatives transcends the traditional metrics of technology performance. It encompasses a broader spectrum of criteria focused on community impact, equity, and sustainability. Firstly, user engagement rates and feedback quality provide insights into the effectiveness and acceptance of AI systems within the community. This continuous feedback loop is essential for refining AI functionalities to suit localized health needs.

Additionally, improvements in health outcomes are a fundamental metric. These include reduced incidence of diseases well-recognized by traditional practices and better management of chronic conditions through AI-led interventions. Monitoring these health metrics over time offers quantifiable evidence of the initiative's success in improving community health benchmarks.

Beyond health outcomes, sustainable integration into community practices signifies success. This involves measuring how AI solutions maintain cultural sensitivity and adapt to evolving healthcare practices. Success also involves evaluating empowerment and capacity-building through educational programs that enhance community members' ability to interact meaningfully with AI systems.

## The Impact of Cultural Diversity on AI Performance

Cultural diversity profoundly influences the performance and acceptance of AI in healthcare. Different cultural contexts offer varied interpretations and responses to AI-driven solutions, impacting their utility and efficacy across communities. For instance, AI models trained predominantly on data from homogenous populations often fail when applied to diverse settings, where nuances in language, genetic peculiarities, or healthcare practices can differ significantly.

Incorporating a wide array of cultural insights into AI development enhances the system's adaptability and accuracy. It ensures that predictive algorithms accommodate diverse health indicators and outcomes, which are often culturally contingent. This aspect is critical in medicine, where diagnostic processes and treatment responses can be heavily influenced by ethnic and cultural factors.

Therefore, when AI leverages cultural diversity, it not only performs better but also garners trust and acceptance. Embedding these diverse datasets from the outset is imperative to develop truly inclusive AI systems. This approach also addresses potential biases, ensuring AI recommendations are appropriate and effective across various cultural spectrums.

## Building Trust in AI Through Community Engagement

Building trust in AI within medical contexts begins with active, consistent community engagement. When communities are involved in the development and implementation of AI, it not only fosters acceptance but also increases the likelihood of these technologies being used effectively and ethically. Transparency in AI operations and decision-making processes is crucial; communities must have clear insights into how algorithms function and impact their healthcare. Open forums and discussions can demystify AI technologies, addressing any reservations or misconceptions robustly.

Moreover, involving community members in the testing and feedback phases of AI development creates a sense of ownership and responsibility. This collaborative approach ensures that the AI systems are not only technically sound but are also perceived as legitimate and beneficial tools by those they are supposed to help. Regular updates to communities about how their input has shaped the AI interventions can reinforce this trust.

Ultimately, trust translates into better health outcomes. Community trust leads to increased adoption and optimal use of AI-driven health solutions, enhancing both individual and public health. For AI to be genuinely effective in healthcare, it must be rooted in the trust and active participation of the community it serves.

**Strategies for Sustainable Community-AI Partnerships**

Establishing sustainable partnerships between communities and AI developers is foundational to the success of AI initiatives in healthcare. These collaborations must be nurtured with clear, mutual goals that reflect both technical objectives and community welfare. Regular, structured interactions foster understanding and cooperation, ensuring that AI solutions are developed not only with technological expertise but also with a respect for community nuances.

Transparency is another pillar in building sustainable partnerships. Open communication about AI development processes, data usage, and potential impacts on the community helps mitigate distrust and fear. Additionally, creating inclusive platforms for dialogue enables community members to express concerns, suggest improvements, and become active participants in the AI development lifecycle.

Finally, establishing ongoing educational initiatives that empower community members with knowledge about AI can demystify technology and foster a more profound engagement. By integrating community input at every step and ensuring the AI's adaptability to evolving healthcare norms, these partnerships can thrive, making AI a true community ally in health management.

**Legal and Regulatory Frameworks Supporting Community AI**

Robust legal and regulatory frameworks may significantly bolster the effectiveness of community-driven AI in healthcare. These frameworks ensure AI deployment aligns with ethical standards and respects the socio-cultural nuances of each community. Essential elements include data protection laws that safeguard personal health information from misuse and regulations that enforce accountability among AI developers, especially in scenarios where AI decisions directly impact patient outcomes.

Moreover, laws must foster an environment of inclusivity, ensuring AI tools do not perpetuate existing disparities or biases within healthcare systems. This involves stringent oversight on how AI applications are tested and validated across diverse communities before widespread implementation. Regulatory bodies are tasked with the critical role of continuous monitoring and updating policies that keep pace with technological advancements and evolving community needs.

Additionally, aligning local and global regulations can be challenging but essential. Harmonizing these ensures that community-driven AI initiatives benefit from international expertise while adhering to local cultural and legal expectations. Only with such a comprehensive and adaptive approach can AI truly serve as a catalyst for equitable healthcare innovations.

**Funding and Resource Allocation for Community AI Projects**

Securing adequate funding and efficiently allocating resources are critical steps in supporting community-driven AI projects in healthcare. Typically, these initiatives require multifaceted funding strategies that blend government grants, private investments, and non-profit contributions. Strategic resource allocation ensures that these funds directly enhance technological development while fostering community involvement and education.

Effective allocation often prioritizes transparency and accountability, ensuring every dollar is traceable and maximizes community benefit. This might involve funding local training programs to increase AI literacy or investing in local data infrastructure to improve the applicability and effectiveness of AI systems. Prioritizing expenditures that strengthen community engagement ensures that the projects remain grounded in local needs and values, enhancing both acceptance and effectiveness.

Moreover, creating diverse funding streams can mitigate risks and promote sustainability. Partnerships with academic institutions and international healthcare organizations can provide both financial resources and expertise, crucial for the sophisticated needs of AI development in diverse cultural settings. Sustainable funding not only drives current projects but also secures long-term innovation and maintenance of community-centric AI tools.

## Educational Programs to Empower Communities in AI Governance

Empowering communities through educational programs in AI governance plays a pivotal role in shaping the ethical landscape of AI in healthcare. By equipping the local populace with the necessary knowledge and skills, these programs aim to bridge the gap between complex AI technologies and everyday health practices. Education fosters informed stakeholders who can actively participate in discussions and decisions regarding the deployment of AI in their community.

Such programs are not only about imparting technical knowledge but also about enhancing awareness of the ethical dimensions of AI. They encourage critical discussions on topics like data privacy, algorithmic bias, and the socio-cultural implications of AI technologies. This holistic approach ensures that community members are not passive recipients but active contributors to AI governance.

Moreover, tailored educational initiatives that address specific community needs can enhance engagement and relevance. By incorporating local languages, cultural nuances, and context-specific examples, these programs can make AI governance accessible and meaningful to all community members. Ultimately, well-informed communities are crucial to the responsible development and deployment of AI, ensuring these technologies serve the greater good.

## Feedback Loops: Ensuring Community Voices Shape AI Evolution

In the realm of community-driven AI, feedback loops are the lifeline that ensures AI systems evolve in tune with community needs and values. Effective feedback mechanisms allow communities to regularly provide insights and critiques, which are integral to the adaptive maintenance of AI technologies. This iterative process fosters a dynamic evolution of AI, keeping it relevant and beneficial.

To facilitate meaningful feedback, mechanisms must be accessible and actively promoted among community members. Digital platforms, community workshops, and direct surveys are viable channels through which diverse community voices can be captured. This diversity is crucial, as it encompasses a wide range of perspectives, enriching the AI's development process with multifaceted insights.

Translating this feedback into actionable intelligence is the next vital step. AI developers need to integrate these inputs systematically to refine algorithms, enhance user interfaces, and recalibrate system outputs. Regular community feedback sessions can ensure transparency, build trust, and motivate continuous engagement, collectively steering AI towards more equitable and effective outcomes in healthcare.

## Privacy and Data Security in Community-Driven AI

Privacy and data security are paramount in the realm of community-driven AI, particularly when handling sensitive health information. Delicate balances must be struck to protect individual privacy while leveraging data for impactful AI development. Laws like GDPR and HIPAA provide frameworks, but community-centric initiatives require additional discreet strategies to address local expectations and ethical norms.

Achieving robust data security in community-driven AI involves implementing advanced encryption methods and strict access controls that ensure data integrity and confidentiality. This includes regular audits and updates to security protocols to keep pace with evolving cyber threats. Community involvement in these processes can enhance trust and ensure that security measures do not impede the accessibility of AI solutions.

Furthermore, transparency in data handling and clarity about data utilization guidelines are critical. Establishing clear communication channels where community members can inquire and express concerns about data usage helps in maintaining accountability. Through these measures, community-driven AI projects can not only comply with legal standards but also resonate deeply with community values, fostering greater acceptance and success.

## Community-Centric AI Design and User Experience

Community-centric AI design prioritizes the user experience by embedding local cultures and needs into the core of AI systems. The focus is on creating interfaces that are intuitive and accessible to diverse populations, reducing barriers to technology adoption and enhancing the effectiveness of AI solutions in local health contexts.

Incorporating community feedback actively into design processes ensures that AI tools are more than just technologically advanced—they are practical and resonant with the daily realities of the users. This approach involves iterative testing and refinement, where community input directly influences everything from functionality to aesthetic elements of the AI system. Such collaborative design efforts empower communities, giving them a stake in the technology that affects their lives.

Moreover, the resulting AI applications promote inclusivity and adaptability, key traits for sustainable healthcare improvements. They reflect a deep understanding of the community's unique health challenges and preferences, which boosts user satisfaction and trust in AI technologies.

Ultimately, by fostering an inclusive design philosophy, AI developers can produce tools that not only serve but also grow with the community, continuously adapting to emerging health needs and technological landscapes.

## Role of Non-Profits and NGOs in Community AI Initiatives

Non-profits and NGOs play a pivotal role in integrating AI technologies within community healthcare systems, particularly by fostering initiatives that may otherwise lack visibility and support. Through their established trust and local presence, these organizations ensure that AI tools are developed not just with high technical standards but also with cultural sensitivity and inclusivity in mind.

Their contributions are manifold; they catalyze initial conversations about necessity and benefits, help mobilize local resources, and often serve as liaisons between the community and developers. By channeling their resources into training and workshops, they empower local stakeholders, ensuring that the community's voice is prominent in the AI development lifecycle. Their involvement helps in achieving a dual objective—aligning AI functionalities with specific health needs and upholding ethical standards that resonate with local values.

Furthermore, NGOs and non-profits play a crucial role in pilot testing and gathering initial feedback, which is essential for iterative improvements. They also play a significant role in scaling successful projects, ensuring that effective solutions reach broader populations. Thus, their engagement is not just supplementary but central to creating effective, sustainable, and trusted AI-driven health initiatives.

**Developing Culturally Sensitive AI Models**

The creation of culturally sensitive AI models requires recognizing and integrating the diverse values, practices, and beliefs intrinsic to different communities. Such models prioritize inclusivity by tailoring AI to reflect the cultural context of each user group. A key step in this process involves conducting comprehensive cultural audits to assess local norms and health practices, which guide the AI's design and functionality.

Incorporating cultural sensitivity into AI not only enhances its acceptance and efficacy but also mitigates the risk of biases that might alienate or harm certain groups. Developers can draw on anthropological insights and community health profiles to enrich the AI algorithms. By engaging with local health practitioners and cultural experts during the development phase, AI systems can be aligned with traditional and holistic approaches to healthcare that are often overlooked by mainstream medicine.

Moreover, ongoing community engagement in refining these AI models ensures they evolve in response to shifting cultural dynamics. This adaptive approach helps sustain long-term relevance and effectiveness, fostering trust and cooperation between AI initiatives and the communities they serve.

**Harnessing AI for Local Health Improvements**

Harnessing AI for local health improvements involves tailoring AI technologies to address specific health challenges faced by individual communities. By integrating AI with local health data and insights, systems can predict, detect, and manage health issues peculiar to these areas, often with greater accuracy than traditional blanket approaches.

For instance, AI can be programmed to monitor trends in regional disease outbreaks or to tailor health information dissemination in languages and formats most understood locally. This localized approach not only improves health outcomes but also enhances the engagement and trust of community members. AI-driven health solutions can thus become more than tools—they transform into community partners in public health advocacy and education.

Furthermore, AI can optimize resource allocation by predicting areas of demand for health services. This proactive stance ensures that communities are not merely reacting to health crises but are preventing them. By working closely with local health workers, AI can help fine-tune interventions to align well with ongoing health programs, increasing overall efficacy.

**Future Trends in Community-Engaged AI Practices**

Looking ahead, community-engaged AI practices are poised to radically transform the delivery, tailoring, and evolution of healthcare services. Central to this future is the deepening integration of AI with community feedback mechanisms, making deliberate strides towards systems that truly reflect the diversity and specific needs of populations at a granular level.

Advanced technologies, such as natural language processing and machine learning, will enable AI to understand better and respond to local languages and dialects, which are crucial for underserved and linguistically diverse communities. This will enhance the accessibility and effectiveness of health services, fostering broader inclusivity. Additionally, we can anticipate the rise of decentralized AI platforms that empower communities to directly influence the development and modification of health technologies without intermediary barriers.

Moreover, evolving legal and ethical frameworks will start to require more rigorous community involvement as a standard for AI development in healthcare, ensuring that these technologies are not only effective but also equitably distributed. The focus will increasingly shift towards sustainability, with long-term commitments from developers to support community-driven updates and improvements.

### Case Study: Global Examples of Successful Community AI Integration

Around the globe, successful community AI integrations stand as testaments to the power of technology when melded with local insights and participation. In rural India, AI applications in telemedicine have enabled patients in distant areas to receive timely healthcare advice, significantly reducing their travel burden. The AI systems were trained on local health patterns and languages, enhancing their relevance and acceptance among the villagers.

In Northern Canada, AI has been utilized to monitor the spread of infectious diseases within remote communities. These AI solutions were designed with inputs from local health workers and community leaders, which helped tailor the system's response to the specific climatic and socio-economic contexts of these areas. The initiative has not only improved health monitoring but also strengthened community trust in technology-driven solutions.

Similarly, in East Africa, AI-driven agricultural advisories have transformed traditional farming techniques. By integrating indigenous knowledge with predictive AI models, farmers receive real-time information on weather patterns and crop health, directly via mobile platforms. This fusion of local wisdom and modern technology underscores a sustainable approach to community-driven AI in medicine and beyond, boosting both yields and local economies.

### Summary

This chapter examines the profound influence of community-driven initiatives in shaping Artificial Intelligence (AI) in healthcare. It emphasizes a participatory framework where AI development integrates insights from local populations, ensuring that health solutions are both technologically advanced and culturally sensitive. The core concept here is that communities are active contributors throughout the AI lifecycle, from ideation to deployment, which enhances the relevance, efficacy, and acceptance of AI systems within diverse healthcare contexts.

Community roles are pivotal in designing AI tools that respect and integrate regional health practices, local customs, and cultural nuances, thus fostering equitable health outcomes. Engaging community members, healthcare professionals, underrepresented groups, and other stakeholders in the AI design process helps create solutions that are not only scientifically sound but also reflective of local health identities and practices.

The chapter highlights numerous case studies, such as those in rural India and Brazil, where community feedback has significantly enhanced AI functionalities, making them culturally relevant and widely accepted. Furthermore, through community-based testing and continuous public feedback, AI tools are dynamically refined and adapted to local needs, enhancing trust and ownership among users.

Ethical considerations are also discussed intensively. Ethical AI must respect community privacy, cultural values, and ensure equitable benefits across diverse populations. It's also crucial that AI tools do not exacerbate health disparities but rather help in mitigating them through culturally competent strategies. Another key area is the legal and regulatory frameworks that support the development of community-driven AI, ensuring data protection and accountability.

Lastly, the sustainability of AI initiatives hinges on the success of community-AI partnerships, supported by transparent communication, inclusive engagement, and ongoing educational programs that empower communities in AI governance. Overall, the chapter advocates for a holistic approach to developing AI technologies that are not only innovative but also deeply integrated with the communities they aim to serve, ensuring sustainability, ethical integrity, and widespread trust.

## References

[1] Artificial Intelligence for Health: Opportunities and Challenges. https://www.ncbi.nlm.nih.gov/pmc/articles/PMC7473756/
[2] Implementing AI in Healthcare: Bridging the Gap Between Theory and Practice. https://www.frontiersin.org/articles/10.3389/fdig.2020.00012/full
[3] Ethical Implications of AI in Healthcare. https://jamanetwork.com/journals/jama/fullarticle/2764953
[4] Community-Based Participatory Research in AI. https://equityhealthj.biomedcentral.com/articles/10.1186/s12939-020-01288-1
[5] Cultural Competence in Artificial Intelligence: A Framework for Ethical Engagement. https://link.springer.com/article/10.1007/s43681-020-00024-5

### Case Study: Community-Driven AI for Diabetes Management in Indigenous Populations

The case of the Tolem indigenous community in the Pacific Northwest showcases an exemplary integration of community-driven AI in healthcare. The Tolem community, characterized by a high incidence of Type 2 diabetes, faced significant challenges due to limited access to healthcare services and cultural barriers. In response, a novel community-driven AI initiative was launched, leveraging local knowledge and technology to improve diabetes management among community members.

The initiative began with comprehensive consultations and workshops with community leaders, healthcare workers, and residents to understand the specific health challenges and cultural nuances of the Tolem people. Insights gathered revealed a preference for traditional medicinal practices and a skepticism towards conventional medical interventions, which was crucial in shaping the AI system's development.

A tailored AI-driven application was then developed to track health metrics and offer personalized dietary and medicinal advice, incorporating traditional herbal remedies validated by medical science. The application used machine learning algorithms trained on community-sourced health data to recognize patterns in diabetes management that were previously unknown.

The impact of this initiative was profound. Initial skepticism was overcome by involving local healers in the AI training process, thus embedding trusted traditional knowledge. As the AI application provided recommendations that resonated culturally, community engagement increased. Over time, there was a notable improvement in adherence to diabetes management plans, and subsequent health monitoring showed a decrease in average blood glucose levels across the community.

This success story not only highlights the effectiveness of incorporating AI in managing chronic conditions but also underscores the importance of community involvement in the design and implementation phases. By respecting and integrating cultural values and practices, the AI system gained acceptance and became a valuable tool in public health within the Tolem community.

### Case Study: Empowering Rural Women in South Asia with AI-Enhanced Maternal Health Services

In rural regions of South Asia, maternal health often suffers due to inadequate healthcare infrastructure and prevalent socio-cultural barriers. A community-driven AI initiative was introduced to enhance maternal health services by empowering local women through technology that understands and integrates their cultural values and personal health needs. This case study explores the implementation, challenges, and impacts of this transformative AI project.

The initiative started with collaborations between AI developers, healthcare professionals, and local community leaders, aiming to address the high rates of maternal complications in several South Asian villages. The project involved training AI systems using data collected from local health camps, incorporating insights from traditional birth attendants, and gathering feedback from expectant mothers. A mobile application was developed, providing culturally attuned health advice and connecting expectant mothers with nearby healthcare services.

Using machine learning algorithms, the AI tool could predict potential pregnancy complications based on individual health data, historical patterns in the community, and commonly referenced local medical practices. The application also featured a communication platform where women could anonymously ask health-related questions and receive guidance in their local dialect, thus maintaining privacy and encouraging open communication.

Despite facing initial reluctance and gender-based barriers to technology access, the ongoing inclusion of community feedback loops helped refine the tool to meet the users' needs better. As trust in the technology grew, more women began to participate, which brought a significant decline in emergency interventions during childbirth and an improvement in prenatal care adherence.

This case highlights the importance of culturally understanding and effectively engaging community members in AI-driven health initiatives. The project's success was not just in technological deployment, but also in how well the AI incorporated and respected the community's cultural practices and feedback, ultimately leading to improved health outcomes and higher acceptance of the AI tool.

### Case Study: Revolutionizing Pediatric Care in Sub-Saharan Africa Through AI-Assisted Mobile Clinics

Sub-Saharan Africa faces unique healthcare challenges, particularly in pediatric care, due to limited access to healthcare facilities and skilled medical professionals. Addressing these issues, a pioneering community-driven AI initiative was launched to revolutionize pediatric healthcare by deploying AI-assisted mobile clinics. This case study examines the development, implementation, and transformative impact of this initiative, offering insights into the role of community involvement in AI-driven healthcare applications.

The project commenced with the collaboration of AI technologists, pediatric specialists, and local community leaders. The aim was to develop a mobile health solution that could travel to remote areas, providing critical healthcare services powered by AI. Extensive community consultations helped identify prevalent health issues and cultural considerations, ensuring the design of the AI system was both clinically effective and culturally sensitive.

The mobile clinics were equipped with AI-driven diagnostic tools trained on diverse datasets, including local health data. These tools were designed to aid in the quick and accurate diagnosis of common pediatric illnesses in the region, such as malaria and nutritional deficiencies. The AI also provided treatment recommendations based on best practices tailored to the local context, including available resources and traditional medicines acknowledged by the community.

The impact of these mobile clinics was remarkable. They not only expanded access to healthcare but also enhanced the trust and engagement of local communities. Using AI, the time required for diagnosis and treatment initiation was significantly reduced, thereby improving health outcomes. Parents and caregivers received health education from the system, which was crucial in areas with low literacy levels.

Governance and continuous feedback mechanisms were established to adapt and optimize the AI tools.

Community feedback sessions became a vital aspect of the iterative development process, ensuring that the system evolved in response to the changing needs and feedback of the communities served. This case study highlights not only technological innovation but also the importance of cultural competence and the need to build trust through active community engagement in AI-driven health initiatives.

## Case Study: Enhancing Mental Health Support in Southeast Asian Communities Through AI

In many Southeast Asian communities, mental health often carries a stigma, and resources are limited, particularly in rural areas. An innovative community-driven AI initiative was designed to tackle these challenges by enhancing mental health support through culturally attuned AI technologies. This case study outlines the intricate processes of implementation, the challenges faced, and the transformative impact of the AI initiative, emphasizing the critical role of community involvement in its success.

The project began with a series of collaborative workshops that brought together mental health professionals, AI developers, local healers, and community representatives. The primary aims were to identify prevalent mental health issues within the communities, understand cultural attitudes towards mental health, and gather data that would inform the development of an AI solution. These initial discussions revealed a strong preference for confidentiality and traditional healing practices, which guided the AI's design and functionality.

A mobile application was developed, equipped with AI tools that can provide initial mental health assessments, personalized coping strategies, and crisis management support. The AI was trained with anonymized mental health data from the region, supplemented with insights into local healing practices and languages. Integration of natural language processing enabled the tool to offer support in regional dialects, dramatically increasing accessibility and user engagement.

However, the deployment was met with initial skepticism. Ongoing community engagement strategies were essential in gaining trust. Monthly feedback sessions were incorporated to address concerns, update functionalities, and educate the community about mental health. These feedback loops allowed the AI system to evolve continuously, resonating more deeply with community needs and reducing the stigma associated with mental health discussions.

The impact was significant, with reported increases in users seeking help and an observable decrease in common stress-related symptoms among regular users. The project's success highlighted the indispensable nature of aligning technological solutions with cultural sensitivity and community involvement, ensuring both practical and socially sustainable AI outcomes.

## Case Study: Integrating AI with Indigenous Agricultural Practices for Disease Prediction

In the expansive agricultural fields of Central America, a pioneering AI-driven project was undertaken in collaboration with local agricultural communities and AI developers focused on predictive analytics for crop diseases. This initiative aimed at integrating traditional agricultural knowledge with modern AI technology to enhance crop yields and disease management. The collaboration was instrumental in creating a culturally sensitive AI model that respects and leverages the wisdom of indigenous practices.

The project began with extensive field visits by AI researchers and several community workshops to gather local farmers' insights on signs of crop diseases and their traditional methods of controlling them. These interactions provided a wealth of data on indigenous knowledge, which was previously undocumented. The AI developers used these insights to train machine learning models that could predict crop disease outbreaks based on weather conditions, soil type, and traditional indicators recognized by the farmers.

Key to the project's success was the development of a user-friendly mobile application that could be used even by farmers with limited technical skills. The application not only forecasted potential disease outbreaks but also suggested culturally accepted management practices and organic treatment options, aligning with the traditional agricultural practices of the community.

However, the adoption of this technology presented challenges. Initially, there was skepticism from the local farmers towards relying on digital tools for farming, a practice they had mastered over generations through hands-on experience. To overcome this, the project team established a continuous feedback system that allowed farmers to report on the accuracy of the AI predictions and the effectiveness of the recommended treatment methodologies.

Over time, as farmers saw tangible benefits in terms of reduced crop losses and increased yields, trust in the technology grew. The AI system continually adapted to incorporate real-time feedback from farmers, refining its predictions and recommendations. This case study highlights the power of blending traditional knowledge with advanced technology and illustrates how AI can be crafted not just to support but actively enhance indigenous practices for sustainable agricultural success.

### Case Study: AI-Driven Public Health Strategies in Urban Slums: A Community-Based Approach

The deployment of community-driven, AI-powered public health initiatives in the urban slums of Southeast Asia provides an illustrative case study on applying artificial intelligence to complex social contexts characterized by high densities, informal economies, and limited healthcare infrastructure. This project aimed to leverage AI to improve public healthcare outcomes by tailoring strategies to the unique needs and behavioral patterns of slum dwellers.

The initiative commenced with the formation of an interdisciplinary team including AI developers, public health experts, community leaders, and local NGOs. Early stages involved meticulous community mapping to gather data on common health issues, demographic factors, and existing healthcare resources. It was imperative to ensure that data collection respected privacy and cultural norms, utilizing community liaisons to foster trust and participation.

An AI system was then designed to analyze the collected data, identifying key health challenges, including infectious disease outbreaks, malnutrition rates, and healthcare access barriers. Machine learning algorithms predicted high-risk areas and times for health issues, enabling the more effective allocation of medical resources and the timely implementation of interventions. Importantly, the AI platform incorporated a feedback mechanism allowing continuous community input to refine its predictions and operations.

On the deployment front, mobile health units equipped with AI-driven diagnostic tools began regular visits to identified high-risk areas, providing screening, vaccines, and basic healthcare services. These units also collected additional health data to inform the AI model, ensuring a dynamic and adaptive public health strategy. Community health workers received training on AI tool interfaces and basic data interpretation, enhancing their role as both care providers and data collectors.

Challenges included initial distrust in AI technologies, logistical issues in data collection, and cultural barriers in the acceptance of certain medical interventions. Overcoming these barriers was achieved through ongoing community engagement, transparent communication about AI processes, and visible improvements in healthcare outcomes. Crucially, adapting public health strategies to incorporate local traditional medicine practices where possible helped in gaining wider acceptance.

### Case Study: AI Tailored Drug Therapies in Diverse Populations

The evolving landscape of personalized medicine in diverse urban populations provides a compelling case study of community-driven AI in healthcare. In one major U.S. city, health disparities among ethnic groups concerning drug efficacy and adverse reactions were notably high due to genetic diversity. In response, a local university partnered with healthcare providers and AI developers to address these challenges by creating a community-driven AI model that tailors drug therapies.

The initiative started with the establishment of a biobank of genetic material voluntarily contributed by a diverse cross-section of the community. Community meetings were held to ensure transparency about how the genetic data would be used and to address concerns about privacy and data use. Insights from local healthcare professionals, coupled with historical health data from the community, provided a preliminary framework for the AI's learning algorithm.

Using machine learning, the AI system analyzed genetic markers that influence drug metabolism and response to treatment. It was designed to provide personalized drug therapy recommendations, potentially reducing adverse drug reactions and increasing the efficacy of treatments. The system was initially tested in a controlled environment, where it successfully recommended alternatives to standard dosages and drug types for individuals with specific genetic markers associated with poor drug metabolism.

However, challenges arose during broad implementation, including resistance from individuals wary of genetic discrimination and the integration of technology into existing health systems. Continuous community engagement was crucial; regular updates, workshops, and open feedback sessions were implemented to educate the public on genetic privacy, the benefits of personalized therapies, and to collect ongoing input to refine the AI algorithms.

Eventually, as the community saw tangible benefits such as fewer adverse reactions and more effective drug treatments, trust in the AI system grew. The project not only highlighted the potential of AI to personalize medicine in genetically diverse populations but also underscored the importance of community involvement in addressing complex ethical and practical challenges.

### Case Study: AI-Assisted Language Adaptation for Healthcare Communication in Multilingual Societies

In the diverse urban landscape of Megacity, with its melting pot of cultures and languages, effective communication in healthcare settings posed a significant barrier. An innovative project was launched to address these challenges, utilizing artificial intelligence to break down language barriers and enhance healthcare outcomes. This case study illustrates the process of AI implementation, the collaboration with local communities, and the significant improvements achieved in patient-doctor communication.

The project began with a collaborative venture between AI developers, healthcare professionals, and linguistic experts, aiming to develop an AI-driven tool that could translate and adapt healthcare communication into several predominant local languages. The initiative also sought to understand and integrate culturally specific expressions and medical terminologies that are particularly challenging to translate directly.

Data was meticulously collected from various local health institutions, alongside input gathered through community workshops and surveys to delineate commonly faced issues in healthcare communication. This data informed the training of an AI model capable of understanding and effectively translating nuanced language, ensuring both medical accuracy and cultural appropriateness. The AI tool was integrated into patient management systems of local clinics as a pilot test, providing real-time translation services during patient interactions.

During the initial rollout, significant challenges were faced, including the reluctance of older healthcare providers to adapt to new technologies and varying dialects that complicated translation accuracy. Continuous feedback mechanisms were established, allowing for rapid iterations of the AI tool based on real-time user experiences. Over time, these adaptations significantly improved the tool's accuracy and user-friendliness.

The impact of this AI-powered communication tool was profound. It led to a notable decrease in misdiagnosis rates, improved patient satisfaction, and a higher rate of treatment adherence among non-native language speakers. This case study serves as a model for how AI can enhance communication in healthcare, resulting in improved outcomes and greater equity in medical service delivery.

## Review Questions

**1. A 55-year-old male patient with chronic back pain visits a healthcare clinic utilizing a community-driven AI system for diagnosis and treatment recommendations. Despite his extensive use of traditional herbal treatments and participation in local spiritual healing ceremonies, the AI system does not recognize these practices and suggests standard pharmacological treatments, which the patient has previously found ineffective. He feels his cultural practices are being overlooked. Which of the following should be integrated into the AI system to accommodate patients like these?**

A) Inclusion of ethnographic and cultural data relevant to the patient's background

B) Enhanced pharmacological database for alternative herbal remedies

C) Upgraded imaging technology for precise anatomical diagnosis

D) Expansion of only biomedically approved treatment options

**Answer: A**

Explanation: Integrating ethnographic and cultural data into the AI system will enable it to recognize and validate diverse healing practices beyond Western medicine, such as patients' use of traditional herbal treatments and participation in spiritual healing ceremonies. This inclusion respects cultural diversity and provides a more personalized and holistic approach to healthcare, potentially increasing the acceptance and effectiveness of the proposed treatments for patients from various cultural backgrounds.

**2. A clinical trial is designed to utilize AI to identify effective interventions for patients with diabetes, leveraging a comprehensive dataset that encompasses both conventional medical treatment outcomes and integrative approaches incorporating traditional Native American herbal remedies. What could be a potential outcome of this AI integration for the diabetes management program?**

A) Development of biased AI models due to overrepresentation of conventional treatments

B) Improvement in personalized treatment plans that incorporate traditional Native American knowledge

C) Decrease in patient compliance due to distrust in AI recommendations

D) Limitation of treatment options to only those that are biomedically proven

**Answer: B**

Explanation: By incorporating traditional Native American herbal remedies into the dataset, the AI can learn from a diverse range of effective treatments. This could lead to improved personalized treatment plans that respect and integrate the cultural and traditional healing practices of Native American patients. Such an approach not only broadens the therapeutic options available but also enhances patient trust and compliance, recognizing the value of their cultural health practices.

**3. An AI system in a multicultural city is tasked with recommending mental health treatment for a diverse population. To ensure cultural competence, what strategy should AI developers use when creating the recommendation algorithms?**

A) Limit the input data to only include treatments backed by strong biomedicine research

B) Incorporate a diverse set of treatment modalities, including spiritual counseling and community-based therapies

C) Focus on developing algorithmic efficiency without considering cultural implications

D) Exclude non-pharmacological treatments to streamline the decision-making process

**Answer: B**

Explanation: Incorporating a diverse set of treatment modalities, including spiritual counseling and community-based therapies, ensures that the AI system can offer culturally appropriate recommendations. This approach respects the healing practices of various cultures represented in the multicultural city, improving the relevance and acceptability of the treatment suggestions. Considering the wide array of cultural beliefs and practices in mental health treatments enhances patient engagement and treatment effectiveness.

**4. A Native American community is seeking to integrate AI into their healthcare system, with a focus on managing traditional herbal treatments. What is an essential consideration for integrating AI to protect the community's interests?**

A) Prioritizing AI algorithms developed by external tech companies

B) Ensuring AI systems are exclusively managed by biomedical professionals

C) Embedding community participation in the development and deployment of AI systems

D) Keeping the traditional knowledge out of AI systems to prevent misuse

**Answer: C**

Explanation: Embedding community participation in the development and deployment of AI systems is crucial for protecting and respecting the community's interests. By involving the community, especially traditional healers and knowledge keepers, in the AI's development, the system will be better tailored to the specific needs and cultural practices of the community. This collaborative approach helps ensure that traditional herbal treatments are represented accurately and used appropriately within AI-enhanced healthcare, safeguarding intellectual property and cultural integrity.

**Case Studies: Successful Integrations of AI and Traditional Medicine**

**Integrating AI with Ayurvedic Medicine: Improvements in Diagnostic Accuracy**

The integration of artificial intelligence with Ayurvedic medicine is revolutionizing diagnostic accuracies, fostering a synthesis of traditional wisdom and modern technology. AI tools are now analyzing vast arrays of herbal combinations and patient data to predict therapeutic outcomes with astonishing precision. This synergy not only enhances the personalization of treatments but also significantly reduces error margins in diagnosis.

Pioneering projects have employed machine learning algorithms to interpret the complex patterns of doshas (body energies) and their imbalances, considered fundamental in Ayurveda. These AI systems learn from historical treatment data, refining their diagnostic models to align with Ayurvedic principles, ensuring that treatments are both tailored and effective.

Moreover, the digitization of ancient texts through natural language processing allows AI to access and utilize centuries-old knowledge. This integration respects the tradition's integrity while opening new avenues for its application in contemporary medical scenarios. As a result, AI is not merely an adjunct but a potent tool that propels Ayurvedic medicine into the digital era, enhancing its global relevance and efficacy.

## Blending Traditional Chinese Medicine with AI for Enhanced Drug Discovery

The fusion of Artificial Intelligence with Traditional Chinese Medicine (TCM) is spearheading a transformation in drug discovery, marrying ancient wisdom with cutting-edge science. By analyzing classical TCM formulations and vast databases of herbal properties, AI is innovating the identification of active compounds that could revolutionize modern pharmacology.

Advanced machine learning models simulate TCM compound interactions at an unprecedented scale, enabling the efficient discovery of potential therapies for chronic illnesses compared to conventional methods. These AI systems not only accelerate the R&D cycle but also reduce costs, making groundbreaking treatments more accessible. Furthermore, by respecting and integrating the holistic TCM approach, these AI models ensure culturally nuanced health solutions that are more likely to be embraced by both practitioners and patients.

Ultimately, this collaboration aims to validate and revive interest in TCM globally, enhancing its credibility and applicability in the international medical community. AI's contribution is pivotal in bridging the gap between traditional therapies and modern clinical needs, leading to a more inclusive global health paradigm.

## AI-Driven Analysis of Indigenous American Herbal Practices

The integration of AI with Indigenous American herbal practices marks a promising frontier in personalized medicine. Utilizing machine learning, researchers have begun to decode complex patterns found in traditional herbal remedies, revealing new insights into their efficacy and potential applications. This AI-driven approach not only helps validate long-held indigenous wisdom but also enhances the accuracy of identifying plant-based treatments specific to individual health needs.

In this analysis, AI algorithms are trained with extensive databases of herbal components, their historical uses, and outcomes noted in various tribal communities. The technology then predicts possible synergies and interactions between herbs, providing a scientific basis for their medicinal properties, which were traditionally passed down orally. This meticulous process respects and preserves the integrity of cultural knowledge while providing a scalable method to explore and potentially expand the use of herbal medicines.

Furthermore, AI's capability to process vast amounts of data rapidly accelerates the research phase, reducing time and cost compared to traditional methods. By linking traditional practices with modern healthcare frameworks, AI facilitates a more holistic approach to medicine, emphasizing preventive care and natural remedies, thereby aligning with global trends towards sustainable health solutions.

## Case Study: AI Applications in Unani Medicine

In a monumental stride towards the amalgamation of ancient wisdom with modern technology, AI applications in Unani Medicine herald a new era of medical diagnostics and treatment. Sophisticated machine learning models are being designed to interpret the principles of Unani, such as the humoral theory (theory of humors or five elements), which is crucial to patient diagnosis and treatment management. These AI systems are trained on extensive data from herbal prescriptions and patient outcomes, thereby enhancing the precision and customization of treatments.

Another aspect involves digital preservation of age-old Unani texts, where natural language processing tools are deployed to translate and decode classical Arabic and Persian texts into actionable medical knowledge. This not only safeguards the historical richness of Unani Medicine but also makes it accessible to researchers and practitioners worldwide.

Conclusively, the integration of AI in Unani practices not only bridges the gap between traditional and modern healthcare but also fortifies the relevance of Unani Medicine in today's digital age. This pioneering approach promises to enhance patient care while respecting and revitalizing a time-honored medical tradition.

**Implementing AI for Better Accessibility of African Traditional Medicines**

The integration of artificial intelligence (AI) into African traditional medicine is transforming accessibility and understanding of time-honored healing practices across the continent. By digitizing and analyzing vast archives of medicinal plants and indigenous knowledge, AI is breaking down barriers between remote, underserved communities and the global health landscape.

AI technology helps catalog various plant properties and their historical uses in African traditional medicine. These digital databases are then utilized to create accessible, user-friendly platforms where practitioners and patients alike can explore and utilize traditional remedies with greater ease and precision. The technology also facilitates the distribution of this knowledge more evenly across regions that may have been previously isolated or underserved.

Moreover, the application of AI in this field supports the standardization and quality control of herbal medicines. AI algorithms help identify optimal harvesting periods, processing methods, and preservation techniques, thereby enhancing the efficacy of natural remedies. Through this thoughtful incorporation of AI, the depth and breadth of African traditional medicine are preserved and celebrated, paving the way for a future where modern technology and ancient wisdom coexist and enrich the global health community.

**Collaboration between AI and Traditional Hawaiian Healing Techniques**

The innovative merging of AI with traditional Hawaiian healing techniques represents a groundbreaking advancement in holistic healthcare. By integrating machine learning algorithms with the rich heritage of native Hawaiian practices, such as Lā'au lapa'au (herbal medicine) and Lomi Lomi (massage), AI is enabling deeper insights into their methodologies and efficacy.

AI systems are trained to analyze patterns within historical healing outcomes, thereby providing a robust framework for predicting and enhancing therapeutic results. This collaboration extends beyond mere data analysis, respecting and revitalizing ancestral wisdom through modern technology. Such initiatives help preserve and propagate these age-old practices globally while ensuring they meet contemporary health standards.

Moreover, the partnership between AI and Hawaiian healers also supports the sustainability of local medicinal plants, utilizing predictive analytics to optimize their usage and conservation. Ultimately, this fusion paves a new path for the symbiosis of technology and tradition, enhancing the accessibility and effectiveness of Hawaiian healing arts.

**Enhancing Naturopathic Medicine with AI-Based Predictive Tools**

The integration of AI-based predictive tools into naturopathic medicine is revolutionizing the approach to natural and preventative healthcare. Harnessing the power of data analytics, these tools enable practitioners to craft highly personalized treatment plans tailored to the individual characteristics and health needs of each patient.

Machine learning algorithms analyze vast arrays of patient data, including genetic information, lifestyle factors, and previous health records, to predict potential health risks and recommend preventive naturopathic interventions. This precise customization enhances the effectiveness of treatments, including dietary changes, herbal supplements, and holistic wellness strategies.

Additionally, AI's predictive capabilities facilitate the early detection of diseases, allowing for timely naturopathic interventions that can significantly alter a patient's health trajectory positively. This fusion of technology and traditional healing not only empowers healthcare providers but also offers patients a more proactive stance in managing their health.

**Successful Integration of AI in Japanese Kampo Medicine**

The integration of artificial intelligence (AI) in Japanese Kampo (Japanese Acupuncture-acupressure commonly practice in Jiu-Jitsu) medicine illustrates a significant advancement in blending traditional practices with modern computational techniques. AI's role in Kampo has primarily been in enhancing the precision of herbal formulations, which are central to this centuries-old medical system. By employing machine learning algorithms, researchers can analyze historical efficacy data and patient outcomes to optimize these formulations for individual needs.

AI tools also assist in deciphering the complex interactions between different herbs. This not only streamlines the development of effective treatment plans but also revitalizes interest in Kampo practices, ensuring they remain relevant in contemporary healthcare settings. Moreover, AI's analytical power helps in identifying potential new applications for traditional herbs, further broadening the scope of Kampo medicine.

Thus, the thoughtful application of AI in Kampo medicine not only preserves but also expands this traditional wisdom, offering refined solutions that uphold both historical significance and modern health standards. This synergy between AI and Japanese herbalism serves as a model for preserving cultural heritage while embracing technological advancements.

**Utilization of AI in Analyzing Traditional Korean Medicine**

The intersection of AI and Traditional Korean Medicine (TKM-AMMA-Altong, Koreo Jin and Su Jok Acupuncture) marks a significant milestone in the globalization of medicine. By leveraging cutting-edge AI, researchers can delve deep into the vast repository of herbal knowledge and diagnostic systems of TKM. Sophisticated algorithms analyze patterns in herbal efficacy and interactions, providing insights that refine and validate centuries-old practices for global application.

Machine learning models also facilitate the translation and interpretation of ancient texts and medical records, making them accessible to practitioners worldwide. This not only enhances the understanding and application of TKM but also ensures its authenticity and adherence to traditional principles. The AI-enabled platforms are becoming crucial in advancing research and developing integrated treatment solutions that respect the holistic nature of Korean medicine.

Furthermore, AI aids in predicting treatment outcomes by correlating traditional methods with modern medical data, essentially bridging the gap between the old and the new. This homogeneous integration fosters a more inclusive approach to health, symbolizing a blend of legacy and progress in the pursuit of well-being.

## AI Strategies That Respect Shamanic Practices

The symbiotic relationship between AI and shamanic healing practices opens transformative avenues in healthcare. By integrating AI into these ancient rites, practitioners can preserve nuanced traditions while enhancing diagnostic and therapeutic precision. AI tools are crafted to analyze ritualistic patterns and outcomes, ensuring respect for the spiritual dimensions of shamanism.

In this context, AI systems are designed with cultural sensitivity at their core, engaging with healers to understand and codify esoteric knowledge without stripping it of its essence. These systems help predict health outcomes based on spiritual and herbal interventions, making them invaluable for remote or underserved communities where such practices are predominant.

Furthermore, AI contributes to the global recognition and validation of shamanic medicine, articulating its efficacy and mechanisms in a scientific language that can be understood worldwide. This not only safeguards these practices but also encourages a respectful integration of global healing traditions.

## Intersecting AI with Islamic Medical Traditions

The fusion of AI with Islamic medical traditions offers a unique blend of historical healing practices and modern computational power. Islamic medicine, rooted in rich prophetic teachings and characterized by holistic approaches such as herbal remedies, dietary regulations, and spiritual care, provides a fertile ground for AI integration. AI tools can analyze traditional prescriptions and patient outcomes to enhance the individualization of treatments.

Furthermore, by leveraging machine learning, researchers explore the efficacy of herbs and dietary recommendations documented in ancient Islamic texts. This could lead to the development of more personalized medicine, respecting both the cultural nuances and the therapeutic integrity of the traditional methods. This intersection also opens opportunities for a greater understanding of the preventive aspects of Islamic medicine, particularly its emphasis on lifestyle and mental health.

Lastly, AI's role in cataloging and validating centuries-old Islamic medicinal knowledge helps preserve it, ensuring that these healing traditions are not lost but rather evolved. Integrating AI thus supports not just the preservation but also the innovative expansion of Islamic medical practices in contemporary settings.

## Bolstering Old Russian Healing Techniques Through AI Tools

The pioneering integration of Artificial Intelligence (AI) into old Russian healing techniques (znakharki Meditsinskie) is redefining the landscape of traditional medicine in Russia. AI tools are now being employed to decipher and enhance the vast array of herbal remedies, therapies, and preventive measures that have been part of Russian folklore for centuries. Through the application of machine learning algorithms, researchers can analyze historical data and patient outcomes to improve the efficacy and specificity of these traditional treatments.

This digital intervention helps standardize and document age-old practices, ensuring their preservation and accessibility. AI's capability to sift through large datasets allows for the identification of patterns that human researchers might overlook, paving the way for innovative applications and the validation of Russian herbal medicine.

Furthermore, AI enhances the customization of treatments to individual needs, integrating traditional Russian practices with modern medical approaches, and fostering a unique healthcare model that respects cultural heritage while embracing contemporary advancements.

The application of AI in South American tribal medicine represents a pivotal endeavor in preserving and enhancing indigenous healthcare practices. This case study explores the collaborative projects that integrate advanced artificial intelligence technologies with traditional healing techniques unique to South American tribes. By utilizing AI, researchers have been able to catalog vast amounts of undocumented medicinal plants and their uses, capturing invaluable ethnobotanical knowledge that was at risk of being lost.

Furthermore, AI systems analyze patterns in treatment effectiveness, correlating traditional remedies with clinical outcomes. This not only validates the medicinal potency of tribal practices but also integrates these solutions into broader healthcare systems, offering a complementary approach to conventional medicine. The engagement also respects the cultural significance of each practice, ensuring that technology serves as an ally rather than a disruptor.

These integrations, spearheaded by both local healers and AI experts, mark a transformative phase in healthcare, where technology enhances the reach and recognition of ancient wisdom in modern medical settings, promoting a nuanced appreciation and application of traditional South American healing modalities.

## Modeling AI Systems to Understand Native Canadian Healing

The integration of AI into Native Canadian healing practices offers a groundbreaking perspective on indigenous healthcare systems. By developing AI models tailored to understand the complexities of these traditional practices, researchers are pioneering a new form of cultural and medical synthesis. These models are designed to analyze historical and contemporary data on herbal remedies, ritualistic practices, and healing ceremonies, uncovering patterns that might otherwise remain obscured.

This approach not only assists in cataloging vast amounts of indigenous knowledge but also in validating the efficacy of Native Canadian healing practices within the framework of modern science. AI systems facilitate a dialogue between traditional knowledge holders and global medical communities, enhancing mutual understanding and respect.

Moreover, the use of AI helps in personalizing healthcare, adapting ancient wisdom to meet individual health needs. This tailored approach promises to significantly improve healthcare outcomes for communities that continue to rely on their ancestral practices. The combination of AI and Native Canadian healing traditions is a testament to the potential of technology to preserve and revitalize ancient wisdom in contemporary contexts.

## AI-Assisted Personalization of Ayurvedic Treatment Plans

AI is revolutionizing Ayurvedic medicine by personalizing treatment plans, fusing millennia-old wisdom with contemporary computational techniques. This seamless integration starts with the diagnostic procedure. Machine learning algorithms interpret the unique physiological and psychological data derived from patients, aligning them with Ayurvedic constitutions (doshas), which govern bodily energy and are crucial to individual health diagnostics.

Bespoke treatment plans are then dynamically configured by AI, taking into account intricate details such as seasonal variations, geographic climatic conditions, and the patient's daily routine. This meticulousness ensures the treatments are finely tuned to the individual's systemic balance, enhancing efficacy and reducing potential side effects. Moreover, AI's predictive analytics help foresee possible adverse interactions between herbal prescriptions and conventional medications when used concurrently.

Finally, AI systems accumulate and learn from each interaction, continuously optimizing and refining treatment protocols. This adaptive learning promotes a deeper understanding and more comprehensive integration of Ayurvedic principles in global healthcare contexts, thereby making personalized Ayurvedic healthcare more accessible worldwide.

## Evaluation of AI's Accuracy in the Context of Zootherapeutic Medicines

The application of AI in the realm of zootherapeutic medicines, which utilize animals or animal-derived substances for healing, is altering perceptions and methodologies in traditional medicine practices. By applying advanced analytical techniques, AI can quantify and validate the efficacy of treatments that have been used ancestrally across various cultures but have often been overlooked by conventional medicine due to a lack of empirical evidence.

AI's role extends to enhancing the accuracy of diagnosing conditions that are traditionally treated with zootherapeutic methods. Through machine learning models, AI can analyze complex patterns of patient responses to treatments, which improves the precision of these traditional remedies. This scientific validation not only bolsters the credibility of zootherapeutic medicines but also facilitates their integration into modern healthcare systems.

Moreover, AI tools assist in safeguarding biodiversity by predicting sustainable harvesting methods of zootherapeutic resources. This ensures that the ecological balance is maintained while leveraging these ancient practices for contemporary medical use, creating a harmonious blend of conservation and healthcare innovation.

## AI as a Tool for Preservation and Validation of Local Medicine in Oceania

In Oceania, where diverse islands are home to unique medicinal knowledge, AI is playing a crucial role in preserving and validating local healing traditions. By digitizing traditional remedies and techniques, AI systems enable the analysis and categorization of indigenous wisdom that was once vulnerable to loss from one generation to the next. This technological embrace is safeguarding ancestral health practices across the vast Pacific.

Moreover, AI's analytical prowess brings rigorous scientific validation to these traditional methods, often based on holistic and environmental considerations unique to each island culture. By bridging the gap between empirical science and traditional know-how, AI is not only affirming the value of Oceanian medicine in the global healthcare landscape but is also enhancing its integration into modern medical practices.

The collaboration between local healers and AI experts fosters a respectful and synergistic exchange, ensuring that these age-old practices are neither exploited nor misrepresented. Through this innovative partnership, AI proves itself as an indispensable ally in the resurgence and legitimization of Oceania's traditional medicine, offering a model for similar initiatives worldwide.

## Using AI to Enhance Traditional Slavic Herbal Treatments

The integration of AI in Slavic herbal treatments marks a significant milestone in the convergence of ancient wisdom and modern technology. By digitizing and analyzing centuries-old Slavic recipes and herbal concoctions, AI is redefining the scope and efficacy of traditional remedies known for their natural healing powers. This process involves the sophisticated use of machine learning algorithms to scrutinize the properties and synergies between different herbs, ensuring a more refined understanding of their medicinal potential.

Moreover, AI assists in customizing herbal treatments to individual patient profiles, considering genetic predispositions and existing health conditions, thereby enhancing both the safety and effectiveness of traditional Slavic medicine. This tailored approach not only preserves cultural heritage but also aligns it with contemporary clinical practices, offering personalized care pathways.

Continued advancements in AI are poised to further enhance the precision of herbal treatment protocols, fostering a resurgence of interest and trust in Slavic herbalism within global healthcare paradigms. Through these sophisticated AI applications, traditional Slavic medicine is not only preserved but also enhanced, making it relevant and accessible in today's medical landscape.

### Case Studies: AI's Role in Facilitating Better Understanding of Māori Rongoā

The intersection of AI with Māori Rongoā, traditional New Zealand healing practices, marks a profound stride toward cultural preservation and medical innovation. By incorporating AI, researchers can decipher complex patterns within the multifaceted knowledge of herbalism and therapeutic rituals among the Māori, providing a clearer understanding of their efficacy and potential applications in modern medicine.

This AI-enhanced approach facilitates a more nuanced analysis of Rongoā practices, which often intertwine spiritual well-being with physical health, offering a holistic overview that conventional medical research methodologies may overlook. The digital modeling of these traditions facilitates the translation of age-old wisdom into actionable data that can enhance health outcomes, while ensuring that these practices are respected and accurately represented within academic and healthcare frameworks.

Moreover, as AI technologies evolve, the potential for these tools to adapt and respect the intricacies of Māori cultural protocols improves, ensuring that the integration of Rongoā into global healthcare respects the values of the source culture. Such applications highlight AI's capacity not only as a technological tool but as a bridge between ancient healing arts and contemporary scientific practices.

### AI-Enhanced Interpretation of Ancient Egyptian Medicinal Practices

The implementation of AI in interpreting ancient Egyptian medicinal practices unveils a fascinating synthesis of historical depth and cutting-edge technology. Machine learning models delve into hieroglyphic prescriptions, translating and correlating them with modern insights in phytotherapy. This process illuminates the sophisticated botanical knowledge that ancient Egyptians utilized, bridging thousands of years in medical evolution.

Moreover, AI tools analyze patterns in recorded treatments, identifying efficacy and potential modern applications. For instance, AI has identified parallels between ancient remedies and the current pharmacological uses of certain plants, lending credibility and uncovering new applications to these age-old treatments. This not only validates the ancient wisdom but also expands the repertoire of contemporary medicine.

Furthermore, virtual simulations created by AI enable researchers to test ancient Egyptian formulations in virtual environments, predicting outcomes without the ethical or logistical complications of real-world testing. These AI-driven explorations are critical in reintegrating historically significant medical knowledge into today's healthcare landscape, offering new perspectives on wellness and treatment.

### AI Integration in the Study of Traditional Tibetan Healing Methods

In the realm of traditional Tibetan healing, the integration of artificial intelligence marks a significant advancement. Utilizing AI to analyze and interpret ancient texts and practices, such as those in *'Sowa Rigpa'*, the science of healing, enhances understanding and application in modern contexts. This involves digitizing old manuscripts and deploying natural language processing to unveil insights previously obscured by language barriers and historical gaps.

AI's role extends further to identifying patterns in patient responses to various treatments. By correlating these with historical efficacy reports, AI creates a database that supports more tailored and effective healing strategies. Such technology not only enriches the practice but also ensures its viability and relevance in the contemporary medical landscape.

Moreover, AI simulations enable predictive analysis, projecting the outcomes of traditional remedies under various conditions. This both preserves and innovates Tibetan medicine, ensuring it's adapted accurately and respectfully, linking ancient wisdom with cutting-edge technology in a seamless fusion that respects heritage while embracing progress.

## Utilizing AI to Bridge Modern Psychotherapy with Traditional Spiritual Practices

The fusion of AI with the spiritual dimensions of traditional healing practices presents a groundbreaking approach in modern psychotherapy. By integrating machine learning with spiritual rituals, AI is equipped to identify and enhance the therapeutic elements inherent in age-old spiritual traditions. This synthesis facilitates a deeper understanding of the psychological impacts of spiritual practices, potentially leading to more effective mental health interventions.

In this realm, AI algorithms analyze data derived from spiritual sessions, discerning patterns that contribute to emotional and mental well-being. This innovative use of technology enables psychotherapists to tailor spiritual practices to individual needs, creating personalized therapeutic plans that balance modern science with traditional wisdom.

Furthermore, these AI-driven insights not only validate the significance of spiritual practices in mental healing but also ensure that such ancient knowledge is preserved and propagated in a manner that aligns with contemporary therapeutic frameworks. Thus, AI acts not just as a tool of innovation but as a bridge that thoughtfully connects the past with the present, enhancing the holistic approach to mental health.

## AI Applications in Central Asian Nomadic Medicinal Knowledge

The adaptation of AI in exploring Central Asian nomadic medicinal knowledge presents a pioneering leap into marrying ancient cures with modern algorithms. Nomadic tribes, known for their deep-rooted herbal wisdom passed down through generations, find a digital counterpart in AI that sifts through vast ethnographic and botanical data. These mapping patterns have been almost forgotten by time.

By implementing Natural Language Processing (NLP), AI deciphers historical texts and oral traditions, transforming them into comprehensive databases. This aids in the resurgence of nomadic recipes, providing a scientific backbone to their traditional uses. It allows a factual basis for integrating these age-old remedies into contemporary medical practices without compromising their essence.

Furthermore, AI simulation models provide predictive analyses on the efficacy of these traditional remedies for various modern-day ailments, ensuring a tailored and effective application. Thus, the symbiosis between AI and Central Asian nomadic medicine not only preserves but revitalizes ancient wisdom in a modern health paradigm.

## Development of AI Systems for Enhanced Effectiveness in Traditional Thai Therapeutics

The integration of AI in Thai therapeutics, particularly in the realm of traditional Thai medicine, represents a significant evolution in healthcare. By applying AI technologies to the ancient wisdom encompassed in Thai herbalism and massage therapies, there is newfound potential to refine diagnostic procedures and expand treatment effectiveness.

AI algorithms analyze herbal combinations and treatment outcomes, providing insights that were previously inaccessible due to the subjective nature of traditional practice assessments. This fusion not only increases the credibility of Thai remedies in the global market but also refines their application, making them more personalized and effective.

The employment of AI further aids in preserving these cultural medicinal practices by documenting, validating, and propagating traditional knowledge in a format that is both accessible and scientifically endorsed. This thoughtful integration ensures that Thai therapeutic wisdom continues to flourish, bridging the gap between age-old practices and modern medical techniques.

## Summary

This chapter explores various case studies where Artificial Intelligence (AI) has been integrated with traditional medical systems worldwide, demonstrating significant enhancements in diagnostics, drug discovery, and personalized treatment. The fusion of AI with Ayurvedic medicine exemplifies a remarkable advancement in diagnostic accuracy, where AI's capability to analyze complex data and historical patterns has enhanced treatment personalization and error reduction. Similarly, Traditional Chinese Medicine (TCM) has seen revolutionary progress in drug discovery through AI's ability to analyze herbal properties and interactions, drastically improving efficiency in identifying new therapeutic potentials. Indigenous practices, such as those from Native American, African, and Oceanian traditions, have also capitalized on AI to preserve valuable medicinal knowledge and integrate it into contemporary medical practices more effectively. AI's role in these integrations typically involves creating extensive databases, utilizing predictive analytics, and enhancing understanding through the digitization of ancient texts and oral traditions. For instance, AI's application in Unani and Kampo medicine has not only recalibrated traditional formulations for modern relevance but also preserved the integrity of these age-old practices through digital translations and modeling. Furthermore, the chapter covers how AI enhances the accessibility and effectiveness of holistic treatments, including those stemming from Hawaiian, Russian, and South American tribal medicine, by aiding in the standardization, quality control, and personalized treatment planning, thus bridging the gap between traditional remedies and modern medical requirements. Through these diverse examples, the chapter illustrates AI's pivotal role in validating, revitalizing, and integrating traditional medical wisdom into the global health system, paving the way for a more inclusive, efficient, and personalized medical paradigm.

## References

[1] Integrating Artificial Intelligence into Traditional Medicine Systems. https://example.com/ai-traditional-medicine
[2] Advances in AI for Traditional Chinese Medicine Drug Discovery. https://example.com/ai-tcm
[3] AI Applications in Indigenous Medicinal Practices. https://example.com/ai-indigenous-medicine
[4] Digital Preservation and Enhancement of Unani Medicine through AI. https://example.com/ai-unani-medicine
[5] AI's Role in Enhancing Traditional Kampo Medicine. https://example.com/ai-kampo

### Case Study: Integrating AI in Enhancing Traditional Balinese Healing Techniques

The island of Bali, Indonesia, renowned for its unique cultural tapestry, is also home to a diverse array of traditional healing practices deeply rooted in local spirituality and the natural environment. A pioneering project that integrates Artificial Intelligence (AI) with traditional Balinese healing techniques offers a captivating case study on the intersection of technology and indigenous medicine. Balinese healers, known locally as 'Balian,' utilize a combination of herbal remedies, massage techniques, and spiritual guidance to treat physical and mental ailments. This multifaceted approach, although effective, often faced challenges in terms of standardization and widespread documentation due to its highly personalized and oral transmission nature.

To address these challenges, a collaborative effort was initiated among local healers, researchers, and AI technologists. The project's first phase involved digitizing and cataloging the various herbal remedies and massage techniques used by the Balian. Utilizing Natural Language Processing (NLP) technologies, the vast amount of qualitative data gathered from the healers was codified into a structured digital format, making it accessible for further analysis.

Following the digitization of the data, AI-powered machine learning algorithms were developed to analyze patterns in remedy effectiveness and patient outcomes. This analysis enabled the identification of the most effective combinations of herbs and techniques for specific conditions, significantly enhancing the personalization of treatments while preserving the essence of traditional practices. Furthermore, predictive analytics were employed to recommend adjustments in treatment plans according to seasonal changes and patient responses, significantly enhancing the adaptability of Balinese healing traditions.

In the concluding phase of the project, an interactive AI-driven platform was launched to disseminate this integrated knowledge, allowing global access while respecting the cultural significance of the healing practices. This platform not only facilitated the education of a new generation of healers but also ensured that Balinese traditional medicine could be preserved and practiced far beyond its geographic origins.

### Case Study: Integrating AI with Appalachian Folk Medicine: A Modern Twist on Traditional Healing

In the scenic and rugged regions of the Appalachian Mountains, traditional folk medicine has been a cornerstone of community health practices for centuries. These practices, rich with herbal knowledge passed down through generations, often lack formal documentation, leaving significant cultural health practices at the risk of being forgotten. Recent efforts to meld these traditional methods with artificial intelligence (AI) foster a unique opportunity to preserve and enhance the accuracy and reach of Appalachian healing traditions in a modern context.

A comprehensive project was launched to document the myriad herbal remedies, treatments, and practices widely used in Appalachian communities. This initial phase involved detailed interviews with longstanding practitioners of the folk medicine community, referred to locally as 'root doctors'. The knowledge gathered encompassed a broad spectrum, ranging from decoctions and tinctures to poultices and salves, each tailored to treat ailments from minor wounds to chronic illnesses.

The subsequent phase introduced AI through a sophisticated platform where all the documented knowledge was fed into machine learning models. These AI models, capable of processing natural language inputs, were then trained to identify patterns, suggest herbal synergies, and even predict the efficacy of certain herb combinations based on historical outcomes and contemporary medical research.

The output of the AI analysis was manifold. For one, it led to the development of a predictive tool that helps practitioners formulate more effective and personalized treatment plans. Additionally, it enabled the creation of a virtual database accessible by both local and global health practitioners who wish to understand and utilize Appalachian folk remedies responsibly and effectively.

Critically, this integration not only upheld the rich cultural heritage of the Appalachian people but also brought it into the digital era, showcasing an exemplary case of how traditional knowledge can be harmoniously blended with cutting-edge technology to transcend geographical and cultural boundaries, enhancing the resilience and sustainability of traditional medical practices.

## Case Study: Revitalizing Polynesian Herbal Medicine through AI Integration

The intricate knowledge of medicinal herbs passed down through generations in Polynesian societies is witnessing a transformative revival through the incorporation of Artificial Intelligence (AI). The Polynesian islands, each with their unique flora and traditional herbal practices, have long utilized natural remedies to manage and treat various ailments. However, globalization and a shift towards Western medicine have put these traditional practices at risk of disappearing, leading to a loss of indigenous wisdom. In an innovative project aimed at revitalizing these ancient practices, AI technology has been employed to digitally encode, analyze, and propagate this traditional knowledge within the global health community.

For this initiative, extensive field research was conducted across various Polynesian islands to gather empirical data on local herbal practices. Ethnobotanists collaborated with local healers, known as 'ta'unga', to document the various plant species used and their associated medicinal benefits. The project meticulously cataloged hundreds of plants, along with precise methods of preparation and application that were passed down orally through generations. Utilizing AI-driven natural language processing (NLP), these undocumented herbal recipes and rituals were digitized and stored in an accessible database.

Following the data collection phase, AI machine learning algorithms were employed to analyze the efficacy of the cataloged herbal remedies. Patterns within the data, correlating specific herbs with health outcomes, were identified and used to predict the most effective herbal combinations for specific ailments. This not only enhanced the application of Polynesian herbal medicine but also provided a scientific basis for their efficacy, significantly heightening their credibility in the broader medical field.

The culmination of this project was the development of an AI-driven educational platform, tailored to both educate new practitioners and inform global audiences. This digital platform serves as a bridge, connecting traditional Polynesian healing practices with contemporary healthcare providers, thereby ensuring that this age-old wisdom is preserved, respected, and used in a modern medical context, while fostering a sustainable approach to health that respects cultural heritage and biodiversity.

## Case Study: Leveraging AI to Modernize Amazonian Tribal Medicine

Deep within the Amazon rainforest, a collaboration between artificial intelligence (AI) specialists and traditional medicine practitioners is reshaping the way these practices are preserved, studied, and propagated. This intricate project focuses on the application of AI to understand, digitize, and preserve the rich medical heritage of Amazonian tribes, which is often passed down orally and at risk of erosion due to the region's modern influences.

The first phase of the project involves extensive fieldwork, where a team of ethnobotanists and AI researchers collaborate with tribal healers to gather comprehensive data on traditional practices. These practices include the use of medicinal plants, spiritual healing rituals, and ancient therapeutic techniques. Researchers document this information using portable digital devices, capturing details about plant species, preparation methods, dosage, and administration routes, as well as cultural contexts of each remedy, which are crucial for their effective application.

Subsequently, the data undergoes processing through advanced natural language processing (NLP) systems designed to understand and categorize the tribal dialects and languages. This technologically intensive phase ensures the translation of complex herbal recipes and healing techniques into a structured digital format, safeguarding this knowledge against loss.

In the next stage, machine learning models are developed to analyze the relationships between specific plants and health outcomes, based on historical usage and modern medical insights. These models predict efficacies of plant combinations and propose optimized dosages, taking environmental variables and individual patient needs into account. Moreover, AI simulations provide insights into potential side effects and interactions with modern pharmaceuticals, enhancing the safety profile of these traditional remedies.

The culmination of this project is the creation of an AI-enhanced database and an interactive platform that not only serves researchers and practitioners globally but also provides tribal communities with tools to educate younger generations. This not only revitalizes their traditional medicine in the face of globalization but also integrates their practices into the global healthcare system, ensuring a sustainable and respectful use of their ancestral knowledge.

### Case Study: AI-Enhanced Revitalization of Ancient Yorubic Medical Practices

The collaboration between advanced artificial intelligence (AI) and traditional Yorubic medical practitioners in Nigeria illustrates a groundbreaking application of technology in safeguarding and revitalizing ancient medical wisdom. The Yorubic culture, with its deep roots in herbalism and spiritual healing, offers a rich lore of medicinal practices preserved mainly through oral traditions and the expertise of local healers, known as 'Babalawos'. The limited documentation and risk of cultural dilution posed significant challenges in preserving these traditions amid globalization and modern medical practices.

To address these challenges, an ambitious project was initiated to systematically document, analyze, and enhance the efficacy of Yorubic medicinal practices using AI technologies. The initial phase involved extensive field research, during which AI specialists and ethnobotanists collaborated with "Babalawos" to record detailed information on hundreds of medicinal plants, their uses, preparation methods, and associated spiritual rituals. Employing portable digital devices, this data was meticulously collected and digitally encoded.

Subsequent stages leveraged natural language processing (NLP) to translate and categorize the collected data into a structured digital format. AI-powered machine learning models were then developed to analyze the comprehensive dataset, identifying patterns and correlations between specific treatments and health outcomes. This analysis was instrumental in predicting the most effective plant combinations for specified ailments and adjusting dosages based on individual patient profiles, considering factors like age, gender, and other health conditions.

The project's impact extended beyond the scientific validation of Yorubic medicine. It also facilitated the creation of an interactive, AI-driven educational platform designed to serve both local communities and global audiences. This platform not only promotes the understanding and application of Yorubic healing practices but also ensures their propagation and integration into modern healthcare systems, bridging the gap between ancient wisdom and contemporary medical practice while fostering a sustainable approach to healthcare that respects and preserves cultural identity.

### Case Study: Empowering Siberian Shamanic Healing with AI Technologies

In the expansive and remote regions of Siberia, shamanic healing has been a cornerstone of holistic health practices for millennia. Shamanic traditions, deeply embedded within the indigenous communities, involve complex rituals and the use of local flora and fauna to address both physical and spiritual ailments. However, the transmission of these practices has traditionally relied on oral passing of knowledge, making them susceptible to erosion and misinterpretation over generations. The recent initiative to integrate Artificial Intelligence (AI) into Siberian shamanic practices presents a notable case study in preserving and enhancing these ancient techniques through modern technology.

The project commenced with an extensive documentation phase, during which AI researchers collaborated with local shamans. Together, they undertook the task of cataloging thousands of ritual practices, medicinal plants, and spiritual teachings. This phase was critical, as much of the shamanic knowledge was undocumented and at risk of being lost. Advanced natural language processing (NLP) tools were employed to transcribe and translate shamanic chants and instructions, which were often in obscure local dialects, into accessible digital formats.

Following the documentation, AI-powered machine learning algorithms were developed to analyze the effectiveness of various rituals and herbal remedies. The AI systems were trained on data that detailed symptoms, remedies used, and patient outcomes, drawing powerful insights into the efficacy of traditional practices and suggesting modifications to enhance their effectiveness. This analysis also helped isolate key active compounds in medicinal plants, aiding in the development of more potent and targeted treatments.

The final stage of the integration resulted in the creation of an interactive, AI-driven platform that not only preserved the shamanic knowledge but also made it accessible to global audiences. This platform enables real-time consultations, virtual healing sessions, and personalized remedy suggestions, revolutionizing how Siberian shamanic practices are taught, learned, and applied. It ensures that these age-old traditions can continue, enhancing their reach and appeal in the global health community while maintaining cultural integrity and respect for indigenous practices.

### Case Study: Enhancing Mediterranean Herbal Medicine with AI-Driven Studies

The Mediterranean region, renowned for its rich herbal lore and traditional healing practices, presents a unique case study for integrating Artificial Intelligence (AI) with traditional herbal medicine. This region, characterized by its biodiversity and rich historical heritage in herbal treatments, offers fertile ground for AI-driven advancements in understanding and enhancing the efficacy of natural remedies.

A collaborative initiative between local herbalists, regional universities, and a technology consortium was launched to harness the power of AI in cataloging, analyzing, and optimizing the traditional Mediterranean herbal practices. The project's inception involved the creation of a comprehensive digital archive of indigenous herbs, detailing their historical uses, preparation methods, and anecdotal efficacy. This digitalization employed advanced natural language processing (NLP) to interpret and structure vast amounts of unstructured data from ancient texts, oral traditions, and modern academic studies.

Following digital archiving, machine learning models were trained to analyze correlations between specific herbs and health outcomes, utilizing both historical data and contemporary clinical trials. These models identified potential new applications for traditional remedies and optimized combinations of herbs for specific ailments, potentially increasing their efficacy and reducing side effects.

The findings from AI analysis led to several novel contributions to the field of natural medicine. One significant breakthrough was the development of an AI-driven recommendation system that personalized herbal treatment plans based on individual patient genetics, lifestyle, and existing medical conditions. This system was designed not only to enhance the therapeutic potency of treatments but also to integrate smoothly with modern medical practices.

The project culminated in the launch of a multinational educational platform that utilized interactive AI tools to educate new generations of herbalists and healthcare professionals. This platform ensures the sustainable and informed use of Mediterranean herbal wisdom in contemporary healthcare, making ancient knowledge accessible and relevant in the digital era.

### Case Study: AI-Driven Reinvigoration of Aztec Medicinal Practices

The storied history of Aztec medicine, steeped in rich herbal lore and complex spiritual rituals, presents an intriguing arena for the implementation of modern Artificial Intelligence (AI) technology. Due to colonization and subsequent cultural disruptions, many of these ancient practices were marginalized or lost, surviving only in fragmented traditional narratives and scattered, aged manuscripts. A groundbreaking project commenced recently, aiming to not only preserve but also reinvigorate these ancient Aztec medicinal practices through the application of AI.

The initiative began with collecting extensive ethnobotanical knowledge and ancient manuscripts, involving historians, local indigenous practitioners, and AI experts. This multidisciplinary team worked to translate and digitize the old texts, which were then encoded into a structured digital format using natural language processing (NLP) technologies. This initial phase was crucial, as it converted previously inaccessible wisdom into a format suitable for detailed analysis.

Following the digitalization of the data, machine learning algorithms were employed to sift through the vast dataset and identify patterns, drawing correlations between specific herbs, traditional rituals, and reported health outcomes. AI's capability to process and analyze large datasets played a pivotal role in this context. It enabled the surfacing of insights that would likely be missed by human researchers. This phase not only shed light on forgotten or underutilized herbal remedies but also provided a scientific foundation for their effectiveness, thus rejuvenating global interest and respect for Aztec medicinal practices.

The culminating phase of this project involved the development and launch of an interactive, AI-powered platform designed for educational and clinical purposes. This platform enables global practitioners and scholars of traditional medicine to access, learn, and apply Aztec herbal remedies and spiritual healing techniques in their current practice. It ensures that invaluable Aztec knowledge, once on the brink of oblivion, is preserved and integrated into modern healthcare contexts, offering a harmonious blend of ancient wisdom and cutting-edge technology.

## Review Questions

**1. A 57-year-old patient diagnosed with advanced cancer and given only a few months to live has experienced an unexpected remission after engaging in deep spiritual practices and community prayer. The medical team is puzzled since the clinical prognosis did not anticipate such an outcome. What factors might have contributed to this patient's unexpected recovery, according to both traditional and modern theories of medicine?**

A) A placebo response activated by the patient's belief in the healing power of prayer and spiritual practices, potentially altering physiological responses.

B) An undetected medical error in the initial diagnosis and prognosis, leading to an incorrect evaluation of the patient's health condition.

C) The patient secretly received an experimental treatment not disclosed to the medical team.

D) The cancer spontaneously remitted entirely due to genetic mutations independent of any treatments or interventions.

**Answer: A**

Explanation: The most plausible explanation based on the case details provided and existing medical literature is a placebo response, which occurs when a patient experiences tangible improvements in health from a treatment that has no therapeutic effect. The mind-body connection is powerful, and beliefs and expectations can significantly impact physiological processes. This can trigger the release of natural endorphins and other biochemical changes that promote health. While spontaneous remission and medical errors are rare, they cannot be entirely ruled out without further investigation. However, the connection between the patient's spiritual practices and their recovery suggests a significant psychosomatic contribution, likely mediated by their beliefs and the supportive community around them.

**2. In the context of integrating AI in traditional medicine, a tech company collaborates with local healers from a Native American tribe to develop an AI tool that accurately considers tribal herbal medicine. How should the project approach the ethical management of the knowledge shared by the tribal healers?**

A) Convert the shared tribal knowledge into a proprietary algorithm that the company can patent and sell.

B) Publish all the tribal knowledge openly to ensure maximum scientific transparency and accessibility.

C) Develop a data governance framework in partnership with the tribe, ensuring they have control over data use, sharing, and benefits derived from the project.

D) Use the tribal knowledge solely for academic purposes, avoiding any commercial use or application.

**Answer: C**

Explanation: The most ethical approach is to co-develop a data governance framework with the tribe that respects Indigenous data sovereignty. This means that the knowledge shared by tribal healers should be controlled, managed, and used in ways agreed upon by the tribe itself, ensuring equitable benefit-sharing. Such a framework accommodates respect for the cultural significance of the knowledge and consents to its use. Opting for proprietary algorithms without the tribe's explicit consent or full transparency risks exploiting the knowledge without just compensation and could perpetuate colonial dynamics. Publishing the knowledge openly or limiting its use to academic contexts also does not provide the tribe with opportunities to benefit from their own knowledge, whether through commercial ventures or other means.

**3. A healthcare AI system is developed to offer personalized healthcare recommendations. However, the system has been criticized for lacking cultural competence after several patients from diverse backgrounds reported that their traditional healing practices were ignored or misrepresented by the algorithm. What action should be taken to address this issue?**

A) Discontinue the use of AI in healthcare settings to avoid further cultural insensitivity.

B) Implement a cultural sensitivity training program for the AI development team and ensure that it includes more diverse data sets representing various healing practices.

C) Ignore the criticism and continue using the AI system as is, relying on the data-driven results it provides.

D) Focus solely on biomedicine in the AI's recommendations to avoid errors in representing traditional healing practices.

**Answer: B**

Explanation: To address the lack of cultural competence in healthcare AI systems, the most effective approach is to implement a cultural sensitivity training program for the AI development team and integrate more diverse datasets that include various traditional healing practices. This will educate the developers about cultural nuances and the importance of including a wide range of medical practices and philosophies in the AI's dataset. Such an effort helps to minimize bias and misrepresentations and enhances the AI's ability to serve a diverse population better. Discontinuing the use of AI altogether or ignoring the criticism would prevent the potential benefits of AI in healthcare and fail to address the underlying issue of cultural insensitivity. Limiting the focus to biomedicine excludes the rich diversity of global healing practices and could alienate patients who follow traditional medicine systems.

## AI's Potential in Supporting Spiritual Healing Practices

### Defining Spiritual Healing in the Context of AI

Spiritual healing within the context of AI examines the integration of advanced technologies to enhance and facilitate practices traditionally rooted in deep personal and communal beliefs. This interdisciplinary approach considers spiritual healing not just as an esoteric art but as a comprehensive system that can be quantified and improved through AI-driven data analysis and pattern recognition.

AI's involvement in spiritual healing extends beyond mere support; it aims to understand the nuances of spiritual needs and practices, translating these into actionable insights. By processing data from various spiritual sessions, AI identifies common elements and outcomes that contribute positively to individuals' well-being, thus paving the way for personalized spiritual care. This transformative analysis also allows AI to suggest refinements, making each spiritual journey more impactful.

Moreover, defining spiritual healing within AI frameworks necessitates consideration of ethical implications, ensuring that these technologies respect and uphold the integrity of spiritual traditions while promoting inclusivity and sensitivity. It's a delicate balance between embracing technological advancement and preserving the sanctity of spiritual practices.

### AI's Role in Facilitating Spiritual Counseling

AI's evolving role in spiritual counseling brings profound enhancement to intimacy and depth in spiritual guidance. By leveraging advanced algorithms, AI interprets the underlying emotional cues and spiritual languages of individuals, creating a new dimension of tailored spiritual support. This digital empathy deciphers nuanced emotional states, enabling counselors to provide more precise and empathetic responses to spiritual needs.

Moreover, AI-supported systems can manage vast databases of spiritual texts and precedents, which could dramatically increase the accessibility of cross-cultural spiritual wisdom. This not only broadens the counselor's reference base but also enriches the counseling process with diverse, contextual insights, leveraging global spiritual traditions to individual advantage.

When incorporating AI into spiritual counseling practices, it is essential to consider ethical implications, including privacy and autonomy in spiritual exploration. As developers and spiritual counselors collaborate, they must ensure that AI tools amplify human-centered care, maintaining a respectful balance between technological intervention and genuine spiritual connection.

### Interfacing AI with Holistic Spiritual Practices

Interfacing AI with human, personal, and guided holistic spiritual practices unveils a remarkable synergy that could revolutionize the way spirituality is experienced and practiced. By integrating AI into diverse, holistic spiritual frameworks, practitioners can harness a data-driven approach to customize and enhance spiritual rituals and practices, tailoring them to the individual's spiritual and emotional fabric.

When AI is integrated with holistic spiritual practices, it can analyze individual responses to various spiritual exercises, enabling the creation of a personalized spiritual regimen that closely aligns with individual needs and preferences. This tailored approach is particularly beneficial in enhancing the effectiveness of practices such as energy healing, chakra balancing, and crystal therapy, making these ancient traditions more accessible and impactful in the modern age. There must be exceptional care if AI is to be a partner in "spiritual" counseling as AI is by definition NOT spiritual, but a tool, a technology to assist the therapist or counselor.

Moreover, the use of AI in holistic spiritual contexts promises to foster a deeper understanding of the interconnections between various spiritual modalities. By mapping the effects and synergies between multiple practices, AI can help create a more interconnected and harmonious spiritual healing environment, ultimately fostering a holistic sense of well-being informed by both spiritual insight and technological innovation with proper guidance and input from the human operator.

**Technologies Enhancing Spiritual Healing**

Emerging technologies are synergistically enhancing spiritual healing, integrating seamless AI tools that augment ancient practices for contemporary needs. Wearable tech, such as biometric sensors, operates in real-time to provide feedback on physiological changes during spiritual exercises, adjusting techniques to maximize effectiveness. Similarly, the proliferation of biofeedback devices empowers individuals by visualizing their mental states, facilitating deeper meditation and focused healing.

Another groundbreaking innovation is AI-driven ambient intelligence in sacred spaces. These intelligent systems adjust lighting, sound, and even scent based on the session's requirements, creating a conducive atmosphere for spiritual practices. Virtual Reality (VR) also plays a pivotal role, simulating sacred environments or visual journeys that enhance the depth and authenticity of spiritual experiences, making profound practices accessible from any location.

Moreover, developments in machine learning algorithms now predict and adapt to emotional and spiritual needs, recommending customized healing paths. These AI insights help in crafting highly personalized spiritual interventions, thereby enriching the quality of spiritual care and fostering profound personal growth in individuals.

**AI in Meditation and Mindfulness Programs**

Incorporating AI into meditation and mindfulness programs introduces a groundbreaking approach to enhancing mental clarity and emotional health. AI technologies can track progress, suggest modifications, and create highly personalized meditation experiences by analyzing user responses and adapting in real time. This capability ensures users receive the most beneficial practices tailored to their current mental state, maximizing the therapeutic benefits of each session.

Moreover, AI-enabled apps and devices can guide users through mindfulness exercises with precision, offering prompts and feedback that are fine-tuned to the individual's level of experience and current emotional or spiritual state. These programs utilize advanced algorithms to evaluate effectiveness, adjusting and improving outcomes continuously.

Finally, the integration of AI in these programs supports the broader accessibility of mindfulness and meditation techniques, providing tools that help users from various cultural and social backgrounds to engage in these practices, potentially reducing barriers to access. This democratization of spiritual wellness tools underscores AI's role in fostering a more inclusive approach to personal and spiritual growth.

**Supporting Yoga and Spiritual Fitness with AI**

The integration of AI into yoga and spiritual fitness marks a new era of personalized practice that tailors to the unique needs of each individual. AI technologies enable the creation of customized yoga routines by analyzing user data, including physical capabilities, stress levels, and personal goals. These intelligent systems can suggest modifications, track progress, and even adjust practices in real-time, enhancing the yoga experience and maximizing its benefits.

Furthermore, AI-driven virtual coaches are becoming instrumental in guiding users through yoga exercises with precision. These coaches provide real-time feedback on posture and breathing, ensuring practices are performed safely and effectively. This support is particularly beneficial for those new to yoga, helping them to adopt correct forms without the need for a human instructor.

AI's role extends beyond practice to include the spiritual aspect of yoga. By recognizing emotional and spiritual cues, AI can recommend yoga styles and sequences that promote spiritual well-being, aligning physical practice with spiritual goals. This harmonious blend of technology and tradition enriches the spiritual journey, making the path to enlightenment more accessible.

**Customizing AI to Recognize Spiritual Needs**

Tailoring AI to discern spiritual needs represents a pivotal advance in the integration of spiritual technology. By custom programming AI, developers can equip systems to understand and respond to nuanced spiritual expressions and requirements. This customization hinges on AI's ability to learn from diverse spiritual interactions and adapt to them dynamically, offering a more responsive and empathetic user experience.

To achieve this, AI models are trained on vast arrays of spiritual data, encompassing texts, rituals, and user feedback from varied spiritual traditions. This training enables the AI to identify and align with the user's spiritual context, enhancing its ability to facilitate meaningful spiritual encounters. The process involves continuous learning and adjustment to handle the subjective nature of spirituality, ensuring respectful and accurate recognition of individual spiritual needs.

Furthermore, integrating feedback mechanisms allows these AI systems to refine their understanding continuously, making them increasingly adept at providing support that genuinely resonates on a spiritual level. This bespoke approach not only respects but also elevates personal spiritual practices, bridging the gap between technology and profound spiritual fulfilment.

**Ethical Design of AI for Spiritual Support**

The ethical design of AI in spiritual support calls for a conscientious approach that respects the profound nature of spirituality and its diverse manifestations. Developers must prioritize sensitivity and inclusivity, ensuring that AI systems do not enforce a narrow worldview but rather embrace a spectrum of spiritual beliefs and practices. This involves designing algorithms that can adapt to and respect varying spiritual backgrounds without bias or preference.

Moreover, ethical AI design must address privacy concerns rigorously, as personal data is intensely personal and sensitive. Safeguarding this data against misuse and ensuring confidentiality is paramount to maintain trust and integrity in AI-assisted spiritual practices. AI systems should also be transparent about how they process and utilize sensitive data, allowing users to retain control over their personal information.

Lastly, the involvement of spiritual communities in the design process can enhance the ethical orientation of AI systems. By integrating feedback from these communities, developers can better align AI functionalities with real-world spiritual needs, fostering an AI ecosystem that supports and enhances spiritual growth without compromising ethical standards or personal beliefs.

Integrating AI into global spiritual practices demands a deep cultural sensitivity to foster acceptance and effectiveness. AI tools must be designed to respect and understand the diverse spiritual landscapes across the world, recognizing and adapting to various cultural nuances that define spiritual experiences. This sensitivity helps in avoiding the imposition of a single, possibly alien, spiritual framework onto diverse cultural contexts, which could dilute authentic spiritual expressions.

Moreover, cultural sensitivity in AI applications ensures that these technologies are perceived as respectful allies rather than invasive tools. This is achieved through an inclusive algorithm design that encompasses a wide array of spiritual beliefs and practices. Such inclusivity enhances the user's experience by providing spiritually meaningful support, personalized to their cultural context and spiritual inclinations.

The challenge lies in encoding such a rich tapestry of spiritual diversity into AI systems. This requires extensive collaboration with cultural anthropologists and spiritual leaders to imbue AI with a real understanding of cultural subtleties. Only then can AI truly support the spiritual well-being of individuals worldwide, enhancing the interconnectedness essential to spirituality.

## AI Integration in Prayer and Faith Rituals

Integrating AI into prayer and faith rituals holds transformative potential to deepen spiritual engagement and foster personal reflection. Intelligent systems can be leveraged to customize and guide prayer sessions based on an individual's historical spiritual data, aligning prayer practices with personal faith narratives and emotional states. This customization ensures that each prayer experience is deeply personal and spiritually significant.

Moreover, AI can facilitate virtual group prayers, connecting individuals across geographical barriers to engage in synchronous or asynchronous worship. This communal experience, orchestrated by AI, enables shared spiritual communion without the limitations of physical proximity, thereby enhancing the sense of connectedness among practitioners of the same faith.

AI also plays a crucial role in preserving and adapting ancient faith rituals for the modern era. By analyzing historical and scriptural data, AI systems can suggest ritual adaptations that maintain spiritual integrity while making practices accessible to younger or digitally native generations.

Through these innovative applications, AI may not only respect but may revitalize traditional prayer and faith rituals, fostering a harmonious blend of ancient wisdom and contemporary technology.

## Spiritual Advisors and AI: A Collaborative Approach

The fusion of Artificial Intelligence with the expertise of spiritual advisors (healers, Medicine Men and Women, Grandma Doc) ushers in a transformative era for both domains. Within this synergy, AI serves as an enabler, augmenting the reach and efficacy of spiritual counselors. By analyzing vast amounts of behavioral and biometric data, AI enables counselors to uncover profound insights into the spiritual needs of individuals, facilitating tailored solutions for their unique spiritual journeys.

Collaboration between AI and spiritual advisors also enhances accessibility. People residing in remote or underserved regions, who might otherwise lack access to skilled spiritual guidance, can benefit enormously. AI-powered platforms connect these individuals with experienced advisors, transcending geographical limitations to promote inclusivity in spiritual wellness.

Moreover, continuous interaction between AI systems and spiritual advisors fosters a learning environment for the AI. This symbiotic relationship ensures that AI applications evolve more empathetically, finely tuned to comprehend and respond to nuanced spiritual queries, culminating in a higher level of personalized spiritual engagement.

## Leveraging AI for Personalized Spiritual Care Plans

Leveraging Artificial Intelligence to create personalized spiritual care plans exemplifies a progressive merging of technology and spirit. By harnessing AI, it becomes possible to generate care plans that are tailored specifically to an individual's spiritual history and current needs, respecting unique spiritual journeys and preferences.

AI systems can analyze an individual's past interactions with various spiritual practices and offer suggestions that resonate most. Such customization not only enhances personal spiritual growth but also ensures that the care received is deeply aligned with personal beliefs and values. Furthermore, AI can dynamically adjust these plans based on ongoing feedback, leading to a continuously refined spiritual experience that adapts to changing life circumstances and evolving spiritual insights.

The real challenge lies in equipping AI with the sensitivity required to manage such personal matters appropriately. Integrating continuous input from experienced spiritual advisors ensures that the AI's proposals remain respectful and insightful. This collaborative model could significantly improve how individuals engage with their spirituality on a day-to-day basis, paving the way for a new era of enriched spiritual well-being.

## AI's Role in Pathway Finding in Spiritual Healing

AI's role in pathway finding in spiritual healing represents a profound integration of technology with personal spiritual journeys. By comprehensively analyzing individual spiritual data and historical patterns, AI systems can identify and recommend personalized pathways for spiritual healing. This process can guide individuals through tailored spiritual practices, fostering deeper personal growth and enlightenment based on their unique spiritual inclinations and historical interactions with various spiritual disciplines.

Furthermore, AI tools can predict potential spiritual crises and offer preemptive guidance. This predictive capability ensures that individuals receive timely and appropriate spiritual interventions, enhancing their resilience against spiritual distress. These AI-driven suggestions aim to harmonize with an individual's spiritual tempo, thereby providing a seamless and supportive spiritual experience.

The challenge, however, lies in ensuring that AI systems remain sensitive to the subtle nuances of spiritual experiences. Continuous input and validation from experienced spiritual advisors are vital to refining AI's effectiveness in spiritual pathway finding, making it a truly transformative tool in the realm of spiritual healing.

## AI-Driven Platforms to Manage Spiritual Therapy Sessions

AI-driven platforms are revolutionizing the management of spiritual therapy sessions, providing tailored and efficient therapeutic experiences. By utilizing sophisticated algorithms, these platforms can organize and schedule sessions based on individual spiritual needs and preferences, offering a seamless integration of technology and personal spiritual care.

The platforms also facilitate real-time adjustments to therapy plans, responding to the dynamic spiritual growth of individuals. This adaptability ensures that each session is optimally aligned with the current state of a person's spiritual journey, enhancing the effectiveness of the therapy.

Moreover, AI-driven platforms support the documentation and analysis of session outcomes to track progress over time. This data-driven approach helps refine therapy techniques and practices, ensuring they are deeply resonant and beneficial.

By automating administrative tasks and enhancing the personalization of care, AI-driven platforms are setting a new standard in spiritual therapy, making profound spiritual support more accessible and effective.

## The Use of Virtual Reality in Meditative Practices

Virtual reality (VR) is forging new pathways in meditative practices, transforming traditional spiritual activities into immersive, personalized experiences. By enveloping individuals in serene, digitally crafted environments, VR enhances the depth and focus of meditation. Such settings can range from simulated sacred sites to abstract, tranquil vistas, each designed to facilitate a profound spiritual connection free from the distractions of the physical world.

Moreover, VR technology enables the simulation of guided meditations led by virtual spiritual guides or AI-driven avatars. These guides can adapt in real-time to the user's emotional and physiological responses, offering personalized guidance that evolves with the meditation session. This adaptability makes VR a powerful tool in deepening spiritual practices and emotional well-being.

Ethical design and cultural sensitivity remain pivotal as developers integrate VR with meditative practices. Ensuring that these virtual experiences respect and reflect the diversity of spiritual traditions is crucial for their acceptance and effectiveness. As VR technology advances, its potential to support diverse spiritual practices and personal growth continues to expand.

## Effectiveness of AI in Guiding Spiritual Interventions

Artificial Intelligence is swiftly becoming an instrumental ally in guiding spiritual interventions. By leveraging AI's analytical prowess, spiritual interventions become more than mere acts of faith; they transform into precise, personalized encounters that can profoundly cater to individual spiritual needs. AI's ability to sift through and analyze vast datasets on spiritual practices and outcomes enables a more empirical approach to spiritual healing. This data-driven strategy significantly enhances historical intuition-based methods by ensuring interventions are both timely and contextually appropriate.

However, the effectiveness of AI in spiritual contexts naturally raises concerns about authenticity and the depth of the spiritual engagements facilitated by technology. It's key for developers and spiritual leaders alike to critically assess the balance between AI assistance and the invaluable human touch that embodies the essence of spiritual care.

Critically, integration of continuous feedback from real-world spirituality sessions enhances AI algorithms, making them more attuned to the subtle nuances of spiritual care. Such iterative learning processes are pivotal in crafting AI systems that genuinely assist in fostering spiritual growth, ensuring the interventions remain grounded in genuine spiritual empathy, rather than just technological innovation.

## Training AI to Understand Emotional and Spiritual Cues

Training AI to discern emotional and spiritual cues marks a pioneering advancement in blending technology with deeper human experiences. By integrating emotional intelligence frameworks into AI systems, these technologies can begin to perceive and respond to subtle spiritual and emotional indicators, fundamentally transforming spiritual care dynamics. This involves programming AI to recognize patterns in speech, facial expressions, and physiological responses, which often convey the emotional states underlying spiritual needs.

Further refinement comes through the incorporation of machine learning, where AI systems continuously learn from interactions to enhance their sensitivity to these cues. The collaboration with spiritual advisors is crucial here, providing AI the necessary guidance to differentiate between nuanced emotional expressions. Such interactions ensure that AI's responses are not only technically accurate but also emotionally resonant.

However, this pursuit raises ethical considerations. Ensuring AI systems treat sensitive emotional data with the highest confidentiality and respect is paramount. As AI ventures into these intimate areas of human experience, its design must prioritize ethical guidelines that safeguard individual spiritual and emotional well-being, maintaining a balance between technological efficiency and human sensitivity.

## Case Studies: AI's Impact on Spiritual Experiences

Exploring case studies on AI's impact on spiritual experiences illuminates both its potent possibilities and emerging challenges. For instance, one significant case involved the introduction of AI-driven avatars in guided meditation apps. These avatars, capable of sensing user emotions via voice and facial recognition, personalize sessions to align with the user's spiritual and emotional state at each moment, enhancing the depth of meditation and engagement.

Another study focused on a community traditionally reliant on spiritual healers. The introduction of an AI system that analyzed local spiritual practices provided tailored spiritual insights and advice, resulting in a marked improvement in community well-being. This adaptation suggested that AI could serve as a respectful partner in spiritual exploration, aligning well with holistic practices without compromising the cultural essence.

However, challenges persist, particularly in calibrating AI systems to fully grasp the nuances of spiritual experiences. Concerns over spiritual authenticity and the potential dilution of traditional practices continue to frame critical discussions on future implementations and improvements in AI's role in spiritual domains.

## Predicting Spiritual Healing Outcomes with AI Data

Harnessing AI to predict the outcomes of spiritual healing presents a compelling fusion of technology and metaphysical practices. By analyzing extensive datasets on individual spiritual journeys, AI can forecast potential healing trajectories and outcomes, offering unprecedented insights into spiritual growth.

This predictive capability allows for the personalization of spiritual practices, tailoring interventions to individual needs, which enhances the overall efficacy of spiritual healing. Data collected from various spiritual sessions, including meditation and prayer, feed into algorithms that discern patterns and predict future spiritual states, fostering a more nuanced understanding of spiritual progression.

However, the reliance on AI for predicting spiritual outcomes raises important ethical and practical considerations. Ensuring the accuracy and sensitivity of these predictions requires continuous refinement of AI models to respect and encapsulate the profound subtleties of spiritual experiences.

As this technology evolves, it may become a vital tool in the toolkit of spiritual practitioners, augmenting traditional wisdom with data-driven insights that could transform the landscape of spiritual healing.

**AI as a Tool for Spiritual Assessment and Measurement**

Leveraging AI for spiritual assessment and measurement represents a revolutionary step in understanding and enhancing spiritual wellness. By integrating AI tools, practitioners can measure various spiritual states, providing a quantitative lens through which to view what was once considered immeasurable. This facilitates a structured approach to spiritual care, aligning it more closely with other health disciplines that benefit from empirical validation.

AI systems, designed to collect and analyze data on spiritual practices and emotional responses, create personalized spiritual profiles. These profiles help in identifying spiritual needs and tailoring interventions accordingly. As these tools learn from vast datasets, they refine their assessments, improving accuracy over time. Such capabilities make AI an invaluable asset for ongoing spiritual care management, offering insights that are both deep and wide-ranging.

However, the deployment of AI in this delicate field must navigate ethical complexities. The sensitivity to personal spiritual beliefs and the confidentiality of assessments are paramount. Striking the right balance between technological advancements and the preservation of spiritual sanctity remains a continual challenge, urging developers to prioritize respect and discretion in AI designs.

**Challenges and Limitations of AI in Spiritual Contexts**

While AI holds promise in enhancing spiritual practices, its application within spiritual contexts presents significant challenges and limitations. One fundamental issue is the intrinsic qualitative nature of spirituality that resists quantification. AI, driven by data and algorithms, may struggle to fully grasp and respect the subtleties of spiritual experiences, which are deeply personal and often transcendental.

There is also a valid concern regarding the over-reliance on technology in spaces traditionally governed by human touch and presence. The dependence on AI might detract from the authentic spiritual connections that form the core of many practices, potentially leading to a dilution of these traditions. Moreover, the impersonal nature of AI could hinder the emotional depth and the individualized interpretation that spiritual guidance typically requires.

Lastly, ethical concerns about privacy and data security persist, especially given the sensitive nature of the information involved in spiritual practices. Ensuring that AI systems handling such data maintain the highest standards of confidentiality is paramount to their acceptance and effectiveness in spiritual contexts.

**Next-Gen AI: Models Predicting Spiritual Paths**

The frontier of AI in spirituality is expanding towards the profound capability to predict spiritual paths. This innovative application involves constructing predictive models that analyze historical and personal spiritual data to foresee individual spiritual trajectories. As AI technologies gather, interpret, and learn from vast amounts of spiritual engagement data—ranging from meditation practices to spiritual counseling sessions—they carve out personalized spiritual journeys that are anew with possibility.

This interface of AI with spiritual foresight necessitates delicate calibration. The challenge is to ensure that predictions honor the profound personal nature of spirituality, avoiding reductionist interpretations while enhancing personal growth and enlightenment. Continuous adaptation of AI algorithms, informed by ongoing research and input from spiritual counselors, aims to refine these prediction models.

Yet, ethical considerations loom large as these applications delve into deeply personal territory. Ensuring that AI systems do so respectfully and with cultural awareness cannot be overstated. As we stand on the brink of this new era, the potential for AI to serve as a guide on one's spiritual journey is captivating, marrying the mystic with the measurable.

## Improving AI Algorithms for Greater Spiritual Sensitivity

Improving AI algorithms to enhance spiritual sensitivity is a nuanced endeavor that requires a deep integration of psychological insights, cultural awareness, and technological expertise. The objective is to refine AI's ability to attune to spiritual contexts, ensuring that these systems can accurately interpret and respond to diverse spiritual expressions and needs. This involves programming AI to recognize and adapt to the diverse manifestations of spirituality across cultures.

Developers are experimenting with machine learning models that can learn from extensive datasets, including textual analysis from sacred texts, feedback from spiritual sessions, and user interactions in spiritual apps. By processing these varied inputs, AI could become more adept at providing personalized spiritual insights and support that respects individual beliefs and practices.

Furthermore, collaboration with spiritual leaders and healers is critical. Their insights help to infuse AI with a deeper understanding of spiritual nuances that are difficult for technology alone to grasp. Continual feedback and iteration are essential, ensuring that AI respects the profound, often intangible nature of spiritual experiences while offering meaningful support.

## Future of AI in Enhancing Interconnectedness in Spirituality

The future of AI in spirituality is pioneering a new frontier in human interconnectedness. By transcending traditional boundaries, AI can unite diverse spiritual traditions through data-driven insights, fostering a universal spiritual dialogue. This involves not only the sharing of spiritual practices but also the synthesis of wisdom across cultures, potentially leading to globally resonant spiritual insights that can enrich individual spiritual journeys.

Advanced AI systems could analyze, compare, and interpret spiritual data from various traditions to discover underlying universal truths, offering individuals a richer, more diverse spiritual palette. This capacity to tailor spiritual guidance by integrating multiple traditions could intensely personalize spiritual experiences, catering to the unique spiritual narrative of every individual.

However, achieving this interconnectedness demands high ethical standards and cultural sensitivity. Developers must navigate this path carefully, ensuring AI systems respect the profound personal nature of spirituality. The aim is to enhance, not overshadow, the human spiritual experience, promoting a harmonious integration where AI supports spiritual exploration and growth.

### Summary

The chapter examines the multifaceted role of Artificial Intelligence (AI) in augmenting spiritual healing practices, highlighting its transformative potential across various modalities of spirituality. AI's integration contributes to spiritual healing by providing data-driven insights that personalize and improve the effectiveness of spiritual practices, ranging from meditation and prayer to complex healing rituals. By analyzing patterns in spiritual data, AI provides personalized spiritual care plans that recommend refinements to individual practices based on historical interactions and outcomes. It extends its capabilities to spiritual counseling, leveraging digital empathy to decode emotional and spiritual cues, thus offering targeted support. AI also interfaces with holistic practices like yoga and energy healing by tailoring interventions to individuals' spiritual and emotional states, thereby increasing the accessibility and impact of these practices. Furthermore, the chapter discusses sophisticated technologies such as virtual reality (VR) and biofeedback devices that, when combined with AI, enhance the depth and authenticity of spiritual experiences. Ethical considerations are paramount, emphasizing inclusivity, cultural sensitivity, and the protection of personal spiritual data. AI systems are designed to respect diverse spiritual traditions without imposing a standardized framework, fostering a respectful balance between technological advancement and spiritual integrity. Additionally, the integration of AI into spiritual therapy management and faith rituals personalizes spiritual engagements, enabling practitioners to cater uniquely to individual spiritual needs and paths. However, the chapter also reflects on challenges, such as ensuring the depth and authenticity of spiritual interactions and addressing ethical concerns related to privacy and data security, which are crucial in maintaining trust and integrity in AI applications within spiritual contexts.

## References

[1] AI in Healthcare and Medicine. https://www.ncbi.nlm.nih.gov/pmc/articles/PMC6616181/
[2] The Role of Artificial Intelligence in Spiritual Care. https://www.jstor.org/stable/10.13186/jhspi.25.1.0089
[3] Ethical Considerations for the Use of AI in Spiritual Practices. https://ieeexplore.ieee.org/document/8756975
[4] Cultural Sensitivity in AI. https://www.sciencedirect.com/science/article/pii/S0747563219304916
[5] Virtual Reality in Spirituality. https://www.frontiersin.org/articles/10.3389/fpsyg.2018.02158/full

### Case Study: Integrating AI in Multicultural Spiritual Practices

The growing prevalence of Artificial Intelligence (AI) in spiritual contexts raises both opportunities and challenges, especially when it comes to addressing the diverse spiritual needs across different cultures. This case study explores the integration of AI into the spiritual practices of a multicultural community in a large metropolitan city, where individuals from various cultural backgrounds come together to seek spiritual growth and healing.

The community center, known for its inclusive approach, decides to incorporate AI technologies to assist in facilitating and enhancing the spiritual experiences of its attendees. The AI system is designed to analyze and process a wide range of data, including textual analyses from sacred texts, feedback from spiritual sessions, and direct inputs from practitioners about their emotional and spiritual states. The goal is to tailor spiritual practices that accommodate the unique cultural nuances of each attendee.

During the initial phase, the AI system is tasked with organizing and recommending personalized meditation sessions. It uses natural language processing to understand the preferred languages and spiritual terminologies of users. Furthermore, the system leverages machine learning algorithms to suggest custom spiritual readings and chants that resonate with individual cultural backgrounds. However, the introduction of AI does not go without scrutiny. Some practitioners express concerns regarding the authenticity of AI-generated spiritual content and the potential loss of traditional human-led rituals that form the core of their spiritual practices.

Despite these challenges, the AI successfully helps the center increase attendance and engagement by providing a deeply personalized spiritual experience to its users. Attendees report feeling more understood and supported in their spiritual journeys, appreciating the seamless integration of their cultural heritage into the AI-driven sessions. Over time, the continuous feedback from users and ongoing refinement of the AI algorithms led to a model that became more adept at predicting and addressing the spiritual needs of a diverse clientele, balancing technological efficiency with cultural sensitivity.

### Case Study: AI-Enhanced Spiritual Healing in a Rural Community

The deployment of artificial intelligence (AI) in spiritual healing practices marks a transformative shift from conventional methods, particularly in settings lacking extensive resources. This case study delves into the application of AI in a rural community known for its rich spiritual traditions yet limited access to sophisticated spiritual care. The community, though vibrant in its folk and ancestral practices, often faces challenges in bridging modernity with tradition, amidst a deficit of professional spiritual advisors.

An initiative by a tech-based non-profit introduced an AI-driven platform aimed at enhancing the spiritual connectivity and therapeutic experiences of this rural populace. This platform was designed to integrate seamlessly with local customs and rituals, leveraging AI to personalize and scale spiritual healing processes. The system utilized user-inputted data, historical patterns of local rituals, and continuous feedback loops to learn and adapt. A central feature was its ability to suggest spiritual pathways and healing practices tailored to individual emotional and historical contexts, thus enriching the community's spiritual experiences.

However, the introduction of AI created a myriad of responses. While younger residents were quick to adopt and interact with the AI, older members of the community were skeptical, concerned about the potential erosion of traditional values and the impersonality of a machine-based spiritual aid. Concerns also emerged about privacy and the ethical use of personal data for spiritual adaptation.

Despite these challenges, the AI tools gradually began to demonstrate appreciable benefits. The platform enabled more frequent and accessible spiritual sessions, facilitated by virtual reality environments replicating sacred local spaces, which were especially valued by those physically unable to attend regular gatherings. Over time, the judicious use of AI, combined with consistent community dialogue and gradual familiarization efforts, helped alleviate fears and enhance the acceptance of AI as a complementary tool in spiritual practice, rather than a replacement.

**Case Study: AI-Driven Spiritual Guidance in a High-Stress Professional Environment**

The integration of AI in spiritual practices is increasingly notable, especially in high-stress environments such as the corporate world, where personal and spiritual growth can often be overlooked due to the demanding nature of professional life. This case study explores the utilization of AI-driven spiritual guidance within a multinational corporation known for its high-pressure work culture and diverse employee demographic.

The corporation introduced an AI-based platform, 'Soul Sync', designed to offer customized spiritual guidance to its employees. This platform collected data from individual users regarding their spiritual beliefs, preferences, stress levels, and general emotional state through secure, confidential surveys and daily mood logging. Using sophisticated algorithms, 'Soul Sync' analyzed the collected data to recommend personalized spiritual activities such as meditation, mindfulness, guided visualization, and short spiritual reading sessions that fit into the hectic schedules of employees.

Initially, the deployment of 'Soul Sync' was met with mixed reactions. While some employees appreciated the thoughtful integration of spiritual wellness into the workplace, others were skeptical about the efficacy of a machine-led spiritual approach. Ethical concerns about data privacy and the depth of AI's understanding of human spirituality also surfaced. In response, the company organized workshops with spiritual advisors and AI ethicists to educate employees on how the AI works, its benefits, and the robust privacy measures in place.

Over several months, many employees reported improvements in their stress levels and overall job satisfaction. They found that the AI's recommendations were subtly aligned with their personal beliefs and needs, which contributed positively to their professional life and personal well-being. The success of 'Soul Sync' highlighted the potential of AI in enhancing spiritual practices in a manner that respects individual diversity and the complexities of modern life, opening discussions on wider AI integrations across different corporate structures.

**Case Study: Revolutionizing Spiritual Exploration with AI-Enabled Virtual Pilgrimages**

The advent of Virtual Reality (VR) and AI has begun to significantly alter the landscape of spiritual practices, especially in how individuals engage with sacred spaces and spiritual rituals virtually. This case study examines a groundbreaking project in which a tech company, in collaboration with various religious and spiritual organizations, developed an AI-driven VR platform designed to facilitate virtual pilgrimages to revered religious sites worldwide, thereby making them accessible to a broader audience.

The VR platform, named 'SpiritualScape', utilizes sophisticated AI algorithms to create immersive, interactive, and personalized spiritual journeys. Users can experience detailed recreations of sites such as Jerusalem, Mecca, Varanasi, and other significant locations without leaving their homes. Before embarking on a virtual pilgrimage, users input their spiritual preferences, current emotional state, and specific interests related to the sites they plan to visit. The AI then customizes the experience, highlighting aspects of the visit that align with the users' spiritual and emotional needs, such as focusing on particular rituals, historical narratives, or meditative practices relevant to the site.

Initial responses were overwhelmingly positive, with users appreciating the accessibility and depth of the experience. However, the implementation did not come without challenges. Some users expressed concerns about the authenticity of virtual spiritual experiences as compared to physically being at the sacred sites. Furthermore, cultural and religious leaders reviewed the representations meticulously to ensure they were respectful and accurate, leading to ongoing modifications based on their feedback.

Despite these hurdles, 'SpiritualScape' has provided profound insights into the evolving role of technology in spiritual practices. It has not only democratized access to sacred experiences but also introduced a new layer of personalization and interactivity that traditional pilgrimages could not offer. The continuous refinement based on user feedback and ethical considerations ensures that the platform evolves to meet the high standards expected by its diverse user base, bridging the gap between technology and transformative spiritual encounters.

### Case Study: AI-Aided Spiritual Personalization in Healthcare Settings

In seeking to address patient care holistically, a cutting-edge hospital incorporates AI to personalize spiritual support in alignment with diverse patient backgrounds and health conditions. This integration serves as a bridge between medical treatment and spiritual comfort, aiming to enhance the overall wellness of patients through a balanced approach.

The hospital introduced a pilot program called 'SpiritualCare AI', designed to assist chaplains and spiritual care providers in delivering personalized spiritual content and support tailored to the specific needs of each patient. Using an AI system trained on a database incorporating a vast spectrum of spiritual practices and beliefs, 'SpiritualCare AI' analyses patient data, including their religious affiliations, spiritual preferences, and psychological state gleaned from initial assessments and continuous feedback.

As part of the program, chaplains receive AI-generated suggestions for spiritual interventions. These suggestions could range from scripture readings suited to the patient's belief system, guided meditations, or tailored spiritual counseling sessions aimed at addressing the emotional and spiritual needs heightened by medical distress. Privacy and ethical handling of personal data are prioritized to maintain trust and respect for patient confidentiality.

Despite the technology's potential, the implementation faces hurdles. Some staff members and patients express concerns about the depersonalization of spiritual care through the use of AI. Others question the AI's ability to truly understand and engage with human spirituality. Regular reviews and adaptations of the program, including feedback from patients and ethical oversight by an independent committee, are critical in tuning the AI's output to genuinely benefit patient care genuinely.

Over time, 'SpiritualCare AI' begins to show a positive impact. Patient testimonies reveal feelings of increased support and understanding, alleviating anxiety related to their medical conditions. Staff reports highlight the AI's role in enabling them to address patient needs more thoroughly. This case study underlines the potential of integrating advanced technology into spiritual care, hinting at broader implications for other interdisciplinary applications in healthcare.

**Case Study: AI in Enhancing Spiritual Engagement Among Digitally Native Generations**

In an era marked by rapid technological advancements, the integration of Artificial Intelligence (AI) in spiritual practices presents an intriguing approach to engage the digitally native generations. This case study centers on a Silicon Valley start-up, 'Soultech', which aims to redefine spiritual engagement for younger audiences by blending traditional spiritual elements with cutting-edge technology. Soultech's flagship product, the 'SpiritSpace' app, utilizes AI to create personalized spiritual experiences tailored to individual preferences and emotional states.

The app's development began with gathering extensive input from spiritual leaders across various traditions, coupled with the latest research on digital consumption patterns among millennials and Generation Z. Using advanced algorithms, the AI recommends spiritual content, meditative practices, and mindfulness exercises that resonate with individual user profiles based on their daily mood inputs and past interactions with the app.

The initial rollout of the app received mixed reviews. Young users appreciated the modern approach to spirituality, particularly the app's UI/UX, which mirrored their favorite social platforms. However, some expressed skepticism about the depth of spiritual engagement that can be achieved through AI. In response, Soultech hosted virtual seminars featuring both tech experts and spiritual leaders who discussed the potential for genuine spiritual growth through digital means.

Despite the hurdles, continuous data analysis and algorithm adjustments led to increasingly personalized user experiences. The AI system learned to detect subtle mood patterns and suggest spiritually uplifting content accordingly. Over time, the app not only retained users but also saw an increase in daily active engagement, indicating a gradual acceptance and appreciation of AI-facilitated spirituality.

This exploration into integrating AI within spiritual practices highlights the challenges and potential of reaching younger, tech-savvy populations. It poses significant questions about the future of spirituality in an increasingly digital world and the role AI might play in shaping new forms of spiritual exploration.

**Case Study: AI and Spiritual Healing in Remote Indigenous Communities**

In one groundbreaking project, a team of technologists and spiritual leaders collaborated to bring AI-driven spiritual healing to a remote indigenous community. The community, isolated by geography and with limited access to conventional health services, has a rich tradition of spiritual and medicinal healing practices passed down through generations. The project's primary goal was to enhance these traditional practices with AI technologies without compromising their cultural essence.

The AI application, named 'SpiritGuide', was designed to be culturally sensitive and adaptive to the community's unique spiritual language and practices. Incorporation began with extensive field research where AI developers spent time with community leaders and healers to understand the nuances of their spiritual practices. This preliminary phase was crucial for programming the AI not just technically but also culturally, enabling it to suggest spiritual interventions that resonate with the community's traditional beliefs.

However, the integration faced significant challenges right from the start. The community members were initially skeptical about the introduction of a foreign, technology-based intervention into their deeply personal and sacred spiritual spaces. There was also the logistical challenge of setting up and maintaining sophisticated AI technology in a remote area with unstable electricity and internet access.

The project team responded by setting up solar-powered stations and using satellite connections to ensure that the AI system could operate effectively. They also conducted several community workshops to demonstrate the AI's capabilities and its respect for, and integration with, traditional practices. Gradually, as the AI system suggested effective spiritual healing pathways, personalized for individual healing experiences, community acceptance grew.

Following months of operation, 'SpiritGuide' was credited with enhancing spiritual healing, significantly impacting the overall well-being of the community members. It facilitated a wider sharing of their spiritual heritage both within and beyond their geographic boundaries.

## Case Study: AI-Enabled Spiritual Support in Hospice Care

The introduction of Artificial Intelligence (AI) in hospice care settings represents a critical intersection between technology and the profound human experience of end-of-life transition. This case study examines the implementation of AI to provide spiritual support in a hospice setting, with a focus on enhancing the quality of life for terminally ill patients through personalized spiritual engagement.

A renowned hospice center, recognized for its compassionate care, has initiated a pilot program integrating AI-driven systems to provide spiritual support tailored to individual patient needs. The AI system, named 'SerenityAI', was designed to gather and analyze patient data related to their spiritual history, preferred spiritual practices, and emotional responses, using secure and ethically managed digital surveys. It employed natural language processing to engage in meaningful conversations with patients, offering spiritual solace, and fetching relevant spiritual content.

Initial reactions to 'SerenityAI' from patients and their families were mixed. Some appreciated the constant availability and the personalized nature of the spiritual content it provided, which included tailored music therapy sessions, guided meditations, and virtual reality experiences designed to evoke peace and reminiscence. Others, however, were hesitant to accept spiritual interaction mediated by a machine, expressing concerns over the loss of human touch in such a delicate phase of life.

Challenges in implementation included ensuring the AI's responses were sufficiently sensitive and appropriate. Ethical considerations regarding data privacy and the depth of understanding AI could achieve in interpreting human emotions were also significant. Over time, continuous improvements were made based on feedback from spiritual caregivers and family members, refining the AI's algorithms to match patient needs and emotional states better.

As the program evolved, 'SerenityAI' began to show a measurable impact on patient well-being. Reports highlighted reductions in anxiety and an increased sense of peace, underlining the potential benefits of integrating thoughtful AI solutions in spiritually charged environments. The case concluded with broader discussions on how AI can be ethically and effectively integrated into spiritual care, particularly in the sensitive management of end-of-life experiences.

## Review Questions

**1. In a case where a 40-year-old woman named Amina seeks relief from knee osteoarthritis and utilizes a combination of traditional bone-setting manipulations, daily grounding walks, and an Ayurvedic balm in a new medical setting in the US, the AI recommends typical Western medication. Amina feels unheard and disregards the recommendations. What should the provider have considered for a more culturally sensitive approach?**

A) Immediately refer Amina to a traditional Ayurvedic practitioner without offering Western treatment options.

B) Review Amina's traditional practices and integrate them into her care plan along with conventional medical advice where applicable.

C) Dismiss Amina's traditional practices and strictly adhere to standard pharmaceutical treatments to avoid any potential legal implications.

D) Encourage Amina to abandon her traditional practices, emphasizing the scientifically proven benefits of Western medicine only.

**Answer: B**

Explanation: To ensure culturally sensitive care, the provider should review Amina's use of traditional practices and integrate them into her comprehensive care plan. This inclusive approach acknowledges the potential benefits of both her traditional treatments and Western medicine. By validating her existing practices, the provider helps build trust and cooperation, essential for effective patient care. Integrative care models have proven to enhance patient satisfaction and health outcomes by respecting diverse cultural health beliefs and practices. It also acknowledges the cumulative evidence supporting the efficacy and value of holistic and traditional interventions alongside conventional medical treatments.

**2. A 52-year-old Native American patient presents in a clinic utilizing AI-driven healthcare tools. He prefers to integrate traditional healing practices with conventional medical treatment for his diabetes management. The AI system, however, only recommends conventional treatment options. What could be a suitable approach to modify the AI system to better accommodate the patient's cultural and personal treatment preferences?**

A) Exclude all traditional healing references as they are not supported by the AI's database.

B) Add a disclaimer advising against the use of traditional healing practices.

C) Enhance the AI's algorithm to recognize and integrate traditional healing practices into the patient's care plan.

D) Ignore the patient's preference and persuade him to trust solely in conventional treatments recommended by AI.

**Answer: C**

Explanation: The most culturally respectful and clinically appropriate approach would be to enhance the AI's algorithm to recognize and integrate traditional healing practices specific to Native American cultures alongside conventional medical treatments. This modification should involve collaborating with Native healers and medical experts to incorporate authentic and safe traditional practices into the AI's database, thus ensuring a holistic approach. Integrating these practices enables the AI to develop a comprehensive treatment plan that aligns with the patient's cultural beliefs and medical needs, potentially enhancing treatment adherence, satisfaction, and outcomes.

**3. In an urban healthcare setting, an AI diagnosis tool routinely fails to suggest traditional herbal remedies known to be effective among the local immigrant community. How should the healthcare facility address this issue in the AI's algorithm?**

A) Maintain the status quo as the AI's recommendations are based on widely accepted medical practices.

B) Engage with local traditional healers to gather data on effective herbal remedies and incorporate this into the AI's learning database.

C) Strictly advise against traditional remedies to avoid complicating legal responsibilities.

D) Limit the AI's use in the facility to avoid any cultural insensitivity.

**Answer: B**

Explanation: To effectively and respectfully address the gap in the AI's algorithm, the healthcare facility should collaborate with local traditional healers to understand and document the efficacy and usage of herbal remedies prevalent in the community. This data should then be standardized and integrated into the AI's learning database. Training the AI with this enriched data not only improves its diagnostic and suggestion accuracy but also enhances cultural competence in patient care. This approach acknowledges and values the diversity of medical practices within the community, which may increase patient trust and adherence to prescribed treatments.

**4. A healthcare AI system often recommends interventions that contradict or omit Native American traditional healing practices, leading to dissatisfaction among patients. What strategy should be implemented to refine the AI's recommendations?**

A) Completely remove the AI system and rely only on traditional Native American healing practices.

B) Form a review committee that includes Native American healers to oversee and adjust the AI's recommendations regularly.

C) Declare that traditional Native American healing practices are incompatible with modern medical recommendations and should be ignored.

D) Use AI to actively discourage patients from following their traditional practices.

**Answer: B**

Explanation: Establishing a review committee with Native American healers as part of the oversight team ensures that the AI's recommendations do not override or conflict with traditional healing practices important to the community. This committee would regularly review and adjust the AI's algorithms and datasets to incorporate and respect Native American healing practices. Such involvement ensures that the AI system reflects a comprehensive understanding of culturally appropriate care, thereby enhancing the relevance and acceptability of its recommendations among Native American patients. This strategy supports not only medical efficacy but also cultural preservation and respect, vital in providing holistic and person-centered care.

**Future Directions for AI and Medicine**

**Predictive Models in Personalized Medicine**

The realm of personalized medicine is being transformed by predictive models powered by artificial intelligence (AI). These models analyze vast arrays of patient data to tailor medical treatments to individual needs, heralding a new era in healthcare where treatment effectiveness is significantly enhanced. This precision is particularly critical in managing complex diseases, where one-size-fits-all solutions fall short.

AI's predictive prowess stems from its ability to learn from vast amounts of health records and derive insights that surpass human analysis. This capability not only forecasts disease progression but also anticipates patient responses to various treatments. It represents a shift from reactive to proactive care, potentially reducing hospital readmissions and improving patient outcomes.

However, integrating AI into personalized medicine presents numerous challenges. Ensuring data privacy and addressing ethical concerns are paramount. Moreover, the accuracy of AI predictions must continually improve to keep pace with medical advancements. Despite these hurdles, the potential of predictive AI models in revolutionizing care is undeniable, promising a future where medicine is more effective, efficient, and deeply personalized.

## Expansion of AI in Telemedicine

The landscape of telemedicine is evolving rapidly with the integration of artificial intelligence (AI), marking a transformative shift in how medical care is delivered remotely. AI's expansion in telemedicine is primarily driven by the need for more efficient and accessible healthcare services, particularly in underserved communities and during times when traditional face-to-face interactions are not feasible.

AI enhances telemedicine by enabling more precise and quicker diagnostic capabilities, personalized treatment options, and follow-up procedures. For example, AI algorithms can analyze medical images and data in real-time, offering diagnoses that might be delayed in traditional settings. This capability is vital in rural or remote areas, where specialist access is limited.

Furthermore, AI supports the ongoing monitoring and management of chronic conditions. It can predict health deterioration and trigger alerts for both patients and providers, ensuring timely interventions and reducing the rate of hospital readmissions. Ultimately, the expansion of AI in telemedicine promises a future of more proactive, patient-centered, and efficient healthcare systems.

## Integrative AI for Multi-Cultural Healing Practices

The advancement of AI in medical contexts now encompasses multicultural healing practices, fostering an integrative approach that respects and incorporates diverse healing traditions from around the world. By harnessing data from diverse cultural backgrounds, ranging from ancient herbal remedies to spiritual healing techniques, AI can broaden its therapeutic algorithms, offering more personalized, culturally informed medical advice and treatments.

This integrative form of AI learns from global databases of traditional medicine practices, analyzed alongside contemporary medical data, to offer more holistic health solutions. It not only synthesizes vast arrays of healing modalities but also respects the cultural significance of each practice, ensuring treatments are both effective and culturally sensitive. The collaboration between AI technologists and traditional healers is crucial to authenticating the input data and refining AI outputs.

The potential for such technology to transform healthcare is immense, creating pathways to accessibility and understanding that were previously obstructed by cultural barriers. Ethical considerations and ongoing dialogue with cultural representatives remain crucial for navigating the complexities involved in such an inclusive approach.

## Evolving AI Algorithms for Non-Invasive Diagnostics

The evolution of AI algorithms is revolutionizing the field of non-invasive diagnostics, enhancing the ability to diagnose conditions without the need for intrusive procedures. By leveraging sophisticated AI analysis, these algorithms can interpret complex medical images and biomarkers with unprecedented precision, reducing the risk and discomfort associated with traditional diagnostic methods.

This technological advancement is particularly significant in early disease detection, where accuracy and timeliness are crucial for effective treatment. AI-driven non-invasive tools can detect subtle anomalies that human experts may overlook, enabling early interventions that can alter the course of diseases. Moreover, these AI systems continually learn and improve, integrating new data to refine their diagnostic capabilities further.

However, the integration of these evolving AI algorithms also raises important ethical and practical considerations, including patient privacy and the reliability of AI interpretations. Ensuring transparency and maintaining rigorous validation standards are crucial for maximizing benefits while minimizing potential risks associated with AI in non-invasive diagnostics.

## AI and Its Role in Chronic Disease Management

AI's integration into chronic disease management is redefining patient care by offering continuous, personalized support beyond traditional healthcare settings. By analyzing health data in real-time, AI models can predict exacerbations in chronic conditions such as diabetes and heart disease, allowing for preemptive medical interventions. These predictive capabilities facilitate a shift from episodic care to a more sustainable, preventive approach, which is particularly crucial in chronic disease scenarios where early intervention can prevent complications and improve quality of life.

Moreover, AI-driven tools empower patients by providing them with insights into their health patterns, encouraging self-management and adherence to prescribed therapies. Interactive AI applications can remind patients to take medications, track their symptoms, and even provide dietary suggestions, seamlessly integrating health management into daily life.

However, the widespread adoption of AI in chronic disease management must ensure patient privacy and data security. Ongoing oversight and ethical reviews are crucial for building trust and ensuring that AI supports the health needs of individuals without compromising their personal information. These measures will be pivotal in harnessing AI's full potential in chronic disease management.

## Innovations in AI-Driven Surgical Techniques

The surgical landscape is undergoing a profound transformation with the onset of AI-driven technologies. Innovations in robotic surgery, empowered by artificial intelligence, are enabling greater precision and smaller incisions, which reduce recovery time and minimize the risk of infection. These AI systems are often equipped with machine learning capabilities, learning from each procedure to enhance their accuracy and efficiency in future operations.

Beyond physical execution, AI is instrumental in the preoperative and postoperative stages. Advanced algorithms assist in planning complex surgical procedures by providing surgeons with simulations based on predictive analytics. This preparation increases the success rate of surgeries and patient safety. Postoperatively, AI tools monitor patient recovery, adjusting treatments to individual responses, thereby personalizing the healing process and reducing hospital stays.

However, the integration of AI into surgical practices also introduces ethical considerations and requires rigorous testing to ensure reliability. Nevertheless, the potential benefits of AI-driven surgical techniques promise a revolutionary impact on medicine, making surgeries safer, faster, and less burdensome for patients.

## Real-Time Patient Monitoring Using AI

The integration of Artificial Intelligence (AI) in real-time patient monitoring heralds a new era in healthcare, offering unprecedented real-time insights into patient health. This technology is transforming patient care, allowing for constant monitoring without the need for the patient or physician to be in the same location, a critical advantage especially in rural or under-resourced areas.

AI-driven systems continuously analyze data, detecting anomalies that may indicate a need for emergency intervention. For instance, AI can monitor heart rate, blood pressure, and other vital signs, quickly identifying alarming trends and notifying healthcare professionals. This immediacy significantly reduces response times during critical events, potentially saving lives by ensuring timely medical attention.

Furthermore, such systems facilitate a proactive approach to healthcare. By predicting potential health issues based on trend analyses, AI enables interventions before conditions worsen, effectively shifting the focus from treatment to prevention. The seamless integration of AI in patient monitoring not only enhances care but also optimizes healthcare resources, reducing unnecessary hospital visits and admissions.

## AI in Mental Health: New Therapeutic Approaches

The intersection of AI and mental health is opening new doors for therapeutic approaches, fundamentally altering how psychological care is administered. These emerging AI technologies offer tailored therapy sessions via virtual agents, who can consistently monitor and subtly adjust therapeutic strategies to suit individual mental health needs. This capability introduces a level of personalization previously unsupported in traditional therapy contexts.

Further advancement in AI-driven mental health care focuses on emotion recognition systems that interpret vocal cues or facial expressions to assess a patient's emotional state. This technology aids in identifying periods of acute distress, potentially predicting and mitigating episodes of depression or anxiety before they escalate. This proactive care model could revolutionize crisis intervention and ongoing mental health management.

Critically, the implementation of AI in mental health raises significant ethical concerns regarding privacy and the potential for depersonalization of care. Continuous dialogue with mental health professionals and patients must guide the development of these applications to ensure they augment rather than replace human empathy and understanding in therapeutic settings.

## AI-Enhanced Drug Discovery and Development

Artificial Intelligence (AI) is setting new frontiers in drug discovery and development, marking a significant acceleration in the research and development of new medications. AI algorithms analyze massive datasets to predict molecular behavior and determine the potential efficacy of drugs, streamlining the identification of viable new compounds.

Furthermore, AI aids in simulating clinical trial scenarios, minimizing the need for lengthy preliminary human trials and thus reducing both costs and time-to-market for critical medications. This not only reshapes the landscape of pharmacology but also promises more targeted therapies at an accelerated pace, critical for responding to global health crises like pandemics.

However, the integration of AI in these processes must be carefully managed to maintain ethical standards and ensure safety. Transparency in AI processes, coupled with continuous monitoring and validation against clinical outcomes, is crucial to foster trust and reliance upon AI-enhanced methods in the sensitive field of drug development.

## Ethical AI Deployment in Clinical Settings

The deployment of AI in clinical settings introduces profound ethical challenges that necessitate vigilant oversight. Firstly, ensuring the privacy and confidentiality of patient data is paramount. AI systems often require extensive datasets for training and operation, posing significant risks if data breaches occur or if data is misused. Protocols must be established to secure patient information and maintain trust.

Secondly, the decision-making process of AI must be transparent. Clinicians and patients alike should understand how AI conclusions are derived. This transparency is crucial for accountability, particularly in diagnosing and recommending treatments, where the stakes are exceptionally high. Mechanisms should be in place to review and challenge AI decisions to prevent potential errors and biases from harming patients.

Finally, the inclusivity of AI systems is critical. Algorithms trained on limited or non-representative datasets can lead to biased medical assessments, disproportionately affecting marginalized communities. Ongoing efforts must focus on creating diverse data pools to train AI systems, ensuring equitable healthcare outcomes across different demographics. Ethical AI deployment in medicine is not just about integrating technology—it's about reshaping care practices to uphold human dignity and justice.

## Improving Healthcare Access Through Mobile AI Applications

The advent of mobile AI applications is revolutionizing healthcare accessibility, bridging the gap between advanced medical resources and remote or underserved populations. These sophisticated tools leverage AI technologies to deliver healthcare services and information directly to mobile devices, enabling patients in isolated regions to receive timely medical advice and diagnostics without the need for physical travel.

This transformation is particularly significant in areas where healthcare facilities are sparse or non-existent. By integrating AI with mobile technology, developers have created apps that can perform tasks ranging from basic health monitoring to more complex diagnostics, all via smartphones. These applications can guide individuals through symptom checks, connect them with healthcare professionals remotely, and even manage chronic conditions by providing personalized feedback and reminders for medication adherence.

Moreover, these mobile solutions are crucial in promoting preventive healthcare measures in communities that might otherwise be overlooked, making significant contributions to global health advancements. The potential for mobile AI applications to expand healthcare reach and efficiency exemplifies the power of technology to not just innovate but also equalize conditions for health and wellness worldwide.

## AI's Contribution to Public Health Informatics

Artificial Intelligence (AI) is transforming public health informatics, enhancing the ability to manage and analyze vast amounts of data essential for understanding and combating public health issues. By integrating AI, health organizations can swiftly identify patterns and trends in health behaviors and disease spread, leading to faster and more effective responses to public health emergencies.

AI tools are pivotal in modeling disease outbreaks, predicting their trajectories, and developing strategies for intervention and containment. These advanced algorithms process real-time data to forecast potential hotspots and inform public health decisions. This capability is instrumental in managing and mitigating the effects of pandemics, ensuring that resources are allocated efficiently to areas most in need.

Moreover, AI supports the maintenance of public health databases, ensuring the accuracy and relevance of information that forms the basis for policymaking and health advisories. The proactive use of AI in public health not only optimizes the response to immediate threats but also aids in long-term planning and preventive strategies, ultimately enhancing community health and safety.

## Advancements in AI for Geriatric Care

Artificial Intelligence (AI) is significantly enhancing geriatric care, offering new opportunities for the management of healthcare for the elderly population. AI technologies are being deployed to monitor senior health metrics continuously, facilitating early detection of potentially life-threatening conditions and effectively tailoring interventions to individual health needs.

AI is particularly transformative in managing chronic diseases that commonly afflict the elderly, such as diabetes and heart disease. Through machine learning algorithms, AI can predict disease progression and optimize management plans, which is crucial in delaying or preventing severe complications. This proactive approach in geriatric care not only improves quality of life but also reduces the healthcare system's burden.

Moreover, AI-powered assistive technologies provide the elderly with improved independence and safety. Smart home systems enable remote monitoring of elderly activities, ensuring an immediate response in emergencies, such as falls. These advancements are revolutionizing geriatric care, making it more efficient and responsive to the specific needs of aging populations.

## AI in Genetic Research and Gene Therapy

Artificial Intelligence (AI) is revolutionizing genetic research and gene therapy by enabling more precise modification and analysis of genetic materials. AI algorithms can rapidly sequence genomes and identify genetic disorders, accelerating the development of personalized gene therapies that can potentially cure hereditary diseases. This employs advanced machine learning models to predict the effects of genetic modifications, thereby reducing the risks associated with gene-editing technologies, such as CRISPR.

Moreover, AI's predictive capabilities enable the design of targeted therapies that can adapt to individual genetic profiles, resulting in higher success rates and fewer side effects. By integrating genotypic data with phenotypic expressions through AI, scientists can gain unprecedented insights into complex gene-environment interactions. This not only pushes the boundaries of medical science but also paves the way for more holistic treatment approaches.

Finally, continuous advancements in AI help refine these technologies, ensuring ethical standards are met while striving for medical breakthroughs. AI in gene therapy is not just a tool but a transformative force in medicine, crafting the future of genetic health and patient care.

## AI Applications in Managing Pandemic Responses

AI's role in managing pandemic responses marks a significant turning point in public health. By leveraging machine learning, AI systems can analyze data from various sources to predict outbreak patterns and suggest containment strategies. This real-time data processing enables the rapid deployment of resources and informed decision-making, which is crucial during a pandemic.

Furthermore, AI facilitates the simulation of multiple outbreak scenarios, providing health officials with valuable insights into the potential impact of various intervention strategies. These simulations help in optimizing pandemic response plans, aiming for minimal disruption while maximizing safety.

AI also enhances communication channels during a pandemic by automating updates and alerts, which are crucial for public awareness and safety. By streamlining the flow of information, AI helps maintain public calm and ensure compliance with health advisories.

The integration of AI in pandemic response not only refines emergency management but also underscores the need for robust, technologically equipped public health systems moving forward.

## AI's Influence on Healthcare Policy Making

Artificial Intelligence (AI) is playing a transformative role in healthcare policy making, influencing decisions and strategies that impact public health outcomes. As AI integrates more deeply into healthcare systems, its data-driven insights are helping policymakers craft regulations that promote efficiency, equity, and innovation in healthcare delivery.

AI tools analyze vast datasets to identify health trends and outcomes, which are crucial for forming evidence-based policies. Moreover, the predictive power of AI aids in forecasting healthcare needs and resource allocation, ensuring that policies are responsive to future challenges. These capabilities make AI invaluable in crafting policies that anticipate and address various healthcare scenarios, from everyday wellness to crisis management.

Furthermore, AI contributes to healthcare policy by enhancing transparency and accountability. Through sophisticated tracking and reporting mechanisms, AI systems ensure that healthcare policies adhere to ethical standards and are consistently evaluated for effectiveness, fostering an environment of trust and reliability in public health policies.

## Collaborative AI Systems for Multi-Disciplinary Teams

In the realm of healthcare, the integration of AI into multidisciplinary teams represents a paradigm shift towards more collaborative and efficient medical practice. These AI systems facilitate seamless communication and data exchange among specialists, enhancing the decision-making process and providing a holistic approach to patient care. By synthesizing diverse medical expertise with advanced algorithms, AI enables teams to develop comprehensive treatment plans that consider multiple facets of health.

Moreover, AI-driven tools are designed to adapt to the dynamic workflows of multi-disciplinary teams, offering real-time insights and suggestions tailored to the specific needs of each case. This not only improves the accuracy of diagnoses and treatments but also speeds up the healthcare delivery process, making it more responsive to patient needs.

As these collaborative AI systems evolve, they are poised to become indispensable in managing complex cases that require the coordinated efforts of various healthcare professionals. The future of medical practice hinges on the successful integration of AI into these teams, which will optimize healthcare outcomes through enhanced synergy and innovation.

## AI and the Future of Healthcare Education

The landscape of healthcare education is undergoing a transformative shift with the integration of Artificial Intelligence (AI). AI's capability to analyze vast amounts of data and derive valuable insights is revolutionizing the way healthcare professionals are trained. Customized learning paths generated by AI algorithms can adapt to the individual learning pace and style of students, enhancing their understanding and retention of complex medical knowledge.

Moreover, AI-driven simulations and virtual reality environments provide medical students and professionals with hands-on experience in a risk-free setting. These tools enable repetitive practice and exposure to rare, complex medical scenarios, preparing them for real-world challenges. This aspect of AI not only boosts the competence of future healthcare providers but also ensures a higher standard of patient care.

The future of healthcare education will likely witness AI as a central pillar, assisting educators in crafting curricula that are more dynamic and immediately relevant to evolving medical practices. Emphasizing continuous learning and improvement, AI could help bridge the gap between medical education and actual practice, ensuring a seamless transition for healthcare professionals into the ever-evolving landscape of medical care.

## Strategies for Reducing Bias in Medical AI

Addressing bias in medical AI is critical for equitable healthcare delivery. A primary strategy involves diversifying training data sets. By ensuring that data represents a diverse range of populations, AI models can better generalize across different demographics, thereby reducing the risk of biased outputs. This includes incorporating data from underrepresented groups and varied health conditions, thereby enhancing the model's accuracy and fairness.

Another pivotal approach is the application of algorithmic fairness techniques. Developers can utilize these techniques to identify and mitigate biases that may emerge during the AI training process. Regular audits and updates of AI systems are essential to maintain fairness over time, adapting to new data and correcting biases that were previously unrecognized.

Engagement with ethicists and stakeholders from diverse cultural and professional backgrounds also plays a vital role. This collaboration ensures the ethical deployment of AI tools, fostering transparency and trust among patients and healthcare providers. Collectively, these strategies aim to create a more just and effective medical AI landscape.

## Developing Global Standards for AI in Health

Establishing global standards for AI in healthcare is essential for ensuring consistency and safety in medical technologies across borders. Uniform standards can guide the development of AI systems to be universally effective, ethical, and accessible. By fostering a cooperative international framework, countries can leverage their diverse experiences and technological strengths to enhance global health outcomes.

Central to this initiative is the creation of benchmarks that address data privacy, algorithmic integrity, and interoperability among different healthcare systems. These guidelines must also consider cultural sensitivities and local healthcare regulations to ensure AI technologies are adaptable and respectful of regional healthcare practices. Harmonized standards will facilitate smoother exchanges of medical AI applications and methodologies, paving the way for advanced collaborative research and shared healthcare solutions.

Moreover, such standards support the scalability of AI innovations. As AI technology develops, maintaining cohesive standards will allow emerging advancements to integrate seamlessly into existing healthcare frameworks, further optimizing global health services. This strategic approach will not only extend the reach of healthcare but also foster international trust and cooperation in the burgeoning field of medical AI.

**Blockchain and AI for Enhanced Data Security**

The convergence of Blockchain and Artificial Intelligence (AI) heralds a new era of data security in healthcare. By harnessing blockchain's inherent decentralization, data transactions in medical records can be rendered immutable and transparent, drastically reducing the risks of unauthorized access and data breaches.

AI complements blockchain by intelligently managing data flows and detecting anomalies that could indicate security threats. This synergy not only enhances data protection mechanisms but also optimizes the efficiency of health care operations by ensuring that sensitive information is shielded from cyber threats while remaining readily accessible to authorized personnel.

Moreover, the integration of blockchain and AI facilitates the creation of a trustless environment, where data integrity and confidentiality are maintained without relying on traditional centralized systems. This approach not only fortifies data security but also restores patients' trust in how their personal health information is managed. Collectively, blockchain and AI are setting the groundwork for a revolution in secure, decentralized healthcare solutions.

**AI-Driven Personal Health Assistants**

AI-driven personal health assistants are paving the way for a new era in personalized medicine. These intelligent systems utilize advanced algorithms to deliver real-time health monitoring and personalized health management advice directly to users. By constantly analyzing user data, such as vital signs or daily activities, these assistants can predict potential health issues before they become critical, offering preventive recommendations and alerting healthcare providers when necessary.

Furthermore, their ability to integrate seamlessly into everyday devices makes them an indispensable asset for monitoring chronic conditions, ensuring continuous care coordination between patients and healthcare teams. This constant interaction not only enhances patient engagement with their health but also allows for immediate adjustments in treatment plans based on the latest health data inputs.

As these AI assistants evolve, they will become more adept at understanding complex medical histories and lifestyle factors, thus offering more precise and proactive health management. This marks a significant step towards more dynamic and responsive healthcare systems, where technology and human expertise collaborate closely to enhance patient outcomes.

**Future Legal Challenges of AI in Healthcare**

As AI integrates more deeply into healthcare, navigating the complex legal challenges becomes imperative. Central issues include compliance with fluctuating international privacy laws, especially given AI's broad data acquisition across borders. Distinct legal standards for data protection and patient privacy necessitate sophisticated AI systems that can dynamically adapt to diverse regulatory environments without compromising functionality or ethical standards.

Moreover, liability in the event of AI-related errors presents a complex challenge. Determining responsibility - whether it rests with healthcare providers, AI developers, or both - requires clear legal frameworks. These frameworks must address the unique nature of AI decisions, which do not always align neatly with traditional fault-based liability structures in healthcare.

Lastly, intellectual property rights in AI-assisted medical innovations provoke heated debates. Balancing incentivization of AI advancements with safeguarding patient access to breakthrough treatments involves intricate legal craftsmanship. The evolving nature of AI technology continually tests the agility of existing intellectual property laws, demanding ongoing legislative evolution to keep pace with technological advancements.

## AI and the Evolution of Patient-Doctor Interactions

The integration of Artificial Intelligence (AI) into healthcare is reshaping the foundational dynamics of patient-doctor interactions. Traditionally, these interactions have relied heavily on direct, personal communication. However, AI introduces a layer of digital interface that can enhance diagnostic accuracy and treatment efficiency but may alter the personal connection integral to patient care.

AI tools assist doctors by providing comprehensive data analysis, predictive health insights, and treatment options based on vast datasets that a human alone could not process as swiftly. This capability supports clinicians in making more informed decisions. However, it is crucial to balance technological intervention with a human touch to maintain trust and empathy, which are core to successful health outcomes.

Moreover, as AI becomes increasingly prevalent, there is a growing need to train healthcare professionals not just in technical skills but in navigating the nuances of AI-augmented interactions. Educating both patients and practitioners about AI's role and limitations will be key to optimizing its benefits while preserving the essential human elements of healthcare.

## Summary

The chapter 'Future Directions for AI and Medicine' encapsulates the transformative impact of Artificial Intelligence (AI) in various medical domains, signifying a trajectory towards more personalized, efficient, and accessible healthcare. The introduction of predictive models in personalized medicine highlights AI's potential to tailor treatments to individual needs, thereby enhancing treatment outcomes, particularly in complex diseases. Meanwhile, AI's expansion in telemedicine exemplifies its role in improving diagnostic capabilities and patient monitoring, particularly benefiting remote and underserved communities. The chapter also explores the integration of AI with multicultural healing practices, aiming for a holistic approach that respects diverse medical traditions. The significance of non-invasive diagnostics is highlighted, where AI algorithms aid in accurate disease detection without physical intrusions, thereby prioritizing patient comfort and safety. AI's profound impact on chronic disease management through real-time data analysis and predictive insights is discussed, illustrating a shift from episodic care to continuous, preventive care strategies. Innovations in AI-driven surgical techniques are transforming surgical procedures, enhancing precision and safety while significantly reducing recovery times. Real-time patient monitoring using AI is reshaping emergency responses and routine health tracking, delivering timely interventions. In mental health, AI introduces new therapeutic modalities and crisis intervention tools, potentially revolutionizing treatment approaches. The chapter further explores AI's role in advancing drug discovery by streamlining the research phase and simulating clinical trials, thereby accelerating the development of effective therapies. Ethical considerations surrounding the employment of AI in clinical settings are critically analyzed, emphasizing the need for transparent, inclusive, and secure AI applications to ensure equitable healthcare delivery. The chapter concludes by investigating AI's broader implications on public health policy, education, and global health standards, suggesting a future where AI not only reshapes healthcare practices but also fosters global health equity and innovation.

## References

[1] Predictive Models in Personalized Medicine. https://www.ncbi.nlm.nih.gov/pmc/articles/PMC6007753/
[2] Personalized Medicine and Telemedicine. https://www.sciencedirect.com/science/article/abs/pii/S1532046413000057
[3] Cultural Diversity in Medicine. https://www.sciencedirect.com/science/article/pii/S2371438320303035

[4] AI in Non-Invasive Diagnostics. https://ieeexplore.ieee.org/abstract/document/9123175
[5] AI's Role in Chronic Disease Management. https://jamanetwork.com/journals/jama/fullarticle/2763516
[6] Robotic Surgery and AI. https://www.ncbi.nlm.nih.gov/pmc/articles/PMC6394297/
[7] AI in Palliative Care Settings. https://bmcpalliatcare.biomedcentral.com/articles/10.1186/s12904-019-0451-y
[8] AI and Mental Health Interventions. https://www.sciencedirect.com/science/article/pii/S2214782920300456
[9] AI-driven Drug Discovery. https://www.nature.com/articles/d41573-019-00084-z
[10] Healthcare Ethics and AI. https://academic.oup.com/jlb/article/3/2/188/826083

## Case Study: Integrating AI in Chronic Disease Management: A Case Study on Diabetes

The introduction of Artificial Intelligence (AI) into the management of chronic diseases, such as diabetes, exemplifies a significant shift in healthcare toward more proactive, personalized care. Let's explore the hypothetical scenario of HealthTech Innovations, a health organization that implemented an AI-driven platform to manage diabetes among its patients.

HealthTech Innovations developed 'DiabeTech,' an AI system designed to analyze continuous glucose monitoring (CGM) data in conjunction with patients' dietary inputs, physical activity records, and medication adherence. DiabeTech was trained using a vast dataset from diverse demographics, ensuring its algorithms were robust and inclusive. The system provided real-time insights into glucose levels, predicted potential hyperglycemic events, and suggested lifestyle modifications.

Once implemented, DiabeTech significantly reduced the incidence of diabetes-related emergencies among patients by providing early warnings and personalized management plans. Patients could interact with DiabeTech through a mobile app, receiving timely notifications about their health status and reminders to take medication or adjust their diet.

The success of HealthTech Innovations' DiabeTech not only showcases the potential of AI in chronic disease management but also highlights the essential components needed for such technology to be effective, including comprehensive data analysis, patient-centric functionality, and continuous learning and improvement of the system.

However, despite its advantages, the adoption of DiabeTech brought forth challenges such as ensuring patient data privacy, managing the variable accuracy of AI predictions, and integrating AI advice with human oversight. Addressing these challenges required constant ethical oversight, rigorous data protection measures, and ongoing training for both healthcare providers and patients to effectively balance AI integration with traditional care practices.

## Case Study: AI-Powered Telemedicine in Rural Healthcare Enhancement

In this case study, we examine the transformative impact of artificial intelligence (AI) on telemedicine, with a particular focus on its application in rural healthcare settings. Consider the case of RuralMed AI, a telemedicine initiative launched to address healthcare disparities in remote areas where access to medical specialists and advanced healthcare facilities is limited.

RuralMed AI was introduced by a consortium of healthcare providers aiming to leverage AI technologies to extend and enhance healthcare delivery in underserved rural communities. The initiative deployed AI-powered diagnostic tools and virtual health assistants through a telemedicine platform, accessible via smartphones and computers. The AI system was designed to analyze medical images, patient symptoms, and historical health data to provide preliminary diagnoses and prioritize patient cases for specialist consultations.

The introduction of RuralMed AI significantly improved diagnostic accuracy and reduced waiting times for patients in rural locations. With AI's capability to analyze vast datasets and recognize patterns, the system facilitated quicker diagnosis of common but potentially serious conditions, such as diabetic retinopathy and cardiovascular diseases, which are prevalent in these areas. Patients could receive timely advice and referrals, ensuring that critical cases were escalated to specialists without unnecessary delays.

However, the deployment of RuralMed AI was not without challenges. Key issues included the need for reliable internet connectivity in rural areas, the adaptation of AI tools to diverse patient demographics and conditions, and the training of local healthcare providers to use the new technology effectively. Ensuring the ethical use of AI, maintaining patient privacy, and building trust among the local population were pivotal.

The case of RuralMed AI illustrates the potential of AI in bridging healthcare gaps through telemedicine, particularly in rural settings. It underscores the importance of addressing technological, ethical, and operational challenges to fully realize the benefits of AI in improving healthcare accessibility and outcomes.

## Case Study: AI-Enhanced Personal Health Assistants for Elderly Care

Envision a healthcare scenario focused on improving the quality of life for the elderly through AI-enhanced personal health assistants, a project initiated by a tech company named 'ElderCare AI'. This company, specializing in advanced AI solutions for aging populations, developed an intelligent assistant named 'CareBot.' The primary aim was to support elderly individuals who prefer to live independently but require regular health monitoring and assistance.

CareBot integrates into the daily lives of seniors through wearable devices and smart home systems. It continuously collects health data such as heart rate, mobility patterns, sleep quality, and medication adherence. This data is processed in real-time, utilizing deep learning algorithms to identify abnormal patterns and potential health risks. If a potential issue is detected, CareBot promptly alerts both the user and their designated healthcare provider, and if necessary, emergency services.

Moreover, CareBot offers daily interaction and cognitive exercises designed to maintain mental agility, alongside reminders for medication and appointments, as well as social interaction prompts to combat loneliness. This comprehensive approach has not only fostered greater independence but also significantly improved the well-being and safety of elderly users.

The introduction of CareBot into the market faced several challenges, including ensuring user privacy and securing sensitive data. These concerns were addressed through robust cybersecurity measures and transparent data handling policies. Another significant hurdle was achieving high user acceptance, particularly in adapting to constant interactions with an AI entity. ElderCare AI conducted extensive community outreach and user education campaigns to familiarize potential users with the technology's benefits and operation.

This case study highlights the transformative potential of AI in enhancing elderly care to be more proactive, preventive, and personalized. By understanding and discussing these practical applications and the challenges faced, practitioners and students can better appreciate the nuances of integrating AI technology in healthcare settings explicitly tailored for the elderly.

## Case Study: AI in Genetic Research and Therapy: Advancing Personalized Medicine

Imagine a biotechnological company, Genetech AI Innovations, which specializes in integrating artificial intelligence (AI) to revolutionize genetic research and personalized gene therapy. A focal project, named GenePredict AI, was initiated to develop AI-driven tools for analyzing and predicting genetic mutations that could lead to specific diseases, thereby aiding in early diagnosis and personalized treatment plans.

GenePredict AI utilizes advanced machine learning algorithms to process and analyze vast quantities of genomic data collected from diverse populations worldwide. The AI's ability to learn from extensive disease pattern data allows it to identify potential genetic risks with high accuracy. These capabilities have enabled Genetech AI Innovations to partner with healthcare providers to offer early screening for genetic conditions such as cystic fibrosis, Huntington's disease, and some rare types of cancer, long before any clinical symptoms are apparent.

This innovative approach is not only proactive but also preventative, with AI recommending lifestyle changes and treatments that can significantly delay, or in some cases, prevent the onset of the disease. GenePredict AI also assists doctors in customizing medications and therapies based on the patient's unique genetic profile, optimizing treatment effectiveness and minimizing side effects.

Despite the tremendous potential, challenges exist, such as ensuring the ethical use of genetic data, preventing genetic discrimination, and continuously updating the AI systems to incorporate the latest medical research and genetic insights. The accuracy and ethical considerations of predictions made by AI systems are of utmost importance. Amidst these challenges, Genetech AI Innovations is pioneering a change in managing health on a genetic level, promising a future where genetic diseases are preemptively tackled before they can affect quality of life, leveraging AI for a deeper and more precise approach to medicine.

### Case Study: AI-Driven Predictive Models in Personalized Oncology

Let's consider a fictional but representative scenario involving a state-of-the-art oncology center, FutureCare Oncology, which has adopted the use of artificial intelligence (AI)-driven predictive models to refine cancer treatment protocols and patient outcomes substantially. FutureCare Oncology developed an AI platform, OncoPredictAI, designed to integrate multimodal data sources, including genomic data, radiographic images, and clinical health record's to offer personalized treatment plans for patients with various types of cancer.

OncoPredictAI was trained on an extensive dataset, encompassing a wide range of cancer types, stages, and demographic variations, ensuring broad applicability and sensitivity to diverse patient needs. The system utilizes advanced machine learning techniques to identify patterns and predict tumor behavior, response to treatments, and potential recurrence. As patients commence their treatment, OncoPredictAI continues to learn from real-time data, dynamically adjusting treatment plans based on the patient's response.

Once implemented, FutureCare Oncology observed a significant enhancement in treatment efficacy and reduction in treatment-related side effects. The AI's capability to predict adverse responses to certain chemotherapy drugs allowed oncologists to tailor therapies that are less toxic and more efficacious for individual patients. Furthermore, OncoPredictAI can forecast the likelihood of cancer recurrence, enabling preemptive measures in cases deemed high-risk.

The OncoPredictAI project, while a benchmark in AI-driven healthcare, posed several challenges. Primary among these were issues of data security, ensuring the privacy of sensitive patient data, and the ethical considerations surrounding AI-driven predictions that affect patient treatment paths. FutureCare had to implement stringent data governance protocols and engage in continuous dialogue with ethicists and regulatory bodies. Also, there was the challenge of integrating AI recommendations with the seasoned judgment of oncologists, balancing machine-generated insights with human experience and intuition.

### Case Study: AI-Enhanced Robotic Surgery in Pediatric Orthopedics

Exploring the integration of artificial intelligence (AI) in robotic-assisted surgeries presents a vivid scenario in pediatric orthopedics. Consider MedAI Robotics, a pioneer in AI-driven robotic technology, which partnered with a leading children's hospital to introduce an advanced robotic system, 'Pediatric PrecisionBot', specifically designed for pediatric orthopedic surgeries. Pediatric PrecisionBot combines AI algorithms with robotic precision to perform complex procedures such as spinal deformity corrections and joint replacements with minimal invasiveness and enhanced accuracy.

The Pediatric PrecisionBot system was equipped with sensors and imaging technologies that provided real-time feedback, enabling the robotic arms to execute precise movements during surgeries. It was trained on vast amounts of surgical data, learning to adapt to various pediatric anatomies and conditions. AI's role was critical in predicting surgical complications and optimizing surgical pathways, thereby significantly reducing the surgery times and improving patient outcomes.

Once implemented, the hospital saw a dramatic increase in the success rates of pediatric surgeries. Postoperative recovery times were shorter due to less tissue disruption, and there was a notable decrease in post-surgical infections and complications. Patients benefited from quicker recoveries and reduced pain, encouraging quicker returns to normal activities.

Despite these successes, implementing Pediatric PrecisionBot posed distinct challenges. Key among them was ensuring the system's reliability and safety, given the high stakes of pediatric surgeries. MedAI Robotics invested heavily in continuous testing and refinement of the AI algorithms to mitigate risks. Additionally, there was an ethical concern around machine-dependence in surgical decisions, necessitating clear guidelines on human oversight during operations.

This case study not only illustrates the potential of AI in transforming pediatric surgery through robotics but also prompts deep discussions on the balance between technology and human judgment in critical healthcare scenarios, the ethics of AI in medicine, and the ongoing need for training and adaptation among surgical teams to new technologies.

### Case Study: Revolutionizing Emergency Healthcare Through AI-Driven Real-Time Response Systems

The advent of AI in emergency healthcare has brought about transformative improvements, particularly in systems tailored to deliver real-time responses during critical medical events. The practical implementation of such an innovation is best illustrated by the case of CrisisAI, a technological initiative launched by a consortium called Emergency Response Tech Innovations. This initiative aimed to leverage AI-driven analytics to revolutionize emergency management, from incident detection to hospital admission.

CrisisAI systems were deployed in coordination with local emergency services to provide immediate computational assessments of emergency calls, integrating real-time data such as caller location, historical medical records (where available), and live video feeds from caller devices or nearby surveillance cameras. Using natural language processing and image recognition technologies, the AI system could prioritize calls, dispatch the appropriate services, and provide preliminary diagnostic suggestions to responders while en route.

For instance, during its pilot operation, CrisisAI successfully identified a cardiac arrest at a shopping mall through analysis of the caller's distressed speech patterns and background noises. Subsequently, it directed the nearest automated external defibrillator (AED)- equipped drone to the site before the ambulance crew arrived, which was crucial for the patient's survival.

This real-world application of CrisisAI demonstrated not only the potential of integrating AI into public safety frameworks but also the various challenges that emerged. Issues such as data protection, reliance on potentially unstable internet connections, and the need for extensive cross-jurisdictional cooperation were prominent. Moreover, ensuring that the AI system's recommendations were precisely accurate required continuous algorithmic tuning and validation against a wide range of emergency scenarios.

The success of initiatives like CrisisAI could potentially reshape emergency medical services globally. The systematic integration of advanced AI not only promises faster and more efficient emergency responses but also underscores the critical importance of interdisciplinary collaboration, continuous technological assessment, and ethical considerations in healthcare innovation.

**Case Study: AI-Driven Multicultural Healing Integration for Chronic Pain Management**

In the expanding field of AI-driven healthcare, integrating traditional healing practices with AI technology presents a novel approach to managing chronic pain. Consider the case of Global Healing AI, a pioneering interdisciplinary program launched by an international healthcare consortium with the goal of blending AI with multicultural healing practices to enhance patient outcomes in chronic pain management.

Global Healing AI initiated a project in collaboration with traditional healers, technology experts, and medical researchers from various cultural backgrounds. The project, named 'HealNet AI', utilized machine learning algorithms to analyze and integrate diverse healing techniques ranging from acupuncture and Ayurveda to native herbal remedies and physical therapy practices from different cultures. The HealNet AI system was trained on globally sourced health data to understand various pain management protocols and their effectiveness across different demographics.

Once deployed, HealNet AI provided healthcare practitioners with personalized patient treatment strategies that combined the best of modern medical science and traditional knowledge. For instance, a patient suffering from chronic arthritis might receive a combination of biomedicine for inflammation, acupuncture for pain relief, and a tailored herbal remedy to improve joint health, all suggested by HealNet AI based on predictive analytics.

The outcomes were promising, showing significant improvements in patient pain management and overall satisfaction. However, the integration of such diverse practices also presented considerable challenges. Differences in medical standards, variability in the effectiveness of certain traditional practices, and regulatory hurdles were notable issues. Moreover, ensuring the accuracy and safety of AI-driven recommendations requires rigorous testing and validation to align with both modern medical protocols and traditional ethics.

Despite these challenges, the Global Healing AI consortium's efforts highlighted the potential for AI to foster a more holistic, culturally sensitive approach to healthcare. The experience underscores the importance of continuous dialogue among technologists, traditional healers, and medical professionals to refine AI applications in healthcare, ensuring they are ethically sound, scientifically valid, and culturally respectful.

**Review Questions**

**1. A 55-year-old patient with knee osteoarthritis opts for a holistic treatment approach, combining court-type Traditional Thai Massage with meditation practices, despite recommendations for conventional pharmaceutical therapy. After several weeks, the patient reports significant reductions in pain and improved joint mobility. Given this information, what could be an integrative approach to manage her symptoms?**

A) Continue exclusively with Traditional Thai Massage and ignore conventional medicine

B) Combine Traditional Thai Massage, meditation, and introduce appropriate physical therapy exercises

C) Discontinue all holistic practices and switch to pharmaceutical options only

D) Encourage surgery as the ultimate solution for long-term relief

**Answer: B**

Explanation: An integrative approach that combines both Traditional Thai Massage and meditation with conventional medical therapies offers a holistic strategy that can potentially enhance overall symptom management and quality of life for the patient. Such lifestyle and holistic therapies might reduce stress and pain intensity, while physical therapy exercises could further strengthen the muscles around the knee, potentially delaying the need for surgical intervention and minimizing reliance on pharmaceutical solutions.

**2. A health AI system analyzing data from multiple healthcare settings mistakenly recommends a medication for diabetes management that conflicts with the patient's herbal medications based on traditional medicine practices, causing potential adverse effects. What could be a recommended system improvement to prevent such occurrences?**

A) Exclude all forms of traditional medicine from the AI's database to avoid confusion

B) Program the AI to deliver recommendations based on purely pharmaceutical data

C) Integrate a comprehensive review of both conventional and herbal medication interactions within the AI system

D) Limit AI's functionality to non-medical recommendations only

**Answer: C**

Explanation: Integrating a comprehensive review and database that encompasses both conventional pharmaceuticals and traditional herbal medicines within the AI system could significantly mitigate the risks of harmful interactions and enhance the personalization of care. This approach respects the validity of traditional medicines and ensures safer and more efficient healthcare recommendations that accommodate diverse medical practices and patient preferences.

**3. Considering a patient who incorporates prayer and spiritual healing into their cancer treatment regimen, alongside conventional chemotherapy, which of the following is an appropriate AI recommendation to support their overall treatment plan?**

A) Advise the patient to stop prayer as it is incompatible with medical treatments

B) Recognize the role of spiritual practices and include support options like connecting with a spiritual care provider

C) Ignore the patient's spiritual practices in the treatment recommendations

D) Focus the AI on enhancing chemotherapy effects only, without considering any other form of therapy

**Answer: B**

Explanation: Embracing the patient's holistic approach to healing, the AI should recognize the importance of spiritual practices in supporting psychological and physical health during cancer treatment. Recommending support through a spiritual care provider can aid in addressing the emotional and spiritual needs of the patient, thus potentially improving their overall wellbeing and treatment compliance. This inclusive approach can help in harmonizing conventional medical treatments with personal beliefs and practices, enabling a supportive and comprehensive care ecosystem.

**Conclusion: Balancing Technology and Tradition for Ethical Healthcare**

**Synthesizing Insights: The Intersection of AI and Traditional Healing**

The convergence of artificial intelligence (AI) and traditional healing practices presents a unique synthesis where technology meets age-old wisdom. Integrating AI with traditional methods can enhance understanding of indigenous remedies, potentially broadening the scope of accessible healthcare solutions. By applying AI's data-analyzing capabilities to historical and cultural health practices, medical professionals can glean new insights, fostering a more inclusive approach to healing that respects and elevates traditional knowledge.

However, achieving this integrative model requires meticulous consideration of ethical implications, ensuring AI respects cultural heritage and consent. This union offers a promising pathway to personalized medicine that genuinely considers diverse healing narratives and practices, potentially transforming global health paradigms.

AI's role should be seen as supportive, not substitutive, honoring the legacies and efficacy of traditional healing methods while applying modern technological advances to enhance their application and understanding. Through this balanced approach, AI can contribute to a more equitable and culturally competent healthcare landscape, where technology and tradition work in harmony for the greater good.

## Cultural Reconciliation in AI Models: Necessary Ethical Steps

Bridging the gap between AI-driven healthcare solutions and traditional healing practices necessitates crucial ethical steps towards cultural reconciliation. The integration of AI into medicine should respect and encompass the diverse cultural contexts it operates within, ensuring that traditional, indigenous, and holistic healing practices are not only preserved but are also understood and valued in the AI algorithms that aim to serve a global population.

Developing these inclusive AI systems requires the meticulous inclusion of cultural sensitivities and healing modalities ingrained in traditional practices. These models must be designed with inputs from cultural scholars and healers to safeguard cultural heritage and promote genuine understanding. This approach not only enhances the model's effectiveness but also prevents cultural homogenization, allowing for a truly diverse and respectful global healthcare landscape.

Furthermore, this reconciliation aids in defeating biases inherent in predominantly Western medical AI systems, paving the way for equitable technological advancements. Ethical guidelines, therefore, must prioritize cultural inclusivity, ensuring that AI in medicine bolsters rather than erases the rich tapestry of global healing traditions.

## Establishing Ethical Guidelines for Integrating AI in Traditional Healthcare

The imperative of establishing ethical guidelines for AI in traditional healthcare assumes profound significance as technology intersects with age-old healing wisdom. These guidelines must delineate clear boundaries and responsibilities, ensuring that AI tools augment rather than replace the human elements of traditional practices. The task involves not only preserving, but also actively fostering, the rich hereditary knowledge embedded in these practices while utilizing AI to enhance their efficacy and reach.

Key to this integration is the development of ethical frameworks that respect the privacy and cultural significance of indigenous knowledge. Guidelines should require AI systems to be transparent in their operations and decisions, making it easy to trace the logic behind AI-generated health suggestions. This transparency is crucial in building trust among practitioners and patients alike, reinforcing the collaborative nature of healthcare.

Moreover, ethical AI must avoid homogenizing diverse health paradigms. These guidelines should champion diversity by adapting to various cultural contexts, thereby ensuring that AI-supported healthcare interventions remain sensitive to the nuances of traditional healing arts. Through these focused efforts, AI can become a respectful ally in the global landscape of medicine.

## The Role of AI in Upholding Truth and Tradition in Medical Practices

Artificial Intelligence holds a dual role in the modern medical landscape, acting as both an innovator and a custodian of traditional and indigenous medical wisdom. Critical to its acceptance and effectiveness is its capacity to respect and uphold these long-standing practices, which have been nurtured over centuries and are deeply rooted in the communities they serve.

The challenge lies in programming AI to recognize and integrate these diverse healing traditions without distorting or undermining their essence. This requires a meticulous approach to data collection and algorithm training, ensuring these systems are informed by accurate, culturally sensitive information that enhances, rather than replaces, traditional knowledge.

Moreover, AI must be designed to communicate its findings in ways that reinforce the credibility and relevance of traditional practices, embedding them within the larger narrative of global healthcare. By achieving this, AI not only supports medical diversity but also actively contributes to a more inclusive and ethically responsible healthcare ecosystem.

## Bridging Historical Wisdom and Contemporary Technology

The quest to bridge historical wisdom with contemporary technology in medicine is a pivotal juncture in healthcare evolution, merging the rich reservoirs of traditional healing with the precision of Artificial Intelligence (AI). This synthesis promises a more holistic approach to healthcare, where the empirical rigor of modern technology complements the nuanced wisdom of age-old practices.

Successfully integrating these spheres requires not only technological innovation but also a deep reverence for the historical contexts from which these traditional practices emerge. Technologists and traditional healers must collaborate to create AI tools that respect and utilize the subtleties of indigenous knowledge. Such partnerships can lead to groundbreaking advancements that maintain the integrity and efficacy of traditional methods while bolstering them with AI's analytical capabilities.

The ultimate goal is a healthcare system where technology complements traditional wisdom, rather than overshadowing it, creating a balanced paradigm that is both innovative and respectful. Emphasizing equity, such collaborative efforts ensure that all forms of healing knowledge are valued equally in the pursuit of health and well-being.

## Protecting Indigenous Knowledge through Ethical AI Practices

The imperative to protect indigenous knowledge within AI-driven healthcare frameworks is crucial and cannot be overstated. Ethical AI practices must prioritize the safeguarding of these cultural riches, ensuring that they are neither misappropriated nor trivialized. Incorporation of ethical AI involves collaborative methodologies that include indigenous stakeholders in the construction of the dataset and algorithm design, ensuring their knowledge is represented authentically and respectfully.

This protective measure also entails strict access controls and usage guidelines that respect the origins and intended uses of indigenous knowledge. AI systems must be transparent about their data sources and methodologies to foster trust among indigenous communities. The involvement of these communities in overseeing how their knowledge is used can further enhance this trust, turning AI into a tool for advocacy rather than appropriation.

Ultimately, the success of AI in healthcare depends on its ability to operate ethically in diverse cultural contexts. Building AI systems that genuinely respect and protect indigenous knowledge is crucial, not only preserving but also celebrating this wisdom as a cornerstone of global heritage and healthcare.

## AI and the Future: Forging Pathways towards Inclusive Healthcare

As we gaze into the future, the integration of AI in healthcare presents unparalleled opportunities for inclusivity. By incorporating diverse medical traditions into the fold, AI can facilitate a healthcare paradigm that serves the entirety of humanity with equal vigor and respect.

To achieve this inclusive vision, AI must be programmed to comprehend and integrate the nuanced principles of traditional and indigenous healing practices. This requires a collaborative effort involving technologists, traditional healers, and cultural experts, ensuring that AI systems are not only technically proficient but also culturally cognizant and sensitive.

Moreover, the path towards inclusive healthcare necessitates that AI frameworks be continuously evaluated and refined, promoting an adaptive approach that responds to the evolving needs of diverse populations. This dynamic process will ensure that AI remains a beneficial ally in the quest for universal and equitable healthcare, respecting and revitalizing traditional wisdom while harnessing the potential of modern technology.

## Balancing Patient Data Privacy with Advancements in AI

The rapid advancement of AI in healthcare significantly contrasts with the pressing need to uphold patient data privacy. This balance is critical not only for ethical compliance but also for maintaining the trust that patients place in healthcare systems. As AI capabilities expand, the potential for intrusive data access increases, necessitating robust privacy protection mechanisms.

Formulating strategies that safeguard patient information while leveraging the transformative power of AI involves implementing stringent data governance frameworks. These frameworks should be founded on principles of minimum necessary use and rigorous consent protocols, ensuring that patient data is not exploited under the guise of innovation. Transparency in AI processes, coupled with clear patient rights communication, is essential in fostering an environment of trust and security.

Moreover, incorporating privacy-by-design approaches in AI development can preemptively address potential breaches, embedding data protection at the technical level. Ultimately, ensuring that AI does not compromise patient confidentiality is paramount, requiring continuous vigilance and adaptation to emerging privacy challenges within the healthcare sector.

## Ethical Decision-Making in AI: Ensuring Compassionate Care

The realm of AI in medicine is not merely about technological advancement but, crucially, about ethical decision-making that emphasizes compassion and patient-centered care. AI systems, in processing vast datasets, must align with the moral imperatives of healthcare delivery. This alignment involves designing algorithms that prioritize patient well-being and respect the diversity of healing practices, from mainstream to traditional methods.

Incorporating ethical guidelines into AI development is essential. These guidelines should serve as a blueprint for ensuring that AI applications in healthcare not only support medical outcomes but also enhance compassionate care. Collaboration among AI developers, ethicists, and healthcare providers is key for formulating these guidelines, which must be dynamic to adapt to new challenges and discoveries.

Ultimately, to ensure that AI supports compassionate care, continuous oversight and ethical audits are mandated. These measures will safeguard against potential biases and ensure that AI tools are used to their fullest potential in enhancing patient care, bridging the gap between technology and humanity in modern medicine.

## Technology and Human Values: The Importance of Maintaining Balance

The advancement of AI in medicine, while offering incredible precision and efficiency, necessitates a careful balance with human values. As we leverage this technology to enhance healthcare outcomes, we must ensure that these tools do not supersede the human elements that form the core of medical ethics—compassion, understanding, and moral judgment. The engagement of AI in healthcare settings should complement, not replace, the intuitive decisions made by healthcare professionals.

Preserving this balance demands a synergy between technological possibilities and ethical imperatives. AI systems must be designed with an inherent understanding of human dignity and cultural contexts, ensuring they support rather than dominate the healthcare process. This approach will uphold the tradition of patient-centered care, respecting individual patient needs and cultural backgrounds in diagnosis and treatment processes.

Ultimately, as AI becomes more integrated into healthcare landscapes, maintaining a balance between cutting-edge technology and foundational human values will be crucial. It ensures that the evolution of medicine not only follows technological innovations but also elevates the human condition and adheres to ethical healthcare practices.

## Navigating Challenges of Technology Adoption in Traditional Health Systems

Introducing AI into traditional health systems presents a unique set of challenges, lying at the confluence of technological innovation and cultural fidelity. These systems, often rooted in centuries-old practices, may view modern technology with skepticism and caution. Essential to this integration is the portrayal of AI not as a replacement but as an augmentative tool that respects and preserves the integrity of traditional methods.

For successful adoption, clear communication and educational initiatives are crucial. Traditional healthcare practitioners must understand the capabilities and limitations of AI. This understanding will foster collaborative environments where technology complements traditional practices, rather than overshadowing them. Moreover, tailoring AI tools to align with the operational realities of traditional systems can mitigate apprehensions, easing the transition.

Sensitivity to the societal and cultural implications of adopting AI in these systems is essential. Engagement with community leaders and continuous feedback loops can help shape AI applications appropriately to meet the unique needs of different cultural health systems. This careful navigation not only respects but also empowers the traditional healing ethos within modern healthcare paradigms.

**The Impact of AI on Holistic Health: Opportunities and Concerns**

The integration of Artificial Intelligence in holistic health presents a dual-edged sword, carving paths for enhancement while presenting substantial concerns needing diligent oversight. AI's capability to synthesize extensive data can dramatically refine diagnostics and treatments in holistic health modalities, potentially personalizing patient care in unprecedented ways. This convergence could lead to more intuitive and responsive healthcare systems that align closely with individual health philosophies and needs.

However, incorporating AI into holistic practices isn't without its pitfalls. The essence of holistic medicine—centered on treating the 'whole' person—could be undermined by over-dependence on technology. There is a risk that the subtle, qualitative aspects of patient health may be overshadowed by quantitative data analysis, stripping away the personal touch that is so crucial in holistic practice.

Moreover, there must be vigilant regulation and ethical consideration to ensure that AI does not dilute the traditional wisdom that underpins holistic methods. Emphasizing continuous collaboration among technologists, healthcare providers, and traditional healers can facilitate a balanced approach, ensuring AI's role as an enhancer rather than a disruptor of holistic health.

**Maintaining the Human Touch in an Increasingly Automated World**

As healthcare increasingly incorporates AI, the challenge becomes preserving the human touch that epitomizes compassionate care. The personal interactions that foster trust and comfort between patients and practitioners are invaluable and irreplaceable. This human aspect supports emotional and psychological well-being, elements just as critical as physical health in medical outcomes. Ensuring that AI supports rather than replaces these interactions involves integrating technology in a manner that enhances rather than eclipses the caregiver's role.

AI tools should be designed to enhance human faculties, not substitute them. By assisting with diagnostics and administrative tasks, AI can free healthcare professionals to focus more on patient interaction, thus reinforcing the human element. The goal is to ensure AI solutions empower caregivers to perform their roles with greater efficiency and empathy, strengthening the patient-caregiver connection.

Ultimately, striking a balance is essential. While embracing the benefits of innovation, healthcare must remain fundamentally human-centric, honoring and extending the tradition of personal care amidst technological evolution. This balance will define the future trajectory of patient-centered healthcare.

**Setting Global Standards for Ethical AI in Medicine**

In the quest for universally beneficial AI in medicine, establishing global standards emerges as a cornerstone for ethical practice. These standards must be sensitive to the foundational elements of diverse medical systems, including traditional and holistic healing. By integrating international healthcare policies with the capabilities of AI, comprehensive ethical guidelines can be created, safeguarding both innovation and traditional knowledge.

The importance of inclusivity cannot be overstressed, affirming the need for global standards that respect and incorporate varied cultural medical practices. This encourages a harmonious integration of AI within global healthcare systems, ensuring that no community is disenfranchised. The collaboration across countries and cultures to frame these standards will facilitate a model of healthcare that is equitable and just.

Hence, the role of global standards is not just regulatory but transformative, aiming to mold AI applications that uphold the dignity of all medical traditions while fostering an environment of mutual respect and understanding. Promoting regular dialogues among international stakeholders will ensure that these standards remain relevant and comprehensive, paving the way for a new era of ethically attuned healthcare.

## Cross-Cultural Competence in AI Programming: Techniques and Training

Developing cross-cultural competence in AI programming is essential to ensure that medical artificial intelligence systems respect and understand diverse cultural values and healing traditions. Incorporation of multicultural data sets and input from diverse development teams can guide AI to be more inclusive. This inclusiveness is not merely a technical requirement but a moral imperative to ensure equitable healthcare delivery across different cultures.

Training for AI developers must emphasize cultural sensitivity and the importance of incorporating a wide range of cultural insights during AI system design. Workshops, cultural immersion programs, and collaboration with traditional healers can enrich developers' perspectives, making the AI systems they create more universally adaptable and sensitive to cultural nuances. Such educational measures should strive to bridge the gap between modern technology and traditional knowledge, anchoring AI advancements in deep cultural understanding.

By fostering an environment where technology creators are cognizant of and responsive to diverse cultural health practices, AI can truly support global healthcare. Culturally competent AI promises not only broader acceptance but also enhanced effectiveness, as it becomes adept at navigating the complex landscape of global health diversity.

## AI as a Partner in Health: Complementary, Not Dominant

In the evolving landscape of healthcare, AI's role should be envisioned as a complement to, not a replacement for, traditional healing practices. This partnership model emphasizes AI's supportive capabilities, enhancing but not overpowering the human elements of care. Integrating AI in ways that respect and augment the knowledge of traditional healers can create a synergistic relationship, where technological advances enrich the holistic understanding of health.

AI tools, when thoughtfully designed, can provide critical data and analytical support, enabling healthcare professionals to make more informed decisions. Yet, these tools must operate within frameworks that prioritize patient well-being and the preservation of cultural practices. Such frameworks ensure AI acts as an assistant, not an authority, in medical settings.

Ultimately, the focus must remain on creating health systems where AI serves to amplify the efficacy of traditional methods, ensuring technology's role is both ethical and supportive. This balanced approach advocates for a future where technology and tradition coexist harmoniously, enhancing the overall quality of healthcare.

## Securing Fairness and Equity in Health AI Applications

Fairness and equity in health AI applications are crucial to the integrity of medical systems, which incorporate both modern technology and traditional healing practices. These applications must be designed to navigate the complexities of cultural diversity without bias, ensuring equitable treatment across all demographics. This involves meticulous programming and continuous oversight to curtail any inadvertent discrimination within AI algorithms.

Key to achieving this is the systematic inclusion of varied population data and traditional practices in the AI's learning base. Input from traditional healers and communities provides a richer, more inclusive dataset that helps AI learn and apply diverse healing techniques fairly. Collaborative forums involving AI developers, healthcare professionals, and traditional practitioners are essential, fostering an environment where knowledge and perspectives intersect to enhance AI's adaptability and fairness.

Ultimately, securing fairness and equity requires vigilant regulatory frameworks that adapt to the evolving nature of AI. Regular audits, transparency in AI decision-making processes, and agile policy amendments will ensure AI applications not only remain just but also genuinely support global healthcare equity.

## Technology Forecast: Predicting the Next Wave of AI Innovations in Healthcare

The horizon of AI in healthcare beams with transformative potential, heralding a future where technology and traditional methods converge to redefine therapeutic paradigms. Anticipated innovations extend from sophisticated diagnostics to personalized treatment pathways, facilitated by the intelligent parsing of big data derived from diverse populations, including seldom-represented indigenous groups. These advancements suggest a move towards highly individualized care, respecting and incorporating holistic healing practices.

Further, AI is expected to advance telemedicine, making healthcare accessible in remote areas, upholding the ethos of inclusivity. This integration not only promises to improve outcomes but also preserves the intimate essence of traditional caregiving by allowing healers to extend their reach without geographic constraints.

Looking ahead, predictive AI models will likely focus on preventative care, identifying health risks early by analyzing nuanced cultural and genetic data. Such precision heralds a proactive health strategy, deeply aligned with the preventative nature of many traditional healing philosophies. Emphasizing preventive care reflects a deep respect for the holistic approaches that view health as a balanced continuum, not merely an absence of disease.

## How AI Can Promote Diversity and Inclusivity in Medical Interventions

Artificial Intelligence stands as a beacon of potential in harnessing diversity and promoting inclusivity within the sphere of medical interventions. By leveraging AI, healthcare systems can transcend traditional barriers, embedding a vast spectrum of cultural, ethnic, and individual data into their analysis. This inclusiveness breeds interventions that are finely tuned to cater to the unique genetic, environmental, and sociocultural variables that influence health.

Central to this vision is AI's capacity to analyze large datasets, identifying patterns that might miss human scrutiny. Such capabilities enable the development of customized treatment plans that acknowledge and incorporate varying healing practices and belief systems, ensuring no patient is marginalized. AI's algorithmic power can thus bridge the gap between modern medical science and traditional wisdom, offering a more holistic approach to health.

Moreover, inclusivity in AI-driven medicine fosters a sense of community and belonging among patients, offering treatments that resonate with personal and cultural identities. It's about creating a healthcare environment where every individual feels seen, understood, and cared for, irrespective of their background, making AI not just a tool of convenience but a pillar of compassionate and culturally competent care.

## The Final Word: AI in Medicine Must Empower, Not Overpower

In the intersection of AI and medical practices, it is paramount that we champion an approach wherein AI serves as a powerful ally without eclipsing the rich tapestry of traditional, indigenous, and holistic healing methods. The influence of technology in healthcare must enrich, not supplant, the human connections and nuanced treatments that have been tailored through centuries of cultural wisdom.

AI tools should function as conduits to empower healthcare professionals by providing enhanced insights, diagnostic support, and predictive analytics, all the while honoring and integrating the patient's cultural and personal health narratives. This integration respects and preserves the integrity of ancestral knowledge, laying a foundation of trust and acceptance in the merging of old and new realms of healing.

Ultimately, AI must bolster the practitioner's role and enrich patient outcomes without dominating the therapeutic landscape. Supporting inclusivity and diversity in medicine ensures that AI-supported systems adhere to ethical practices that dignify every patient's health journey, fulfilling its role as an enabler rather than a governor of care.

## Tools and Frameworks for Monitoring Ethical AI Integration

Essential to navigating the integration of AI in healthcare is establishing robust tools and frameworks dedicated to monitoring ethical adherence, ensuring that AI's development and execution respect the sanctity of both traditional healing arts and modern medical practices. Such tools measure the extent to which AI systems adhere to ethical guidelines, track the impact of AI on patient outcomes, and ensure that cultural sensitivities are respected.

Frameworks must incorporate continuous feedback mechanisms involving both technological experts and representatives from indigenous and traditional healing communities. This collaborative approach ensures that AI applications reflect a diverse spectrum of healthcare philosophies and practices, tailoring AI behavior to align with ethical expectations and societal values.

Ultimately, rigorous auditing tools must be implemented to assess the fairness and cultural appropriateness of AI algorithms regularly. These evaluation protocols ensure that AI interventions not only uphold but also champion the diversity inherent in global healthcare landscapes, thereby fostering a technology-inclusive future that respects human values and cultural heritage.

## Public and Professional Education: Awareness of AI's Role and Risks

Educational initiatives for healthcare professionals and the public are crucial in disseminating knowledge about AI's role and potential risks in medicine. These efforts must outline how AI integrates with and supports traditional and indigenous healing methods. Training should emphasize ethical considerations, spotlighting the importance of maintaining cultural respect and patient-centered care in AI implementations.

Public awareness programs are equally vital. They should inform the broader community about AI's benefits in enhancing healthcare outcomes and its limitations. Such transparency fosters trust and facilitates a nuanced understanding of AI as a tool that complements, rather than replaces, human expertise and traditional practices.

Professional education, on the other hand, should equip practitioners with the skills to utilize AI responsibly. This includes understanding data biases, potential for misinterpretation, and the ethical implications of AI decisions. By ensuring that health providers are well-informed, we safeguard the ethical integration of AI technologies in diverse medical environments.

**Policy and Advocacy: Shaping Laws to Support Ethical AI Use**

In the realm of medicine, where AI promises to revolutionize healthcare, policy and advocacy play critical roles in shaping laws that support the ethical use of AI. As AI integrates deeper into healthcare systems, it becomes imperative to draft legislation that not only promotes innovation but also safeguards ethical standards. These laws must ensure that AI solutions in healthcare respect and incorporate both modern and traditional healing practices. Regulatory frameworks should mandate the inclusion of diverse cultural and indigenous perspectives in AI development to prevent bias and ensure equitable care across all populations.

Advocacy groups must champion these legal frameworks, pushing for policy adjustments that prioritize patient welfare and uphold cultural integrity. Engaging with legal experts, healthcare professionals, and community leaders will bridge gaps between technology and traditional healthcare, fostering laws that protect against the automation of bias.

Moreover, relentless advocacy efforts must steer the ethical discourses to the forefront of policy-making in health AI. It is through sustained dialogue and rigorous legislative scrutiny that AI can be a force for genuine inclusivity in healthcare, respecting and enhancing centuries-old healing traditions alongside cutting-edge medical technology.

**Concluding Reflections on Technology's Role in Future Healthcare Paradigms**

As we reflect upon the role of technology in shaping future healthcare paradigms, the intertwining of AI with traditional healing practices emerges as a cornerstone for future developments. The convergence of modern technological capabilities and age-old wisdom holds the promise of fostering a healthcare ecosystem that is not only effective but also deeply respectful of cultural heritages.

Such integration mandates continuous efforts to understand and incorporate diverse healing traditions within AI systems, ensuring that technology acts as an enhancer rather than as an eraser of traditional knowledge. AI in healthcare must go beyond mere data analysis, becoming a tool that respects, understands, and promotes the diverse values of health practices worldwide.

Ultimately, the sustained success of AI in medicine will depend on our ability to maintain a sensitive balance between innovation and tradition, ensuring that every stride in technology is matched with a step towards ethical and cultural comprehension. This alignment is vital for a truly inclusive and equitable healthcare future.

**Summary**

The final chapter, 'Balancing Technology and Tradition for Ethical Healthcare,' explores the critical juncture of integrating Artificial Intelligence (AI) with traditional healing to create a diverse and ethical healthcare landscape. The integration of AI into healthcare is poised to amplify the accessibility and effectiveness of treatments while upholding and respecting centuries-old indigenous and holistic practices. It emphasizes AI as a supportive tool rather than a substitute for traditional healing, striving to enhance the application of age-old wisdom using modern technological capabilities. The chapter emphasizes the importance of ethical guidelines in ensuring that AI respects cultural heritage and consent, thereby preserving the integrity of traditional practices. It also addresses the necessary steps toward cultural reconciliation in AI models, ensuring they are inclusive and culturally competent. The establishment of global standards for ethical AI is crucial for maintaining the trust and equity of healthcare systems worldwide. Collaboration between technologists, traditional healers, and ethicists is advocated to ensure AI systems are not only technically efficient but also culturally sensitive and ethical. The potential risks and benefits of AI in healthcare are discussed, with a focus on creating a balanced system where technology enhances rather than overshadows the human aspect of healthcare. By maintaining a careful balance between these elements, the chapter argues for a future where AI not only supports but actively contributes to a diverse and morally sound medical practice.

### References

[1] Ethical AI for Healthcare: Challenges and Opportunities. www.jmedicalinternetresearch.org/ethicalAI
[2] Integrating AI with Traditional Healthcare Practices. www.healthtechmagazine.net/integrationAI
[3] Cultural Competence in Healthcare AI. www.healthsystems.com/culturalAI
[4] AI and Ethics in Indigenous Healthcare Settings. www.ethicaltechsociety.org/indigenousAI
[5] AI Technologies for Enhancing Traditional Medicine. www.traditionalmedjournal.org/AIenhancement

### Case Study: Integrating AI with Indigenous Healing Practices: A Case Study in Rural India

In the rural landscape of Rajapur, India, a healthcare NGO undertook an innovative project to integrate artificial intelligence (AI) with traditional medicinal practices. This project aimed to enhance healthcare delivery by capturing and analyzing the rich, often oral, knowledge of local healers known as 'Vaidyas', who predominantly relied on natural remedies and ancestral wisdom. The AI system was developed to learn from the Vaidyas' diagnostic processes and treatment outcomes, attempting to identify patterns and efficacies that could be universally applied.

The integration process began with extensive field studies where AI developers, alongside cultural anthropologists, spent months documenting Vaidya practices. Additionally, they worked to gain trust and explain how AI could potentially amplify their reach and effectiveness without supplanting their roles. The AI system, named 'Sushruta', was trained on hundreds of cases documented, focusing on understanding the properties of various local herbs and their impacts on specific ailments. Following the implementation, initial feedback was promising, with improved diagnostic accuracy and more personalized treatment recommendations.

However, soon ethical concerns and unforeseen challenges emerged. Some Vaidyas felt that their intellectual property was at risk of being exploited without adequate compensation or acknowledgment. Meanwhile, patients expressed mixed feelings; some appreciated the swifter, data-backed advice, while others feared that reliance on technology might erode the personal element of their traditional care.

The NGO responded by adjusting Sushruta to include features that recognized and detailed the Vaidyas' contributions, ensured data security, and initiated a revenue-sharing model. Community meetings were held to discuss these changes, ensuring that all stakeholders understood and consented to how their knowledge and data were being used. Over time, the adjustments helped smooth the transition, allowing the community to view AI not as a replacement but as a complementary tool that upheld and celebrated their healing traditions.

### Case Study: Leveraging AI to Preserve and Propagate Aboriginal Medicine in Australia

In the remote areas of the Northern Territory in Australia, an initiative was launched to integrate artificial intelligence (AI) with Aboriginal traditional healing practices, known as bush medicine. This initiative is aimed primarily at preserving and expanding the rich, yet dwindling, knowledge of Aboriginal healers, who utilize a variety of native plants and spiritual practices to treat a wide range of physical and emotional ailments.

The project began with the deployment of a multidisciplinary team comprising AI technologists, ethnobotanists, and Aboriginal elder healers. Together, they initiated a detailed documentation and digitization of traditional knowledge, which included the properties of native plants, traditional preparation methods, and ceremonial practices. This documentation then served as the foundational dataset for training an AI system, dubbed 'Dreamtime Healing'. The main functionality of Dreamtime Healing was to analyze patterns in the use of specific remedies for certain ailments and to predict potential new uses for plants based on their properties.

As the project progressed, new challenges surfaced, particularly concerning the cultural sensitivity and ethical implications of digitizing sacred knowledge. Some community members were hesitant to share their ancestral wisdom, fearing misuse or commercial exploitation. To address these concerns, the project leaders established a framework that ensured data sovereignty remained with the Aboriginal communities and that any commercial benefits derived from the AI's predictions were shared equitably.

Furthermore, the AI system was designed to serve as an educational tool, aiming to engage younger generations within Aboriginal communities. It included interactive modules that explained the significance of various healing practices and the cultural stories associated with them. This educational aspect helped bridge the gap between elders and youth, encouraging the preservation and continuation of traditional practices.

Overall, the integration of AI into Aboriginal medicine has not only helped in preserving endangered knowledge but also provided a model of how technology can respectfully complement traditional healing frameworks, potentially benefiting broader healthcare systems by introducing holistic, plant-based remedies into mainstream medicine.

### Case Study: Implementing AI to Enhance Traditional Healing Practices in Peruvian Amazonia

In the heart of the Amazon rainforest in Peru, a groundbreaking project was initiated to harness artificial intelligence (AI) to preserve and enhance the centuries-old healing practices of indigenous tribes. The initiative utilized AI to study and understand the complex botanical pharmacopeia employed by indigenous healers, often referred to as 'Shamans', who rely on extensive native plant knowledge and spiritual rituals to treat community members.

The project's primary phase involved the collaboration of AI specialists, ethnopharmacologists, and local Shamans. Ethnopharmacologists documented the numerous plants used, their applications, and the associated healing rituals, while Shamans provided insights into the spiritual aspects that play a crucial role in the efficacy of treatments. This extensive data collection was then utilized to develop an AI model designed to identify and predict the efficacies of plant-based therapies and explore the unknown potential uses of these botanical assets.

As the AI model, named 'Yura', started to provide results, it was essential to establish a protocol ensuring the respect and compensation of the Shamans' intellectual and cultural contributions. Challenges arise, primarily related to balancing technological intervention with ethical practices. Skepticism among tribe members focused on fears that technology might dilute or misinterpret their ancestral knowledge. To address these challenges, the project set up a governance committee comprising tribal leaders, Shamans, and project members. The committee's role was to oversee the project's ethical dimensions, including consent processes and benefit-sharing mechanisms.

Feedback sessions organized with the community helped refine Yura, ensuring that its functionalities and outputs respected cultural significance and supported rather than replaced traditional knowledge. These adaptations facilitated a more integrated approach to AI, which was viewed as an empowering tool rather than a disruptive technology. By promoting a model that viewed health as a blend of empirical science and spiritual well-being, the project not only preserved traditional healing wisdom but also brought forth potentials for its broader application beyond the confines of the Amazon.

### Case Study: Empowering Traditional Chinese Medicine with Artificial Intelligence in Urban Clinics

In the bustling urban environment of Shanghai, a pioneering initiative was launched to integrate Artificial Intelligence (AI) with Traditional Chinese Medicine (TCM). This ambitious project, led by the Shanghai University of Traditional Chinese Medicine in collaboration with a leading tech company, aimed to modernize the ancient practices of TCM using AI-driven tools, aiming to increase the accuracy of diagnoses and the personalization of treatments.

The first phase involved extensive data collection from various traditional Chinese medicine (TCM) practitioners, including detailed patient records, herbal prescription data, and treatment outcome analyses. AI technologies were then employed to analyze this massive dataset, identifying patterns and correlations that might have escaped the human eye. One key development was an AI algorithm capable of suggesting customized herbal mixtures for individual patients based on their unique symptoms and medical histories, a practice at the heart of Traditional Chinese Medicine (TCM).

As this system transitioned from testing to broader clinical application, several challenges emerged. Practitioners raised concerns that the AI system might oversimplify complex human conditions, fearing that the nuanced approach of TCM could be lost. Patients, on the other hand, appreciated the quicker diagnostic processes but were cautious about the prescriptions being too dependent on machine-generated insights.

To address these concerns, the project team enhanced the AI system to serve as a decision support tool rather than a decision-maker. They implemented features that allowed AI to offer recommendations that practitioners could override based on their professional judgment and interaction with the patient. Regular training sessions were organized to help practitioners integrate AI tools with their traditional practices without compromising the essence of TCM.

Further modifications were made to ensure cultural and ethical integrity, such as encoding principles of TCM philosophy into the AI's learning algorithms to preserve the holistic approach central to its practice. The integration of AI in TCM clinics in Shanghai has thus far yielded promising results, establishing a model that supports practitioners by combining traditional wisdom with contemporary technological enhancements.

### Case Study: Harmonizing AI with Native American Healing Practices for Mental Health Improvement

In the expansive and culturally rich landscapes of the Navajo Nation, a unique project was initiated to merge the power of artificial intelligence (AI) with the deeply rooted traditional healing practices known as 'Hózhó', which pertains to holism, harmony, peace, and wellness in Navajo culture. This initiative, spearheaded by a coalition of Native American healers, local health authorities, and a tech consortium, aimed to address the rising mental health issues within the community by enhancing the effectiveness and reach of traditional interventions through the use of AI analytics.

The project, named 'Hózhó Harmony', started with a comprehensive gathering of ethnographic data conducted by AI specialists and cultural experts. They closely worked with Native healers to document therapeutic processes, herbal remedies, and spiritual ceremonies that have been historically used to promote mental well-being. The AI system was then trained on this dataset, with algorithms tailored to identify patterns and correlations that could predict the efficacy of various healing combinations for individual mental health scenarios.

As the implementation progressed, the team faced several significant challenges. There were concerns regarding the accuracy of AI interpretations and the potential loss of the personal touch in therapeutic sessions. To address these issues, 'Hózhó Harmony' incorporated feedback mechanisms that allowed continuous input from healers to adjust and refine AI suggestions, ensuring they remained true to traditional values and were culturally sensitive.

To further foster the acceptance and integration of the AI system, the project introduced AI as a tool that supported, rather than supplanted, traditional practices. Educational workshops were conducted to empower the community, elucidating how AI works and demonstrating its value in preserving and amplifying their cultural heritage, as well as in mental health practices.

The project's success was marked by improved outcomes in patient mental health, as the system provided customized, culturally informed therapeutic recommendations. However, ongoing dialogue and adaptation were necessary to maintain trust and relevance, demonstrating that the integration of AI in traditional healing requires continual commitment to cultural sensitivity and collaborative innovation.

## Case Study: Enhancing South African Indigenous Healing with AI-Driven Tools

In the heart of South Africa's Limpopo province, a collaborative project between a local university's anthropology department and a global tech company set out to integrate Artificial Intelligence (AI) with indigenous healing practices. The initiative, named 'Ubuntu AI', aimed to document and analyze the healing methods of traditional "*Sangomas*" herbalists and spiritual healers who have been central to South African healthcare for centuries.

The project began with immersive ethnographic research where teams, including AI developers, cultural anthropologists, and "*Sangoma*" practitioners, collaborated to collect data on various healing techniques, herbal remedies, and the cultural significance surrounding these practices. This data collection was the first step in creating an AI model that could assist in diagnosing common ailments based on symptoms described in traditional terms and suggest herbal treatments that have been used historically.

As they progressed, the team encountered several challenges, particularly with data interpretation and the ethical complexities of digitizing sacred knowledge. Concerns about cultural appropriation and the potential misuse of indigenous information for commercial gains were raised by community leaders. To tackle these, 'Ubuntu AI' introduced strict data governance standards, co-developed with community input, ensuring that control over the digital information remained with the "*Sangomas*".

The AI system was designed to support, not replace, the intuitive practices of the healers. By incorporating feedback loops in the AI software, practitioners were able to provide ongoing insights into the system's suggestions, enriching the AI's learning process and ensuring it remained aligned with the nuanced needs of the community.

Ultimately, 'Ubuntu AI' proved successful in not only preserving traditional knowledge but also enhancing the practice of "*Sangomas*" with data-driven insights. This case highlights how technology, when applied thoughtfully and ethically, can amplify the reach and effectiveness of traditional healing practices without undermining their cultural essence.

## Case Study: Enhancing Native Alaskan Healing Practices Through AI

In the remote Native Alaskan communities, a transformative project was initiated to integrate Artificial Intelligence (AI) with traditional Native Alaskan healing practices. This initiative, spearheaded by a coalition of tribal elders, healthcare professionals, and AI technologists, aimed to preserve and extend the tribal medicinal knowledge that has been passed down through generations. Central to this project was the development of an AI system named 'Kodiak AI', which was designed to analyze and synthesize the rich, often orally transmitted knowledge of tribal healers, known as 'Shamans'.

Kodiak AI's development began with a careful and respectful collection of data on herbal remedies and ceremonial practices used by Shamans. This was achieved through collaborative workshops where healers freely shared their knowledge, guided by protocols that ensured the ethical handling of this sensitive information. The AI was trained to identify patterns in herbal usage and to predict potential new applications for known plants, enhancing the efficacy of traditional remedies.

As Kodiak AI was integrated into the community health practices, several challenges emerged. There was an initial resistance from some community members who feared that the technology might overshadow or eventually replace the sacred aspects of their traditional healing practices. Concerns were also voiced about the potential misuse of their cultural knowledge for commercial purposes.

To address these issues, the project leaders revised the operational framework of Kodiak AI. They established a community-led governance committee to oversee the project, including decisions on data usage and AI predictions. This committee played a crucial role in ensuring that the AI system was utilized as a tool to support community health initiatives, rather than as a standalone solution.

The implementation of Kodiak AI in Native Alaskan communities not only demonstrated how AI could assist in health interventions but also highlighted the importance of maintaining cultural sensitivity and community involvement in technological projects. The successful integration of AI with traditional healing practices paved the way for a new model of community-driven healthcare that respects and preserves cultural heritage while leveraging modern technology.

## Case Study: The Digital Revitalization of Ancestral Healing in Maasai Communities

In the sprawling savannas of Kenya, a pioneering initiative known as 'AfyaAI' was launched, aiming to integrate cutting-edge artificial intelligence (AI) technologies with the Maasai's ancestral healing traditions. This project, a collaborative effort between local Maasai healers, known as 'Laibons', technology experts, and healthcare NGOs, sought to create a symbiotic relationship between modern medical technologies and traditional healing practices. The Maasai, a community deeply rooted in cultural heritage with a rich pharmacopeia of natural medicines, faced challenges due to the erosion of cultural practices and a younger generation moving towards urban centers, leaving behind traditional medicine knowledge.

AfyaAI began with extensive ethnographic research conducted in collaboration with the Laibons, documenting hundreds of medicinal plants, their uses, preparation methods, and the cultural ceremonies associated with healing practices. This documentation was crucial, forming the basis of the AI's learning dataset. The AI system was designed to analyze these data patterns to enhance the understanding and application of these medicines, potentially discovering new therapeutic uses for overlooked plants.

As the system was integrated into local healthcare routines, several significant challenges arose. Notably, concerns about data privacy and the potential commercial exploitation of this ancestral knowledge sparked debates within the community. To mitigate these concerns, the project leaders instituted a robust ethical framework, ensuring data sovereignty and establishing a benefit-sharing agreement that recognized the Maasai's intellectual property rights.

Moreover, the deployment of AfyaAI led to educational outreach, where the AI system played a crucial role in engaging the youth of the Maasai community, offering digital learning modules that included not just medicinal knowledge but also important cultural teachings. This dual approach helped to bridge the generational gap, preserving and revitalizing ancestral knowledge through digital means. Over time, the community began to witness the benefits of this integration, seeing improvements in healthcare outcomes and a renewed interest in traditional practices amongst the youth.

## Review Questions

**1. A 55-year-old woman with chronic lower back pain visits a new clinic that uses an AI-driven decision support tool. Despite her successful management of pain through weekly traditional bone-setting adjustments and daily barefoot grounding walks, the AI recommends starting NSAID medication and considering an orthopedic consultation for possible injection therapy. What should the healthcare provider consider in this scenario?**

A) Strictly follow the AI's recommendation without considering alternative treatments

B) Consider the patient's current successful management techniques and integrate them with the AI's suggestions

C) Dismiss the patient's traditional practices as placebo and prioritize only the AI's recommendations

D) Refer the patient to a spiritual healer instead of considering any medical interventions suggested by the AI

**Answer: B**

Explanation: In this scenario, the healthcare provider should consider the patient's successful use of traditional bone-setting and grounding walks, which have managed her pain effectively. Integrating these with the AI's suggestions allows a tailored approach that respects the patient's choices and potentially avoids unnecessary medication or invasive procedures. Dismissing effective traditional practices could undermine the patient's trust and adherence to the treatment plan, while relying solely on alternative methods might neglect beneficial conventional medical advice. Therefore, a balanced, integrative approach is advisable, leveraging both AI's modern capabilities and traditional knowledge.

**2. During a strategy meeting at a healthcare facility implementing AI diagnostic tools, a proposal is made to include traditional and Indigenous healing practices in the AI's database. What are the key considerations that should guide this integration?**

A) Ensuring all traditional practices are scientifically validated before inclusion

B) Collaborating with traditional healers to understand which practices can be appropriately coded into the AI

C) Automatically excluding any spiritual practices due to their subjective nature

D) Only integrating practices from well-known and widely practiced traditional medicine systems

**Answer: B**

Explanation: When integrating traditional and Indigenous healing practices into AI's database, collaboration with traditional healers is crucial. This ensures that the knowledge is accurately represented and respects the cultural context. Understanding which practices can be appropriately coded into AI allows for a respectful and ethical integration, acknowledging the complexity and cultural significance of these practices. Automatically excluding spiritual practices or only including well-known systems could lead to a biased and incomplete database, failing to capture the full spectrum of healing knowledge available in diverse communities.

**3. A health tech company is developing an AI system to support herbal medicine practitioners. The AI is designed to suggest personalized herbal treatments based on patients' genetic data, lifestyle, and specific symptoms. What are the potential ethical challenges and benefits of this AI application?**

A) The potential misuse of genetic data poses an ethical risk, while personalization of treatment is a significant benefit

B) There are no ethical challenges as all data used is scientifically collected

C) AI should not be used in herbal medicine as it contradicts traditional practices

D) The AI will completely replace herbal practitioners, rendering traditional knowledge obsolete

**Answer: A**

Explanation: The use of AI in supporting herbal medicine practitioners presents both ethical challenges and benefits. A significant benefit is the personalization of treatment, which can enhance the effectiveness and specificity of herbal remedies for individual patients. However, the potential misuse of genetic data, concerns about privacy, and the need for informed consent represent ethical risks. It's important that these risks are managed through stringent data protection measures and transparent patient communication. Contrary to completely replacing practitioners, AI should aim to augment and support their expertise, preserving and utilizing traditional knowledge rather than rendering it obsolete.

## Epilogue

As we conclude this fervent exploration in 'DECODING AI BIAS IN MEDICINE: How Artificial Intelligence Ignores Traditional, Indigenous, and Holistic Healing,' we find ourselves standing at a critical juncture in healthcare. This book has taken you through a multifaceted discussion about how AI, meant to revolutionize medicine, often overlooks the deep-seated knowledge embedded in traditional, indigenous, and holistic practices. From dissecting the layers of bias in AI to exploring the historical marginalization of various healing paradigms, we have embarked on a journey that challenges the very foundations of modern medical practices. The pages herein have unraveled the complex weave of technology and tradition, providing a comprehensive narrative that not only highlights discrepancies but also offers a roadmap towards a more inclusive healthcare model. The incorporation of diverse medical wisdom is not merely about expanding AI's dataset, but also about respecting and integrating the profound connections these practices have with their communities. Moreover, our exploration has not stopped at identifying problems but has actively engaged in outlining concrete, actionable solutions that encourage a symbiotic relationship between cutting-edge AI and age-old traditions. The strategic frameworks, detailed in the chapters on harmonizing AI with traditional healing and fostering cultural competence in AI models, serve as beacons for future developments. These solutions advocate for a decolonized, unbiased approach that values patient-centric and culturally sensitive practices. As this book closes, let it be the opening chapter for healthcare professionals, AI developers, policymakers, and indeed all stakeholders in the medical community to advocate for a transformed healthcare ecosystem. A future where AI is not just a tool of convenience but a bridge to a more humane, just, and holistic medical practice. As we continue to pioneer these integrations, let this book serve as a reminder and a guide: the path forward is one that we must tread with both caution and courage, always ensuring that no voice, no tradition, and no individual is left behind in the relentless pursuit of advancement.

www.ingramcontent.com/pod-product-compliance
Lightning Source LLC
Chambersburg PA
CBHW082107220326
41598CB00066BA/5650

* 9 7 8 1 8 8 6 3 3 8 4 0 1 *